Design and Analysis of Time Series
Experiments

Design and Analysis of Time Series Experiments

RICHARD McCLEARY,

DAVID McDOWALL,

AND

BRADLEY J. BARTOS

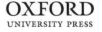

OXFORD

UNIVERSITY PRESS

Oxford University Press is a department of the University of Oxford. It furthers
the University's objective of excellence in research, scholarship, and education
by publishing worldwide. Oxford is a registered trade mark of Oxford University
Press in the UK and certain other countries.

Published in the United States of America by Oxford University Press
198 Madison Avenue, New York, NY 10016, United States of America.

Library of Congress Cataloging-in-Publication Data

ISBN 978-0-19-066155-7 (Hbk.)
ISBN 978-0-19-066156-4 (Pbk.)

9 8 7 6 5 4 3 2 1

Paperback printed by Webcom, Inc., Canada
Hardback printed by Bridgeport National Bindery, Inc., United States of America

CONTENTS

List of Figures and Tables vii
Preface xiii

1. Introduction 1

2. *ARIMA* Algebra 25

3. Noise Modeling 83

4. Forecasting 166

5. Intervention Modeling 186

6. Statistical Conclusion Validity 231

7. Internal Validity 273

8. Construct Validity 315

9. External Validity 333

References 345
Index 361

LIST OF FIGURES AND TABLES

1.1 Annual Skirt Widths (Richardson and Kroeber, 1940) 4

1.2 Canadian Homicides (Silverman and Kennedy, 1987) 5

1.3 Cotton Prices and Lynchings (Hovland and Sears, 1940) 6

1.4 Annual Rorschach and MMPI Citations (Polyson et al., 1986) 7

1.5 Cincinnati Directory Assistance Calls (McSweeney, 1978) 8

1.6 Self-Injurious Behavior (McCleary et al., 1999) 9

1.7 Campbell (1957) Evolves into Cook and Campbell (1976) 13

1.8 Quarterly U.S. Gonorrhea Cases 16

1.9 Self-Injurious Behavior (McCleary et al., 1999) 17

1.10 Co-proxamol Prescriptions, England and Wales
     (Hawton et al., 2009) 18

2.1 Four Time Series 27

2.2 White Noise Time Series 29

2.3 Two $MA1$ ACFs 35

2.4 Two $AR1$ ACFs 36

2.5 Two $MA2$ ACFs 43

2.6 Two $AR2$ ACFs 44

2.7 Two $ARMA$ ACFs 45

2.8 $Y_t = a_t + a_{t-1} + \cdots + a_{t-k}, E(a_t = 0.00)$ 54

2.9 $Y_t = a_t + a_{t-1} + \cdots + a_{t-k}, E(a_t = 0.20)$ 55

2.10 Sample $ACFs$ for Two Simulated Random Walks 57

2.11 $X_t: \mu_X = 0, \sigma_X \propto t$ 59

2.12 $Y_t: \mu_Y = 0, \sigma_Y \propto sin^2 t$ 59

2.13 Sample $ACFs$ for X_t and Y_t 61

3.1 The Iterative $ARIMA$ Modeling Strategy 84

3.2 β-Particles 89

3.3 South Carolina Homicides (King, 1978) 89

3.4   Sample *ACF*s, β-Particles and South Carolina Homicides 90

3.5   Cumulative Normal Distributions 92

3.6   Canadian Inflation Rate 95

3.7   Sample *ACF*s, Canadian Inflation Rate 96

3.8   U.K. Growth in Real GDP 99

3.9   Sample *ACF*s, U.K. Growth in Real GDP 100

3.10 Weekly Pediatric Trauma Admissions 101

3.11 Sample *ACF*, Weekly Pediatric Trauma Admissions 102

3.12 Beveridge's Wheat Price Time Series 104

3.13 Histogram, Annual Wheat Prices 104

3.14 Variance for $-3.5 < \lambda < +2.5$ 105

3.15 Transformed Wheat Price Time Series 106

3.16 Annual Zurich Sunspot Numbers (Yule, 1921) 112

3.17 Variance, $-2 < \lambda < +4$ 112

3.18 Transformed Annual Zurich Sunspot Numbers 113

3.19 Kroeber's Skirt-Width Time Series and its First Difference 116

3.20 Differenced Annual Tuberculosis Cases per 100,000 118

3.21 Annual Tuberculosis Cases per 100,000 119

3.22 Variance, $-1 < \lambda < +1$ 119

3.23 Log Annual Tuberculosis Cases per 100,000 120

3.24 Differenced Log Annual Tuberculosis Cases per 100,000 120

3.25 Sample *ACF*s, Log Annual Tuberculosis Cases per 100,000 121

3.26 Average Monthly Precipitation, Anchorage 123

3.27 Variance, $-1 < \lambda < +2$ 124

3.28 Transformed Average Monthly Precipitation, Anchorage 124

3.29 Sample *ACF*s, $Prcp_t^{1/4}$ 126

3.30 Monthly Atmospheric CO_2 128

3.31 Quarterly Australian Traffic Fatalities 131

3.32 Variance, $-1 < \lambda < +3$ 132

3.33 Quarterly Australian Traffic Fatalities, Square Roots 132

3.34 Nested vs. Unnested Models 136

3.35 Foreign Visitors to Japan 148

3.36 Box-Cox Functions for Two Time Series 152

3.37 $LL(\hat{\mu}|\hat{\phi}_1 = 0.61, \hat{\sigma}_a^2 = 7.47)$ for an *AR1* Model of *Admit$_t$* 157

3.38 $LL(\hat{\phi}_1|\hat{\mu} = 22.01, \hat{\sigma}_a^2 = 7.47)$ for an *AR1* Model of *Admit$_t$* 158

3.39 $LL(\hat{\theta}_0|\hat{\theta}_1 = -0.22, \hat{\sigma}_a^2 = 2.74)$ for an *MA1* Model of *UKGDP$_t$* 159

3.40 $LL(\hat{\theta}_1|\hat{\theta}_0 = 1.46, \hat{\sigma}_a^2 = 2.74)$ for an *MA1* Model of *UKGDP$_t$* 160

4.1   Forecast Profile for a White Noise Time Series 176

4.2   Forecast Profile for an *AR1* Time Series 178

4.3   Forecast Profile for a Random Walk Time Series 179

4.4 Forecast Profile for an $MA1$ Time Series 181
4.5 Forecast Profile for a Seasonal Time Series 182
5.1 Four Useful Impact Models 187
5.2 Directory Assistance Calls (McSweeney, 1978) 189
5.3 Weekly Productivity Measures, PRD_t 192
5.4 Sample $ACFs$, PRD_t, and ∇PRD_t 193
5.5 Surgical Site Infection Rates (Garey et al., 2008) 194
5.6 Surgical Site Infection Rates, Residual $ACFs$ 195
5.7 New Hampshire Medicaid Prescriptions (Wagner et al., 2002) 196
5.8 Sample ACF and $PACF$ for $\hat{a}_t = Prescrip_t - 5.21 + 2.4I_{t-11} - 1.3I_t$ 197
5.9 Percent "Clean" Urine Samples (Kirby et al., 2008) 200
5.10 Sample ACF and $PACF$, $\hat{a}_t = Clean_t - 21.2 - 12.8IA_t - 16.6IB_t$ 201
5.11 First-Order Transfer Functions of I_t, $0 \leq \delta_1 \leq 1$ 203
5.12 Monthly British Traffic Fatalities (Harvey, 1989) 208
5.13 "Talking Out" Incidents (Hall et al., 1971) 211
5.14 Identification, $\hat{a}_t = Talk_t - 19.3 + 6.8(1 + .56)^{-1}I_t$ 213
5.15 Cholera Deaths Near the Broad Street Pump, 1854 (Lai, 2013) 214
5.16 Gallup Quarterly Presidential Popularity 215
5.17 First-Order Transfer Functions of ∇I_t, $0 \leq \delta_1 \leq 1$ 216
5.18 Daily Self-Injurious Behavior for Two Patients 218
5.19 Australian Divorce Rates (Ozdowski and Hattie, 1981) 221
5.20 Monthly Public Drunkenness Arrests, Washington D.C. 223
5.21 Variance, $-4 \leq \lambda \leq 3$ 224
5.22 Log-Transformed Monthly Public Drunkenness Arrests,
     Washington D.C. 225
5.23 Residual ACF and $PACF$ (Model 1, Table 5.17) 226
6.1 Critical Regions for Two-Tailed and One-Tailed Tests of H_0 240
6.2 Monthly Sales Before and After a Broadcast (Coleman and
     Wiggins, 1996) 241
6.3 Statistical Power for a Time Series Experiment, Effect Size 243
6.4 Statistical Power for a Time Series Experiment, Post-Intervention
     Observations 243
6.5 Boston Armed Robberies 252
6.6 Logarithms, Boston Armed Robberies 253
6.7 Hyde Park Purse Snatchings 254
6.8 Histogram: Days with Exactly M Purse Snatchings 255
6.9 Bedtime Disruptions for a Three-Year-Old Boy
     (Friman et al., 1999) 259
6.10 Annual Physician Expenditures from Two Sources
     (Meltzer et al., 1980) 263
7.1 Annual U.S. Motocycle Fatality Rates (Ross and McCleary, 1983) 276

7.2 Weekly Productivity in the Bank Wiring Room
     (Franke and Kaul, 1978) 277
7.3 Tucson UCR Burglaries (McCleary, Nienstedt, and Erven, 1981) 278
7.4 Diabetes Mortality Rates (Mausner and Kramer, 1985) 279
7.5 Connecticut Motor Vehicle Fatalities, Annual Means 282
7.6 Connecticut Motor Vehicle Fatalities, Monthly Totals 282
7.7 British Breathalyzer Experiment (Ross et al., 1971) 285
7.8 Analgesic Poisoning Suicides in England and Wales
     (Hawton et al., 2009) 286
7.9 European Puerperal Death Rates (Legge, 1985) 287
7.10 UCR Property Crimes in 80 Cities (Hennigan *et al.*, 1981) 288
7.11 Per Capita Cigarette Sales, California vs. All Other States 299
7.12 Per Capita Cigarette Sales,California vs. Synthetic California 300
7.13 Motor Vehicle Fatality Rates, California vs. 41 Donor States 304
7.14 Motor Vehicle Fatality Rates, California vs. Synthetic California 304
7.15 Post-Intervention Change (Annual Fatalities per 100,000) 307
7.16 Post-Intervention *MSPE* 308
8.1 Monthly California Prison Admissions, 1980–2007 319
8.2 Patients Treated for Gunshot or Knife Wounds, Calendar Months 321
8.3 Patients Treated for Gunshot or Knife Wounds, 28-Day Months 321
8.4 Sri Lankan Neonatal Tetanus Death Rates (Veney, 1993) 326
8.5 Impact Defined by Changes in Levels and Slopes 329
8.6 Readmissions to a State Psychiatric Hospital: Change-in-Level
     Model 330
8.7 Readmissions to a State Psychiatric Hospital: Change-in-Slope
     Model 330
9.1 U.K. Standardized Prescriptions by Practitioner 341
9.2 U.K. Standardized Prescriptions by Antibiotic 341

TABLES

1.1 Four Validities (Shadish et al., 2002) 14
2.1 Three Basic Autocovariance Functions 34
2.2 Rules and Definitions 70
2.3 Four Example Sequences 72
2.4 Rules for Evaluating Series 73
3.1 Sample *ACFs* 90
3.2 Estimation and Diagnosis 91
3.3 Goodness-of-Fit Statistics for β-Particles and South Carolina
     Homicides 94

3.4 Estimation and Diagnosis, $Infltn_t$ 96

3.5 Estimation and Diagnosis, $UKGDP_t$ 100

3.6 Estimation and Diagnosis, $Admit_t$ 102

3.7 Identification, $Wheat_t^{-1/2}$ 107

3.8 Estimation and Diagnosis, $Wheat_t^{-1/2}$ 110

3.9 The Box-Cox Transformation Function 111

3.10 Identification, $Sunspot_t^{1/2}$ 113

3.11 Estimation and Diagnosis, $Sunspot_t^{1/2}$ 114

3.12 Identification, $Skirt_t$ 116

3.13 Estimation and Diagnosis, $Skirt_t$ 117

3.14 Estimation and Diagnosis, $Ln(Tubrc_t)$ 121

3.15 Identification, $Prcp_t^{1/4}$ 125

3.16 Estimation and Diagnosis, $Prcp_t^{1/4}$ 127

3.17 Identification, $CO2_t$ 129

3.18 Estimation and Diagnosis, $CO2_t$ 130

3.19 Identification, $AuFtl_t^{1/2}$ 133

3.20 Estimation and Diagnosis, $AuFtl_t^{1/2}$ 133

3.21 Model Selection Criteria 137

3.22 Critical Values for the Unit Root Test Statistics 143

3.23 Unit Root Test for $Infltn_t$ 146

3.24 Unit Root Test, $Ln(Tubrc_t)$ 147

3.25 Unit Root Test for $Infltn_t$ 147

3.26 ARMA Model Score Functions 161

4.1 π-Weight Identities of ARIMA Models 171

4.2 ψ-Weight Identities of ARIMA Models 173

4.3 Forecast Profiles 183

5.1 Directory Assistance Calls, Identification 190

5.2 Estimation and Diagnosis, $Calls_t$ 191

5.3 Estimation and Diagnosis, ∇PRD_t 193

5.4 Surgical Site Infection Rates, Estimation and Diagnosis 195

5.5 Medicaid Prescriptions, Estimation and Diagnosis 198

5.6 Estimation and Diagnosis, $Clean_t$ 201

5.7 Australian Traffic Fatalities, Estimation and Diagnosis 204

5.8 Impact of the Australian Seatbelt Law 207

5.9 British Traffic Fatalities, Identification 209

5.10 British Traffic Fatalities, Estimation and Diagnosis 210

5.11 "Talking Out," Estimation and Diagnosis 213

5.12 Impact of the "Talking Out" Intervention 213

5.13 Self-Injurious Behavior, Estimation and Diagnosis 219

5.14 Impact of a Placebo Intervention 219

5.15 Australian Divorces, Estimation and Diagnosis 222

5.16 Impact of the 1975 Family Law Act 222

5.17 Log Public Drunkenness Arrests, Estimation and Diagnosis 225

5.18 Decriminalization Impact in the First Year (1969) 226

6.1 Threats to Statistical Conclusion Validity (Shadish et al., 2002) 232

6.2 The Modern Hypothesis Test as a Jury Trial 238

6.3 Monthly Sales, Estimation and Diagnosis 242

6.4 The Bayesian Vocabulary 246

6.5 Interpreting Bayes Factors (Raftery, 1995, Table 6) 248

6.6 Threats to Statistical Conclusion Validity 251

6.7 Poisson Parameter Estimates, Hyde Park Purse Snatchings 256

6.8 *ARIMA* Models, Hyde Park Purse Snatchings 257

6.9 Useful Facts and Formulae 271

7.1 Threats to Internal Validity (Shadish et al., 2002) 274

7.2 Model Selection, Connecticut Crackdown on Speeding 283

7.3 Medical Marijuana Laws by State and Five-Year Period 303

7.4 Results of a "Discard-a-State" Test 310

7.5 Results of "Discard-a-Segment" Test 310

7.6 Synthetic California Constructed from Predictors 311

8.1 Threats to Construct Validity (Shadish et al., 2002) 317

8.2 Threats to Construct Validity for Time Series Designs 318

8.3 Patients Treated for Gunshot or Knife Wounds,
     Various Aggregations 322

8.4 Estimation and Diagnosis for Two Trauma Patient Time Series 323

8.5 Estimation and Diagnosis, $Tetanus_t$ 327

8.6 Parameter Estimates for Pandiani and Girardi (1993) 331

9.1 Threats to External Validity (Shadish et al., 2002) 334

Two of us began serious work on this book in 2009. Prior to 2009, we had granted university copy centers permission to freely reproduce our earlier work. That seemed to satisfy the classroom demand for an accessible treatment of time series experiments—perhaps fifty to 300 copies per year—as well as our ability to field readers' inquiries about the examples used in this work. So before jumping into this project, we debated two questions. First, did the world need another book-length treatment of time series experiments? Second, did we have the time and energy to master the intricate details of a new set of examples? The answer to the first question is, obviously, Yes. The answer to the second question—No—explains the presence of a co-author who will field complaints, suggestions, and questions.

Our affirmative answer to the first question reflects the ever-increasing interest in time series experiments, especially in the health sciences, as well as some of the emerging ways to draw causal inferences from quasi-experimental results. It is not much of an exaggeration to attribute the time series experiment per se to Donald T. Campbell and collaborators Thomas D. Cook, Gene V. Glass, George C. Tiao, and others. Campbell's approach to validity, which guides the development of this book, is *implicitly* causal. An intervention is presumed to *cause* a change in the level of a time series if the enumerated threats to validity can be ruled out—or rendered implausible. Most psychologists are taught the design of time series experiments from Campbell's perspective and it has served them well.

A newer way to think about the design of time series experiments is due to Donald B. Rubin and collaborators Paul W. Holland, Guido W. Imbens, Paul R. Rosenbaum, and others. Rubin's approach is *explicitly* causal. If the unobserved counterfactual part of an impact can be inferred from the observed factual part, then a *causal* relationship can be inferred. The inferential process is more complicated than this simple statement, of course. Rubin causality extends valid causal inference to *non*-experimental time series designs, however—or time series quasi-experiments as they are called—and that development was a major stimulus for this book.

The potential of Rubin causality was first realized and exploited by economists working in program evaluation. Our development of this material retains the major features of Campbell's approach while integrating the central feature of Rubin's approach. In our opinion, the approaches of Campbell and Rubin are parallel and complementary. A few differences between the two approaches are obvious, nevertheless, especially in the way that control time series are chosen and analyzed. This major difference between the two approaches cannot be ignored.

Over the years, we have benefitted from discussions with and feedback and criticism from many. Needless to say, errors in our thinking cannot be attributed to any of these individuals. The influence of our teachers, including Howie Becker, Dick Berk, Don Campbell, Tom Cook, Ken Land, and George Tiao, may be apparent. We also benefitted from interactions with colleagues, including Tim Bruckner, Ray Catalano, Keith Hawton, Ross Homel, Val Jenness, Tom Kratochwill, Lon-Mu Liu, Colin Loftin, Mike Maltz, Cheryl Maxson, Errol Meidinger, Curt Sandman, Nick Scurich, Will Shadish, Dean Simonton, Sheldon Stone, Bryan Sykes, Alex Wagenaar, and Brian Wiersema. We also benefitted from interactions with our students, of course, especially Tanya Anaya, Chris Bates, Nicholas Branic, Mitch Chamlin, Christine Champion, Jun Chu, Jason Gravel, Michelle Mioduszewski, Carol Newark, Matt Renner, Sanjeev Sridharan, and Doug Wiebe.

Several people made explicit contributions to the project. Tim Bruckner, Ray Catalano, Keith Hawton, Will Shadish, Sheldon Stone, Bryan Sykes, Alex Wagenaar, and Doug Wiebe provided time series data and comments on early drafts. Unbeknownst to them, many of these individuals also tutored us on alcohol and traffic injury epidemiology (Alex Wagenaar), demography (Bryan Sykes), social epidemiology (Tim Bruckner and Ray Catalano), nosocomial disease (Sheldon Stone and Doug Wiebe), and general causal inference (Will Shadish). Bill Lattyak of Scientific Computing Associates was exceptionally generous with his time and counsel, even to the point of modifying our software on several occasions.

Two people made implicit contributions. First, this book would not have been written without Tom Cook's early support and intellectual nurturing. We have tried to convey his notions of causality in this book and to express them in his narrative style. To the extent that the book succeeds, thank Tom Cook. Second, if it is not obvious, the title of this book is an *homage* to Gene Glass, a constant vicarious source of inspiration. Although the meaning of "design" has changed drastically in the 40 years since Glass et al. (1975), the design–causality connection is unchanged.

This project could not have succeeded without the support of our universities. We are grateful for the long-term support of colleagues and staff at Albany and Irvine, especially Mary Underwood. Finally, this project would have failed without the sustained encouragement and support of our families. For that, we are indebted to Alex, Angela, David, and Kaitlin McCleary; to Cynthia and Alexandra McDowall; to John and Susan Bartos; and to Natalie Bock: "When you are old and grey and full of sleep, and nodding by the fire, take down this book . . ."

Design and Analysis of Time Series Experiments

Introduction

The "pretest-posttest" experimental design has never been highly regarded as an experimental technique in the behavioral sciences and for good reasons.
— GLASS, WILLSON, AND GOTTMAN (1975)

The "pretest-posttest" design referred to so dismissively by Glass et al. is the design that Campbell and Stanley (1966, pp. 7–12) call the "one-group pretest-posttest." Using the conventional notation where observations and interventions are represented by Os and Xs respectively, this design is diagrammed as

$$O_{pre} \quad X \quad O_{post}$$

In a treatise aimed at unifying experimental and quasi-experimental designs, Campbell and Stanley relegate the pretest-posttest design to a special category: Along with the "one-shot case study" and "static group comparison," it is a pre-experimental design. Our view of the pretest-posttest design is more qualified. Though agreeing with Campbell and Stanley and Glass et al. that the pretest-posttest design is utterly without merit, we must add that, to our knowledge, no peer-reviewed social science research has actually used this design. The pretest-posttest design is used almost exclusively for didactic purposes, especially for demonstrating the validity, utility, and flexibility of the time series designs that are the focus of this book.

Now of the hundred or so time series books published each year, most focus on forecasting. These books are aimed at students in business and engineering. Our book is distinguished not only by its focus on the design and analysis of time series experiments but by its intended audience of behavioral, biomedical, and social scientists. Our focus and audience dictate an idiosyncratic approach. We develop epistemological issues, such as causality and validity, and statistical issues, such as estimation and uncertainty, as an integrated whole. Some readers may find this approach exasperating, especially if their purpose is to acquire a superficial "how-to" understanding of an application. Our approach aims to demonstrate not only "how to do" a time series experiment but also, how to interpret the analytic results.

Although this present book builds on and extends our prior work (McCleary et al., 1980; McDowall et al., 1980), it takes a more eclectic view of the topic. Due largely to the work of Campbell (1957, 1969; Campbell and Stanley, 1966; Cook and Campbell, 1979; Shadish et al., 2002),"time series experiment" (or more properly, "quasi-experiment") has come to mean a simple contrast of pre- and postintervention time series levels. While this narrow definition simplifies the explication of design issues, especially validity, it obscures the statistical problems shared by all longitudinal analyses.

Since virtually all confirmatory time series analyses confront the same set of obstacles, we expand "time series experiment" in this book to include three design variations: the descriptive time series experiment, the interrupted time series experiment, and the concomitant time series experiment. Purely descriptive time series designs do not support valid causal inference. We use that design to illustrate some of the principles of design. Valid causal inference requires a well-designed interrupted or concomitant time series experiment.

Time series designs are distinguished from other designs by the properties of time series data and by the necessary reliance on a statistical model to control threats to validity. In the long run, a time series is a realization of a latent causal process. We represent the complete time series as

$$\ldots Y_{-1}, Y_0, [Y_1, Y_2, \ldots, Y_N], Y_{N+1}, \ldots$$

The observed time series $[Y_1, Y_2, \ldots, Y_N]$ is a probability sample of the complete realization whose sampling weights are specified in a statistical model. For present purposes, we write the full model in a general linear form as the sum of "noise" and "exogenous" components:

$$Y_t = N(a_t) + X(I_t)$$

The a_t term of this model is the tth observation of a strictly exogenous innovation time series with the "white noise" property,

$$a_t \sim \text{iid Normal}(0, \sigma_a^2)$$

The I_t term is the tth observation of a causal time series. Although I_t is ordinarily a binary variable coded for the presence or absence of an intervention, it can also be a purely stochastic time series. In either case, the model is constructed by a set of rules that allow for the solution,

$$a_t = N^{-1}[Y_t - X(I_t)]$$

Since a_t has white noise properties, the solved model satisfies the assumptions of all common tests of significance. In the context of an appropriately specified design, moreover, the results of these tests can be interpreted causally.

1.1 THREE DESIGNS

We elaborate on the specific forms of the general model and on the set of rules for building models at a later point. For present purposes, the general model allows three design variations: (1) descriptive time series designs, (2) correlational time series designs, and (3) experimental or quasi-experimental time series designs.

Descriptive Designs. The simplest time series design, which we call a "descriptive" design, consists of decomposing the series into elementary components, such as trends and cycles, and then interpreting the time series components. Informal descriptive analyses often precede formal hypothesis testing. But lacking any interpretation—no hypothesis tests about trends or cycles, i.e.—we are reluctant to call this activity an experiment. When hypotheses about trends or cycles are tested, in contrast, descriptive analyses qualify as primitive time series experiments. Early historical examples include Wolf's (1848; Yule, 1927; Izenman, 1983) investigation of sunspot activity and Elton's (1924; Elton and Nicholson, 1942) investigation of lynx populations. In both examples, time series analyses revealed cycles or trends that corroborated substantive interpretations of the phenomenon.

Kroeber's (1919; Richardson and Kroeber, 1940) analyses of cultural change illustrate the unsuitability of descriptive time series designs to many social and behavioral phenomena. Kroeber (1969) hypothesized that women's fashions change in response to political and economic variables. During stable periods of peace and prosperity, fashions changed slowly; during wars, revolutions, and depressions, fashions changed rapidly. Since political and economic cataclysms were thought to recur in long historical cycles, Kroeber tested his hypothesis by searching for the same cycles in women's fashions.

Figure 1.1 plots one of Kroeber's annual fashion time series: 150 years of mean skirt widths collected by Richardson and Kroeber (1940) from museum fashion plates. The time series appears to have two distinct trends. Until 1860, skirts get wider. Thereafter, skirts get narrower. Kroeber (1969) argued that this pattern was not two trends but, rather, a cycle. In his view, women's fashions were

Skirt Widths

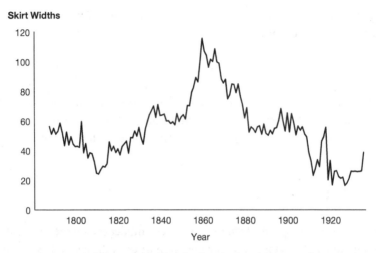

Figure 1.1 Annual Skirt Widths (Richardson and Kroeber, 1940)

stable – or trendless – over time. In those rare periods when fashions did change, the causal agent was a complex construct called "sociocultural unsettlement" that could be inferred from historical events such as wars, revolutions, and depressions. Since episodes of cultural unsettlement were thought to recur cyclically, Kroeber reasoned that fashions would change in the same broad cycles. When the deterministic components are removed from this series, as Kroeber predicted, the residuals during periods of cultural unsettlement are larger than expected.

Kroeber (1969) argued that simple descriptive time series experiments of this sort are an ideal means of testing causal hypotheses. If a pattern of change is not due to chance, then it must have empirically discoverable causes. The descriptive time series experiment, in this sense, distinguishes anthropology from history. Readers with a survey knowledge of stochastic processes might find Kroeber's argument difficult to accept, of course. Wholly random processes can and do generate ostensibly non-random patterns of change. The apparent cycle in Figure 1.1 is not much different than what would be realized from a sequence of coin flips.

Figure 1.2 shows a second example of the descriptive time series experiment. These data are annual proportions of Canadian homicides where the offender and victim are married ("Spouse") and where the offender and victim are strangers ("Stranger"). Silverman and Kennedy (1987) argue that these two types of homicide follow distinctively different trends. There is a theoretical basis to this claim. Whereas spousal homicides often result from routine interactions between intimates, stranger homicides result from impersonal social disintegration processes. From their visual inspection of these two time series, Silverman and Kennedy conclude that spousal homicides are falling while stranger homicides

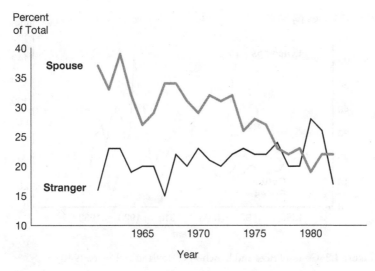

Figure 1.2 Canadian Homicides (Silverman and Kennedy, 1987)

are rising. The spousal homicide time series does seems to trend downward but the trend is not obviously significant. To our eyes, moreover, the stranger homicide time series is not trending upward. Like beauty, of course, trend is in the eye of the beholder. In fact, the difference in the trends of these two time series is not significant.

Whereas other time series designs treat $N(a_t)$ as a "nuisance" function whose sole purpose is to control the threats to statistical conclusion validity posed by cycles and trends, the descriptive design infers substantive explanations from $N(a_t)$. As these examples demonstrate, however, it is difficult if not impossible to infer causal relationships from trends and cycles. The inferential problems inherent to descriptive time series experiments parallel those of the "one-shot case study" design (Campbell and Stanley, 1966). As in the one-shot case study, most descriptive time series designs are unable to rule out alternative rival hypotheses. As a consequence, most descriptive time series experiments are uninterpretable. There are exceptions, of course, but for the most part, this simplest, most primitive time series design is unlikely to uncover valid causal relationships. Although the statistical models and methods developed for the analysis of descriptive designs are applied for exploratory purposes (see Mills, 1991), they are currently not widely used for null hypothesis tests.

Correlational Designs. A second type of time series experiment attempts to infer a causal relationship between two series from their covariance. Historical examples include Chree's (1913) analyses of the temporal correlation between sunspot activity and terrestrial magnetism and Beveridge's (1922) analyses of the temporal correlation between rainfall and wheat prices. The validity of

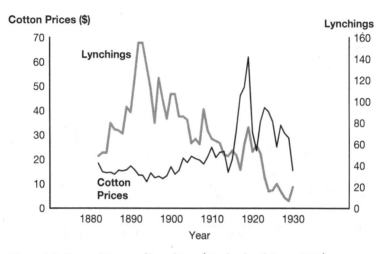

Figure 1.3 Cotton Prices and Lynchings (Hovland and Sears, 1940)

correlational inferences rests heavily on theory, of course. When theory points to a single causal effect operating at discrete lags, as in these natural science examples, correlational designs support unambiguous causal interpretations. Lacking a strong theoretical specification, however, correlational designs do not allow strong causal inferences. Two social science examples illustrate this point.

Hovland and Sears (1940) used the cotton price and lynching time series plotted in Figure 1.3 to test the frustration-aggression hypothesis (Dollard et al., 1939). Hovland and Sears hypothesized that aggressive acts such as lynchings would rise in bad economic times and fall in years of prosperity. To test this hypothesis, Hovland and Sears estimated the Pearson product-moment correlation between the number of lynchings and cotton prices during the 1882–1930 period. Assuming that the correlation would be zero in the absence of a causal relationship, Hovland and Sears interpreted a statistically significant correlation as corroborating evidence. Due to common stochastic time series properties, however, especially trend, causally independent time series will be correlated. Controlling for trend, Hepworth and West (1989) report a small, significant negative correlation between these series but warn against causal interpretations. The correlation is an artifact of the war years 1914–18 when the demand for cotton and the civilian population moved in opposite directions (McCleary, 2000). Excluding the war years, the correlation is not statistically significant.

The time series plotted in Figure 1.4 shows a more recent correlational time series experiment. Polyson et al. (1986) argue that because the Minnesota Multiphasic Personality Inventory (MMPI) and Rorschach tests are based on competing approaches to personality assessment, citations for the two tests should be negatively correlated—a productive year for one test should imply

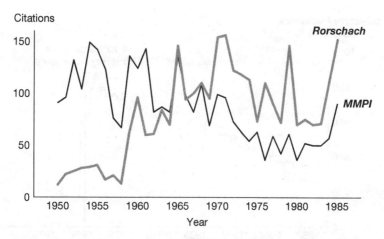

Figure 1.4 Annual Rorschach and MMPI Citations (Polyson et al., 1986)

an unproductive year for the other. As predicted, the Pearson product-moment correlation coefficient between the two series is negative and statistically significant. Estimating a correlation between two time series is more difficult than one might think, however. It is tempting to treat the two time series as if they were cross-sectional samples. And if time series observations had white noise properties, any statistic could be estimated by simply plugging the data into the appropriate cross-sectional formula. Time series observations are seldom independent, however, and given any trend or cyclical behavior, the estimated correlation coefficient between two series will invariably overstate their true relationship. Controlling for their common trend, O'Grady (1988) shows that the correlation reported by Polyson et al. is an artifact.

Where theory supports strong specification, correlational time series designs continue to be used. Other than limited areas in economics and psychology, however, social theories will not support the required specification. Even in these areas, causal inference may require the narrow definition of "Granger causality" (Granger, 1969) to rule out plausible alternative interpretations.

Interrupted Time Series Designs. The third type of time series design infers the latent causal effect of a temporally discrete intervention, or treatment, from discontinuities or interruptions in a time series. Campbell and Stanley (1966, pp. 37–43) call this design the "time series experiment" and its use is currently the major application of time series data for causal inference. Historical examples of the general approach include investigations of workplace interventions on health and productivity by the British Industrial Fatigue Research Board (Florence, 1923) and by the Hawthorn experiments (Roethlisberger and Dickson, 1939). Fisher's (1921) analyses of agricultural interventions on crop yields also relied on variants of the time series experiment.

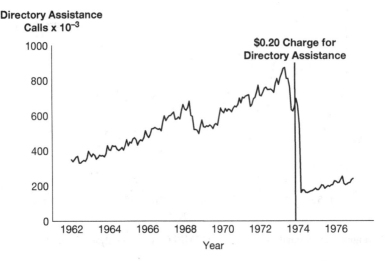

Figure 1.5 Cincinnati Directory Assistance Calls (McSweeney, 1978)

In the simplest case of the design, a discrete intervention breaks a time series into pre- and post-intervention segments of N_{pre} and N_{post} observations. For pre- and post-intervention means, μ_{pre} and μ_{post}, analysis of the experiment tests the null hypothesis[1]

$$H_0: \omega = 0 \quad \text{where} \quad \omega = \mu_{post} - \mu_{pre}$$

against the alternative

$$H_A: \omega \neq 0$$

Rejecting H_0, H_A attributes ω to the intervention. In practice, however, treatment effects are almost always more complex than the simple change in level implied by this null hypothesis.

The time series plotted in Figure 1.5 is typical in one sense, atypical in another. Monthly calls to Cincinnati Directory Assistance (McSweeney, 1978) rise steadily, beginning in 1962. When Cincinnati Bell begins to charge for these calls, the monthly number of calls drops abruptly to a new, lower level. Since abrupt interruptions are not a natural feature of time series processes, the interruption can be interpreted as the causal effect of the exogenous intervention. The magnitude and abruptness of the effect renders all other interpretations implausible. Not all time series quasi-experiments can be interpreted so confidently.

---

1. Some readers may quarrel with this early description of hypothesis testing, especially our use of H_0 and H_A and p-values. We return to this topic in Chapter 6 where we discuss statistical conclusion validity.

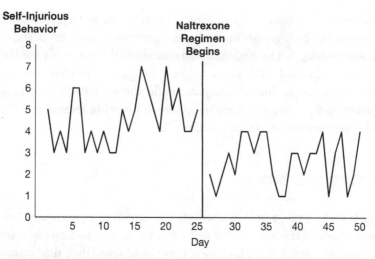

Figure 1.6 Self-Injurious Behavior (McCleary et al., 1999)

Figure 1.6 is a more typical example. These data are 50 daily self-injurious behavior counts for an institutionalized patient (McCleary et al., 1999). On the 26th and subsequent days, the patient is treated with naltrexone, an opiate blocker. The plotted time series leaves the visual impression that the opiate blocker has reduced the incidence of self-injurious behavior. Indeed, the difference in means for the 25 pre- and 25 post-intervention days amounts to a 42 percent reduction in self-injurious behavior. Visual evidence can be deceiving, of course, and that is why we need statistical time series analyses of the sort described in this book.

The most obvious difference between the Directory Assistance and self-injurious behavior experiments is the relative magnitudes of their effects. In the Directory Assistance experiment, the proportion of variance due to the intervention dwarfs the proportion due to trends, cycles, and background noise. A statistical analysis might be superfluous. In the self-injurious behavior experiment, on the other hand, the proportion of variance due to the naltrexone intervention is more modest. A statistical analysis might be recommended. Another apparent difference is less important than some readers would suspect. Whereas the self-injurious behavior experiment is a true experiment, the Directory Assistance experiment is, strictly speaking, a quasi-experiment. In other contexts, experimental manipulation of an intervention controls powerful threats to internal validity. In a time series design, however, the most plausible threat to internal validity —"maturation"—cannot be controlled by design but, rather, must be controlled by a statistical model.

The necessary reliance on a statistical model to control common threats to internal validity distinguishes time series designs from cross-sectional and simple before–after designs. The randomization procedures that are widely used to control threats to internal validity in these other designs may be counterproductive in time series designs. Indeed, compared to the threats to statistical conclusion, construct, and external validities, the common threats to internal validity play smaller roles in a time series experiment.

1.2 FOUR VALIDITIES

Suppose that a large sample of scientists was invited to a professional meeting organized around the topic of "validity." Most attendees would have little interest in the general topic. Left on their own, they would spend their time connecting with colleagues to discuss the core phenomena of their disciplines: molecules, cells, population dynamics, etc. In fact, in what Kuhn (1996) might call the "normal science" disciplines, scientists have neither an interest in nor a practical need to understand the nuances of validity. A minority of attendees at our hypothetical meeting would be drawn to sessions focused on specific applications. Some psychologists and some physicists might attend sessions dealing with measurement, for example, while scientists who design and conduct randomized controlled trials might attend sessions on decision making. A smaller group might be drawn to sessions focused on synthetic review methods and though it would be their second choice, any of the attendees might wander in and out of sessions focused on causality.

The point of this fable is that validity comes in four natural flavors: statistical conclusion, internal, construct, and external. There is no a priori reason why the number of flavors should be fixed at four, much less these specific four. The four natural flavors have survived many practical tests, however. The alternative validity flavors that are proposed from time to time make only minor contributions, on the other hand, and are often cumbersome and difficult to apply. In that respect, the four natural validity flavors are Aristotelian supergenera from which less general flavors can be derived. Attempts to reduce the four natural flavors into components have also proved unsuccessful. Upon inspection, proposed component flavors turn out to be attempts to relabel the four natural flavors. Even Campbell (1986) tried to rename internal and external validity. Although the four natural validity flavors could benefit from shorter, more descriptive names, relabeling them would be wasteful and, probably, futile. We will use the accepted names and definitions that are familar to most readers.

The proximal ancestor of the four-validity system is the two-validity system proposed initially by Campbell (1957) and then elaborated upon by Campbell and Stanley (1966). Nearly three decades after his initial proposal, Campbell (1986) explained the two-validity system as a reaction to the over-reliance, in psychology, on analog experiments:

> In the 1950s, the training in research methods ... was dominated by Fisherian analysis of variance statistics, as though random assignment to treatment were the only methodological control that needed to be taught ... In dialogue with this lopsided and complacent emphasis, we wished to point out that ... there were a lot of threats to validity that randomization did not take care of and that the teaching of research design should be expanded to cover these other threats, which we classified as issues of external validity. It was against the overwhelming dominance of Fisher's randomized assignment models and an implicit, complacent assumption that meticulous care in this regard took care of all experimental validity problems that we were reacting. (Campbell, 1986, p. 67)

Though defined as a residual category, Campbell (1957, p. 297) associated external validity with the "representativeness, or generalizability" of an observed result. Having found an effect, in other words, "to what populations, settings, and variables can this effect be generalized?" Campbell (1957) also acknowledged the potential trade-off between internal and external validity in that "the controls required for internal validity often tend to jeopardize representativeness." Both ideas were integrated into the popular, commonsense understanding of external validity.

Given the salience of causality in Campbell's (1957) thinking, internal validity came to acquire a *primus inter pares* status. In response to what was seen as a narrow focus on specific situations, Cronbach (1982) proposed an alternative validity system that emphasized the generalizability of results. In Cronbach's view, interactions between treatments and local contexts limited the generalizability of experimental results; and if a result could not be generalized beyond the immediate context, then internal validity was irrelevant. Absent control of the treatment–context interactions, an observed result amounted to mere ideographic description.[2]

2. Although the source is obscure, the nomothetic–ideographic distinction is important to psychological science. At the end of the 19th century, Windelband (1894; cited by Mayr, 1997, p. 276) proposed the nomothetic–ideographic dichotomy to distinguish between disciplines whose phenomena were interchangeable or repeatable and disciplines whose phenomena were not. Because hydrogen atoms are indistinguishable or interchangeable and because Newton's mechanical laws describe the path of a falling object no matter how many times it is dropped, chemistry and physics were nomothetic disciplines. But because historical phenomena are not repeatable, history is an ideographic discipline.

Since Campbell had addressed treatment–context interactions as threats to external validity, Cronbach's alternative validity system might be dismissed as a relabeled version of Campbell's. That would be a mistake. Acknowledging Cronbach's critique of the two-validity system, at least as it was popularly understood, Campbell (1986) proposed a more accurate label for internal validity: "local molar causal validity."

> By molar we connote recognition that the treatment is often a very complex hodgepodge put together by expert clinical judgment, not on the basis of the already proven efficacy of its theoretically pure components ... By local we indicate the strategy illustrated in pilot testing. Let's see if it really works in some one setting and time ... Molar and local could both be taken as implying no generalization at all. The causal relationship would be known locally and molarly but there would be no validated theory that would guide generalization to other interventions, measures, populations, settings, or times. This is, of course, an exaggeration. The theories and hunches used by those who put the therapeutic package together must be regarded as corroborated, however tentatively, if there is an effect of local, molar validity in the expected direction. Nonetheless, this exaggeration may serve to remind us that very frequently in physical science (and probably in social science as well), causal puzzles (that is, effects that are dependable but not understood) are the driving motor for new and productive theorizing. We must back up from the current overemphasis on theory first. (Campbell, 1986, pp. 69–70)

Despite its more accurate representation of Campbell's views, "local molar causal validity" never caught on.[3] Campbell did not expect the new label to replace the old, of course, but rather wanted to acknowledge Cronbach's concerns and comment on the reductionist causal explanations commonly favored by social scientists.

In collaboration with Campbell, Thomas D. Cook attempted to generalize the two-validity system to applied social science reseach, especially program evaluation. Several of the new threats to internal validity described by Cook and Campbell (1976) blurred the sharp boundary between internal and external validity. To solve this boundary problem, the two new validities were defined. Threats to statistical conclusion validity addressed questions of confidence and power that had been included implicitly as threats to internal validity. Threats to construct validity addressed questions of confounding that had been included implicitly as threats to external validity.

---

3. No wonder. Campbell's suggested label was actually "local molar (pragmatic, atheoretical) causal validity."

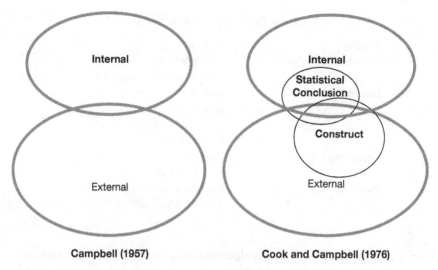

Figure 1.7 Campbell (1957) Evolves into Cook and Campbell (1976)

Figure 1.7 depicts this most obvious difference between the old and new systems. Though less obvious, other differences are worth noting. Whereas the two-validity system was simple and easily mastered, for example, mastering the four-validity system requires great patience and tolerance for ambiguity. Part of this difference is due to the older system's presumed dichotomous logical structure. Under the two-validity system, anything that is not a threat to internal validity is necessarily a threat to external validity and vice versa. This straightforward deductive property comes in handy when we analyze trade-offs between internal and external validity. The design features that strengthen internal validity weaken external validity in a straightforward way. Analyzing the trade-offs among four validities, on the other hand, requires imagination and hard work.

In practice, unfortunately, it is not always possible to partition the validities into discrete collections of threats. When we represent the validities by Venn diagrams as in Figure 1.7, we must allow each validity to overlap its peer validities. These overlaps arise from and reflect minor disagreements on the proper attribution of specific threats. A threat might belong to one validity under one set of circumstances, that is, but to another validity under another set of circumstances. We present examples of these threats in later chapters. For the present, overlaps among the validities are small, inconsequential, and ignorable.

Table 1.1 lists the four validities and their associated threats as described by our authority, Shadish, Cook, and Campbell (2002). Whereas Shadish et al. necessarily pay attention to a wide range of designs, our attention will be narrowly focused on the subset of threats that are endemic to time series designs. Some of

Table 1.1. FOUR VALIDITIES (SHADISH ET AL., 2002)

Validity	Threat
Statistical Conclusion	*Low statistical power*
	Violated assumptions of the test
Internal	*History*
	Maturation
	Regression artifacts
	Instrumentation
Construct	*Reactivity*
	Novelty and disruption
External	*Interaction over treatment variations*
	Interaction with settings

the Shadish et al. threats to validity are irrelevant or even implausible in time series designs. We also describe "new" threats to validity that apply uniquely to time series designs. Finally, some threats to validity that are particularly troublesome in time series designs do not fit neatly into one of the natural categories. With that said, in detail:

Statistical Conclusion Validity. Shadish et al. (2002, p. 45) identify nine threats to statistical conclusion validity or "reasons why researchers may be wrong in drawing valid inferences about the magnitude of covariation between two variables." Although the consequences of any particular threat will vary across settings, the threats to statistical conclusion validity fall neatly into categories involving misstatements of the Type I and Type II error rates. For both Type I and Type II errors, uncontrolled threats to statistical conclusion validity distort the nominal error rates, leading to invalid inferences.

Internal Validity. Under some circumstances, all nine of the threats to internal validity identified by Shadish et al. (2002, p. 55) might apply to a time series experiment. Typically, however, only four threats are plausible enough to pose serious difficulties. History and maturation, which arise from the use of multiple temporal observations, can threaten virtually any application of the design. Instrumentation and regression can also be problems, but only for interventions that involve advance planning. For unplanned interventions—what Campbell (1963) called "natural experiments"—these threats are much less realistic.

Construct Validity. Shadish et al. (2002, p. 73) identify 14 "reasons why inferences about the constructs that characterize study operations may be incorrect." One of the 14 threats to construct validity, novelty and disruption, is especially relevant to time series designs. Regardless of whether an intervention has its intended effect, the time series is likely to react or not react to the novelty or disruption associated with it. If the general form of the artifact is known, it can be incorporated into the statistical model.

External Validity. Time series experiments typically consider the effect of an intervention on only one time series, and this makes it highly vulnerable to external validity threats. External validity considers whether findings hold "over variations in persons, settings, treatments, and outcomes" (Shadish et al., 2002, p. 83) and threats to it are always plausible when analyzing a single series. Ruling out external validity threats necessarily requires replicating the quasi-experiment over a diverse set of conditions.

Although we treat the four validities as discretely partitioned categories, this treatment has two limitations. First, since the four-validity system is an imperfect construct, common threats may leak across categories. An analogous dilemma arises in a multiple-choice test when a question has two or more correct answers. In that situation, students are instructed to choose the "best" correct answer. We will follow that instruction here but admit, nevertheless, that sometimes a threat can belong to two validity categories depending on circumstances and context. Second, we recognize that there are trade-offs among validities. Threats to internal validity are controlled by manipulating the intervention or treatment, for example—or by doing something that has the same effect. Internal validity comes at the expense of external validity, unfortunately. Threats to external validity are controlled in principle by replication. Replication raises common threats to statistical conclusion and construct validities, however. Some of the validities are more plausible in single-subject designs where the intervention is controlled and masked. Other validities are more plausible when the intervention is planned. These trade-offs suggest that the four validities are not independent or, in other words, that they lack the essential properties of discrete categories and, hence, that the four-validity system is a fallible construct. Accepting that, we point out that the four-validity system is nevertheless a useful construct.

1.3 WHEN TO USE A TIME SERIES DESIGN—OR NOT

To demonstrate the strengths and weaknesses of time series designs, we resurrect the simple before–after design that Campbell and Stanley (1966) call the "one-group pretest-posttest" quasi-experiment:

$$O_{pre} \quad X \quad O_{post}$$

Now the "one-group pretest-posttest" quasi-experiment is rarely used for any purpose at all. We use it strictly for didactic purposes here. With that said, the analogous time series design,

$$\dots \quad O \quad O \quad O \quad X \quad O \quad O \quad O \quad \dots$$

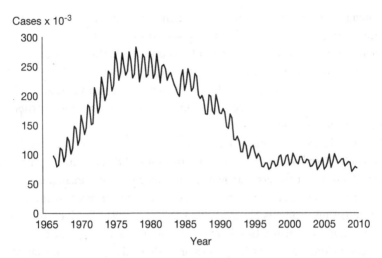

Figure 1.8 Quarterly U.S. Gonorrhea Cases

demands a relatively greater investment of time and effort to collect data. This added cost is the salient weakness or disadvantage of time series designs. When a simpler, less expensive before–after design offers an acceptable degree of validity, it is difficult to justify the added expense of a time series design. In many realistic situations, unfortunately, simple before–after designs perform inadequately or, sometimes, fail categorically. In these situations, time series designs are the only reasonable option.

The most common situation that warrants the expense of a time series design occurs when the underlying phenomenon is complex. Figure 1.8 illustrates this type of situation. Like many public health time series, the quarterly time series of U.S. gonorrhea cases rises steadily between 1965 and 1975 but then levels off between 1975 and 1985. Beginning in 1985, the time series falls steadily, though with one or two interruptions, until 1995. After 1995, the time series levels off again. The seasonality in this time series is also complex. Prior to 1980, the time series peaks each summer in a predictable annual cycle. The summer peaks become more variable after 1980, fading entirely in some years. Considering trend and seasonality together, this time series has the "look and feel" of a composite time series with segments cobbled together from disparate sources. That is what we mean by a "complex" time series.

It may be difficult to believe that this time series is the realization of one underlying process throughout 1965–2009. But it is. Segments of this time series have been used to evaluate the effectiveness of screening programs (Schnell, Zaidi, and Reynolds, 1989; Fox et al., 1998) and analogous time series have been used to evaluate the effectiveness of public health interventions (Wong et al., 1998; for a review, see Shahmanesh et al., 2008). In each instance, the effect

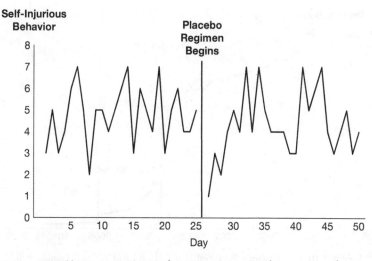

Figure 1.9 Self-Injurious Behavior (McCleary et al., 1999)

of the planned intervention is obscured by the phenomenon's complex trend and seasonality. The statistical time series model untangles the effects of the intervention from the confounding effects of trend and seasonality, allowing for a powerful test of the intervention effect. Ignoring the confounds of trend and seasonality poses serious threats to several validities.

Another common situation that warrants the expense of a time series design occurs when the effect of an intervention is realized dynamically. The time series plotted in Figure 1.9 illustrates one type of dynamic effect. These data are daily self-injurious behavior counts for an institutionalized patient who receives a placebo intervention (McCleary et al., 1999). The level of this patient's self-injurious behavior drops abruptly on the first post-intervention day but then returns gradually to its pre-intervention level. Since institutionalized patients commonly react to any environmental disruption, including a placebo, this patient's response is not unexpected. A simple before–after contrast of the pre- and post-intervention means of this time series might lead to the invalid inference that the placebo treatement was effective. The placebo effect would probably be smaller than the effect of the opiate-blocker intervention (Figure 1.6), of course, but that might be only a minor consolation. Analyzed in a time series design, on the other hand, the dynamic effect of the placebo can be modeled explicitly.

The time series plotted in Figure 1.10 illustrates another type of dynamic impact. These data are the quarterly number of co-proxamol prescriptions written in England and Wales from 1998 through 2010 (Hawton et al., 2009). Co-proxamol was a highly effective analgesic, widely used to treat arthritis

Prescriptions

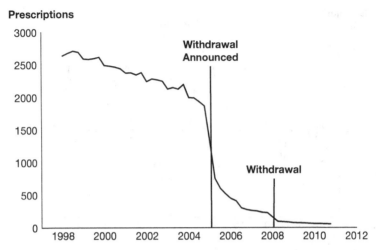

Figure 1.10 Co-proxamol Prescriptions, England and Wales (Hawton et al., 2009)

pain. Concerns for patient safety had been voiced since the early 1980s, however, especially for suicide. In January 2005, the U.K. Committee on Safety of Medicines recommended that co-proxamol be withdrawn from general use. To allow patients to move to alternative pain treatments, the Committee delayed its recommendation for two years. In those rare cases where effective alternatives would not be available, patients would be allowed to continue on co-proxamol after January 2007.

The co-proxamol prescription time series declines smoothly until the fourth quarter of 2004 when—apparently in anticipation of the Committee's announcement—it drops abruptly. In the following quarter, when the Committee's anouncement is made public, the time series again drops abruptly. The time series level continues to decline gradually in successive quarters, approaching a new, much lower post-intervention level. The time series level drops one more time in January 2007, when the withdrawal takes effect, and then continues a slow, smooth decline. If this time series were analyzed as a simple before–after design, the dynamic nature of the intervention would be obscured, leading to a biased estimate of the magnitude of the effect.

Situations where the added expense of a time series design is warranted fall into two overlapping categories. The first category consists of situations where the nature of the underlying phenomenon is obscured by trends and cycles. A well-constructed time series model may reveal the nature of the underlying phenomenon. The second category consists of situations where a known intervention and an appropriate control time series are available. In those situations, a well-designed time series experiment can support explicitly causal inferences that are not supported by less expensive before–after designs.

1.4 OUTLINE OF THE BOOK

As the title implies, subsequent chapters of this book focus on the design and analysis of time series experiments, but not in that order. Whereas it might make sense in some methodological areas to treat design and analysis as distinct, severable topics, that distinction makes little sense here because, after all, time series designs are distinguished by their necessary reliance on a statistical model to control common threats to validity. Issues of design and analysis are inseparable. Our integrative approach is not novel, of course, but builds on the approach established by Cook and Campbell (1979) and articulated by Shadish et al. (2002).

Readers who are familiar with our earlier work (McCleary et al., 1980; McDowall et al., 1980) may notice several differences in this work. These differences reflect the natural evolution of the field and of our thinking. Some ideas have not changed; for example, the idea that the threats to validity arise from four common research tasks. Like any other social construct, the system of four validities may someday be discarded. But until then, it is a useful construct. Other ideas have changed gradually in the last three decades. Now to be sure, many ideas that seemed promising failed to deliver in some way or another. Catastrophe models (Cobb and Zacks, 1985) and chaos models (Granger, 1993) come to mind. Other ideas proved durable and, in the long run, left an ecology of thought that Donald T. Campbell might not recognize, much less endorse. Some of these newer ideas relate to the way that nonstationary time series are modeled and, more generally, to the way in which model adequacy is assessed and significance tested. Other ideas relate to the way that "causality" is defined and tested.

Thirty years ago, the workhorse statistical models for time series experiments were the AutoRegressive Integrated Moving Average (*ARIMA*) models of Box and Jenkins (1970; Box and Tiao, 1975). In succeeding years, the utility of these models has become apparent, so the *ARIMA* model algebra developed in Chapter 2 has changed little. Our feelings would not be hurt if readers who are familar with our earlier treatments of this material decide to skip this chapter. Be warned, however, that in response to classroom experience and student feedback, our current presentation has changed significantly. To accommodate a range of tastes and backgrounds, we continue to relegate technical, mathematical material to appendices. In this instance, brief (and, we hope, accessible) introductions to expected values and infinite sequences and series follow as appendices to Chapter 2. Some students become *ARIMA*-"literate" with little explicit knowledge of this material. But students who understand expected values, sequences, and series will acquire deeper insights into *ARIMA* algebra.

Chapter 3 develops the methods or strategies for building *ARIMA* noise models. At one level, the iterative identify-estimate-diagnose modeling strategy proposed by Box and Jenkins has changed little in 40 years. At another level, however, the collective experience of time series experimenters has led to several minor modifications of the strategy. Most of these modifications are aimed at solving practical problems. Compared to the 1970s, for example, modelers pay more attention to transformations and place greater emphasis on the usefulness and interpretability of an *ARIMA* model. Otherwise, we cover the typical range of models, beginning with stationary *ARMA* models, moving on to nonstationary *ARIMA* models, and ending with multiplicative *ARIMA* models for seasonal time series.

The style of our current treatment of modeling or model building is unchanged. We demonstrate the *ARIMA* modeling strategy by analyzing a range of time series experiments. The analyses are presented in a step-by-step format that parallels the actual analytic steps. The examples were selected to illustrate not only a broad range of applications—ecology, management, psychology, public heath, etc.—but also the range of practical problems that our students and colleagues have encountered over the years. One of the most common problems involves the Normality assumption. The *ARIMA* modeling strategy assumes that the time series observations are drawn from a Normal distribution. When this assumption is unwarranted, as it often is, a Normalizing transformation is required. An introduction to the prevailing theory of transformations is included as an appendix to Chapter 3 along with an introduction to the principles of maximum likelihood estimation.

Chapter 4 develops the models and methods of *ARIMA* forecasting. Although this material lends great insight into the dynamics of *ARIMA* noise models, our development is cursory. Students who have an interest in forecasting can consult other sources. Over the years, a number of students have "discovered" a new way to test time series null hypotheses: Compare the post-intervention time series segment to forecasts estimated from the pre-intervention segment. To put it mildly, this can lead to grave errors. After demonstrating the problems with this attractive misuse or misapplication of forecasting, we move on to the more important topic and material implied in the title of this book.

Chapter 5 introduces *ARIMA* impact modeling. In simple terms, an *ARIMA* impact model is the sum of a noise and an impact component that we wrote earlier as

$$Y_t = N(a_t) + X(I_t)$$

The noise component, $N(a_t)$, describes the behavior of the time series in its equilibrium state. For a stationary time series, specification of $N(a_t)$ consists of a set of parameter estimates including the mean, variance, and autocovariances of Y_t. For a nonstationary time series, specification of $N(a_t)$ would include as well a list of transformations and differences that were used to make Y_t stationary. The specification of $N(a_t)$ allows critics to replicate our analysis. It serves no other purpose. Although the specification may involve esoteric, technical concepts and terms, the structure of $N(a_t)$ is meaningless. After $N(a_t)$ is built and running, we have no reason to explain its structure. All any critic needs to know is that it "works."

The impact component, in contrast, requires an explanation. The $X(I_t)$ component describes what happens to the time series when the intervention drives it out of its equilibrium state. There are only two possibilities: The time series can either move to a new equilibrium state, characterized by a new level, or it can return to its pre-intervention equilibrium state. We encourage readers to think of these two possibilities as permanent or temporary changes in level. It seems reasonable, furthermore, to expect that the post-intervention change, whether permanent or temporary, will be either abrupt or gradual in onset. Crossing these two dichotomies leads to four possible impacts:

	Permanent Change	Temporary Change
Abrupt Onset	*Abrupt-Permanent*	*Abrupt-Temporary*
Gradual Onset	*Gradual-Permanent*	*Gradual-Temporary*

The *Gradual-Temporary* impact component is not theoretically or practically useful, so we do not consider it. The other three impact components are both theoretically and practically useful. All three are predicted by widely accepted theories of social interventions. Examples described in Chapter 5 come from a wide range of applied fields. As a practical matter, moreover, because three impact components correspond to distinct nested sub-models of a general $X(I_t)$, tests of significance and interpretation of results are straightforward. These practical advantages assume a strong intervention theory, of course, and lacking that foundation, statistical and substantive interpretations are not possible. This is because $N(a_t)$ and $X(I_t)$ are invariably correlated. If both $N(a_t)$ and $X(I_t)$ are allowed to be arbitrary, every intervention has an impact. We resolve this problem by relying on a substantive theory of the intervention to limit the number of possible impacts to three. This introduces our threshold consideration.

Our discussion of validity begins in Chapter 6, which deals with statistical conclusion validity. The advent of relatively inexpensive computers in the late 1970s and early 1980s changed the nature of social science research. In light of this change, Cook and Campbell (1979) divided the threats to internal validity into threats that could be controlled in principle by design—control groups, random assignment, and so forth—and threats that could not be controlled by design. This latter group of threats were transferred to the new statistical conclusion validity category.

Reflecting the status quo of those times, most of the threats to statistical conclusion validity involved misstatements of the Type I and Type II decision error rates in null hypothesis significance tests. The conventional null hypothesis significance test has become controversial since then, of course, especially in its "hybrid" form (Gigerenzer et al., 1989). Critics of the status quo urge us to abandon the null hypothesis significance test in favor of some alternative. Wilkinson et al. (1999) recommend that we report effect sizes and confidence intervals instead of p-values, for example, while Rindskopf (1997) recommends Bayesian hypothesis tests.

Although we favor Bayesian approaches and agree with most critiques of the conventional null hypothesis significance test, it seems unlikely that the status quo will be overthrown soon. Kruschke, Aguinis, and Joo (2012) use revolutionary rhetoric to describe the move toward Bayesian methods in genetics, ecology, and particularly psychology. We develop the fundamentals of Bayesian thinking in Chapter 6 and conduct a simple Bayesian hypothesis test. We trust in the inevitability of a Bayesian revolution but doubt that it will occur soon or that it will end painlessly. Frequentist notions continue to dominate.

Chapter 7 covers internal validity, which, Campbell and Stanley (1966) tell us, is the "basic minimum without which any experiment is uninterpretable." Internal validity occupies an honored position among the validities. Threats to internal validity are easily taught and even more easily learned. The common threats to internal validity are also easily controlled, at least in principle, by random assignment. Given the lack of controversy, what more could be said about internal validity?

There is always more. Chapter 7 adds two novel bits of acquired knowledge. Most authorities agree that there are four plausible threats to the internal validity of a time series design: history, maturation, instrumentation, and regression. We remove the threat of regression from this list. Campbell (1957) used a "one-group pretest-posttest" design to demonstrate regression as a threat to internal validity. Whereas regression to the pre-intervention mean is always plausible in a simple before–after contrast, however, it is implausible in a long interrupted time series. Campbell and Ross (1968; Glass, 1968) describe a regression artifact in the "Connecticut crackdown on speeding," but this appears to be the only report of a regression artifact in a long interrupted time series. Our reanalysis of the Connecticut traffic fatality time series corroborates the descriptive finding of Campbell and Ross but not the statistical finding. Based on our analysis, we drop regression from the list of the plausible threats to internal validity.

After dropping regression from the list of plausible threats to internal validity, we add selection. Since selection is plausible only when the design includes an untreated control time series, the addition rests on the underlying methodological principles and practices. In principle, control time series can serve either of two purposes. First, control time series can be used to render plausible threats to internal validity implausible (Campbell, 1957; Campbell and Stanley, 1966). Ruling out the common threats to internal validity establishes a relationship between the observed effect and the intervention but not necessarily a causal relationship. That requires a strict—and perhaps a restrictive—definition of causality. Under the strict definition of Rubin causality (Rubin, 1974; see also Holland, 1986), however, and given an appropriate control time series, we can interpret an observed before–after difference as the *causal* effect of an intervention.

This introduces the second novel bit of acquired knowledge. Over the years, "design" has taken on three slightly different meanings. The first and earliest meaning refers to the allocation of subjects to treatment and control groups in a way that optimizes the efficiency of an experiment. The second meaning, which entered the social science lexicon about 30 years later, refers to the use of quasi-experimental contrasts to rule out threats to internal validity. The first and second meanings are associated with Fisher (1935) and Campbell (1957). The third and newest meaning refers to the a priori use of statistical models and methods to derive causal inferences from non-experimental or observational data. The sense of this third meaning is conveyed by Rubin's (2008) dictum: "For objective causal inference, design trumps analysis."

Although the choice of control time series is only one aspect of a priori design, it is often the most salient aspect. Ideally, the choice is dictated by theory. The fact that appropriate control time series are not always available can pose an obstacle to causal interpretation. Given a collection of less-than-perfect control time series, however, it is sometimes possible to construct an appropriate control. The "synthetic control" methods associated with Abadie, Diamond, and Hainmueller (2010) are the most widely used methods at this point. In a worst-case scenario, the synthetic control time series may not be very "good." In a best-case scenario, on the other hand, a synthetic control contrast can establish a valid causal relationship between an intervention and an impact. In every case, of course, constructing a synthetic control time series forces us to think about what we mean when we say that a particular control is "appropriate." We discuss synthetic control designs in Chapter 7 and work through an example to illustrate the methodological issues.

On general validity questions, we defer to Shadish et al. (2002) and its progeny. Should the reader find what appears to be an irreconcilable difference between our treatment of an issue and theirs, trust Shadish et al. To avoid the confusion of perceived differences, our treatment focuses on validity threats that are specific to—or even unique to—time series designs. We have relatively less to say about construct and external validities as consequence. This does not mean that construct and external are the least important of the four validities but, rather, that relatively fewer threats to construct and external validities are specific to time series designs.

Of the 14 distinct threats to construct validity described by Shadish et al. (2002), five apply to time series designs. We have renamed and articulated these five to emphasize their role in the validity of time series experiments. Two of the five are associated with the construction of the time series Y_t. In the ideal situation, we would construct Y_t to conform with the latent process that it purports to measure. Period—monthly, quarterly, etc.—and timeframe would be obvious considerations. In less-than-ideal situations, we must work with time series that are already constructed. In those situations, we must remain sensitive to the consequences of the constuction. Three additional threats are associated with misspecification of the impact component, $X(I_t)$. These threats include "fuzzy" onsets, "fuzzy" responses, and confusing the detection of an impact with modeling the impact.

Finally, Chapter 9 focuses on external validity. Threats to external validity are difficult to define in general, much less as applied to time series designs specifically. Fortunately, *all* threats to external validity are controlled by replication across persons, populations, settings, contexts, treatment variations, historical periods, and so forth. The external validity of a time series design is not exceptional in this respect and our treatment of this last validity is, thus, quite general. This is not to say that external validity is the "least important" of the four validities. On the contrary, external validity is the queen of validities for one reason: We learn nothing new by controlling a threat to statistical conclusion, internal, or construct validity. When an uncontrolled threat to external validity allows an unexpected result to emerge, on the other hand, we learn something new. Controlling a threat to external validity is not a mystery, however, at least not in a time series experiment. So our discussion of external validity is necessarily brief and general.

2

ARIMA Algebra

The fools who write the textbooks of advanced mathematics—and they are mostly clever fools—seldom take the trouble to show you how easy the easy calculations are. On the contrary, they seem to desire to impress you with their tremendous cleverness by going about it in the most difficult way.

—THOMPSON (1914, P. IX)

Keeping Thompson's words in mind, think of the process Y as a machine that generates realizations (or outputs, or observations) at discrete time-points. Using subscripts to denote these discrete time-points, the realizations of Y are written explicitly as

$$Y_{-\infty}, \ldots, Y_{-1}, Y_0, [Y_1, Y_2, \ldots, Y_N], Y_{N+1}, Y_{N+2}, \ldots, Y_{+\infty}$$

Realizations stretch back into the infinite unobserved past and forward into the infinite unobservable future. The observed realization string or time series, Y_1 through Y_N, is only one of the many infinitesimally small possible samples of Y.[1]

The relationship between the process Y and the time series $Y_1, Y_2, \ldots, Y_N$ is analogous to the relationship between a population and its samples in one sense: In longitudinal and cross-sectional cases alike, a subset—a time series, a sample, etc.—of the whole—a process, a population, etc.—is used to build a model of the whole. Just as distinct populations can yield nearly identical samples, distinct processes can generate nearly identical time series. Analyses of short time series,

---

1. Some authors use T for the length of a time series; for example, "the sum of Y_t from $t = 1$ to $t = T$." We use N instead of T to reinforce the analogy between cross-sectional and longitudinal sampling and, also, to stick with the legacy notations of Cook and Campbell and Glass et al.

like analyses of small cross-sectional samples, are problematic for this reason. As time passes, however, more and more realizations are observed and, as it is made longer, the time series begins more and more to resemble its parent generating process.

A time series model is an abstract representation of Y. Analyses of two time series often lead to similar models and, in such cases, it is reasonable to assume that the time series were generated by similar processes. To say that two processes are "similar" implies that they share properties, parameters, or characteristics. The goal of this chapter is to derive the properties of several common processes and, based on these properties, to develop a general scheme for classifying processes.

As it happens, an important class of processes that we call stationary are fully determined by their means and autocovariance functions, μ_Y and γ_k, defined as

$$\mu_Y = E(Y_t) \quad \text{and} \quad \gamma_k = E(Y_t Y_{t-k})$$

Conceptually, μ_Y is the "average level" or "central value" about which the process fluctuates. An estimate of μ_Y is

$$\hat{\mu}_Y = \frac{1}{N} \sum_{t=1}^{N} Y_t$$

This estimator has more or less the same properties and interpretation as any arithmetic mean. The covariance function γ_k, is estimated as

$$\widehat{\gamma}_k = \frac{1}{N-k} \sum_{t=k+1}^{N} (Y_t - \hat{\mu}_Y)(Y_{t-1} - \hat{\mu}_Y) \text{ for } k = 0,1,2,\ldots$$

The covariance function has an equally straightforward, though less obvious, interpretation. We call k the "lag" in this and all other contexts. It is, simply, an integer measure of the temporal distance between two realizations. Y_{t-k} for example, is the kth lag or lag-k of Y_t. In particular, when $k = 0$,

$$\widehat{\gamma}_0 = \frac{1}{N} \sum_{t=1}^{N} (Y_t - \hat{\mu}_Y)(Y_t - \hat{\mu}_Y) = \widehat{\sigma}_Y^2$$

where $\widehat{\gamma}_0$ is an estimate of the process variance. Otherwise, when $k > 0$, $\widehat{\gamma}_k$ is an estimate of the covariance between observations separated by k time-units.

Having defined a stationary process as one fully determined by μ_Y and γ_k, we must explain "fully determined." No two stationary processes have the same

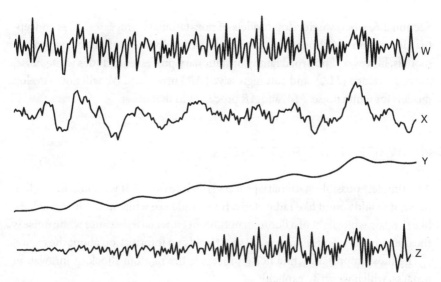

Figure 2.1 Four Time Series

means and covariance functions. If two processes, X and Y, have identical means and covariances,

$$\mu_X = \mu_Y \quad \text{and} \quad \gamma_k(X) = \gamma_k(Y)$$

then X and Y are the same process. This applies only to the stationary family of processes. For the equally important family of nonstationary processes, μ_Y and γ_k are undefined.

The four time series plotted in Figure 2.1 illustrate the concept of process stationarity. Series W_t and X_t are both "flat," fluctuating about a fixed mean with constant variance. Experienced analysts might guess that Y_t and Z_t belong to the nonstationary family. They belong to two distinct branches of the nonstationary family, however. Y_t has a secular trend and, thus, is nonstationary in mean. Z_t appears stationary in mean but nonstationary in variance. Ignoring the particular type of nonstationarity, mean or variance, these two series are "different" from W_t and X_t, the two stationary series. Y_t and Z_t are "similar" in this sense: Both are realizations of nonstationary processes.

If μ_Y is estimated from the Y_t shown in Figure 2.1, the value of μ_Y grows systematically throughout the course of the series, so Y_t is nonstationary in mean. Similarly, Z_t is nonstationary in variance and σ_Z^2 consequently depends on the particular subset of realizations used in the estimate. W_t and X_t, in contrast, are stationary, so μ_W and σ_W^2 and μ_X and σ_W^2 do not depend on the subset of realizations used in the estimates.

Now one picture is worth a thousand words and Figure 2.1 illustrates the concept of process stationarity. But it is not a definition; this must wait until

Section 2.6, when we develop models of nonstationary processes. This conceptual illustration of stationarity is adequate for a development of stationary process models, however. The broad family of stationary processes includes white noise, moving average (MA), and autoregressive (AR) processes. We will now develop models for white noise, MA, and AR processes in that order.

2.1 WHITE NOISE PROCESSES

The simplest possible stationary process is "white noise." If we could hear white noise, it would sound like radio static. If we could see white noise, it would look like the pale white light of a fluorescent tube. In either case, because white noise is the outcome of a random process, its past holds no information about the future.

The most important white noise process is the random shock or innovation process, which we write explicitly as

$$a_{-\infty}, \ldots, a_{-1}, a_0, [a_1, a_2, \ldots, a_N], a_{N+1}, a_{N+2}, \ldots, a_{+\infty}$$

Random shocks have zero mean and constant variance:

$$\mu_a = E(a_t) = 0 \quad \text{and} \quad \gamma_0 = E(a_t^2) = \sigma_a^2$$

But the property that makes a_t white noise is serial independence:

$$\gamma_{k>0} = E(a_t a_{t-k}) = 0$$

Random shocks are the "most important" member of the stationary white noise family for a simple reason: They are the inputs that drive other processes.

Figure 2.2 shows three time series, X_t, Y_t, and Z_t, each generated from the same white noise input. The three time series have different means and variances.

$$\mu_X < \mu_Y < \mu_Z \quad \text{and} \quad \sigma_X^2 > \sigma_Y^2 > \sigma_Z^2$$

Differences among the three time series are obvious. X_t is "noisier" than Y_t, for example, and Y_t is "noisier" than Z_t. Each series belongs to the same stationary white noise family, however, and this similarity is more important than the differences in means and variances.

To illustrate how these time series were generated, think of X, Y, and Z as machines with outputs X_t, Y_t, and Z_t. In each case, the process inputs are the same random shock a_t. But due to differences in the structures of X, Y, and Z, the outputs X_t, Y_t, and Z_t are quite different. In each case, this transformation is accomplished by the sequential operation of two "black box" filters. In the first filter, multiplication by constants σ_X/σ_a, σ_Y/σ_a, and σ_Z/σ_a transforms the

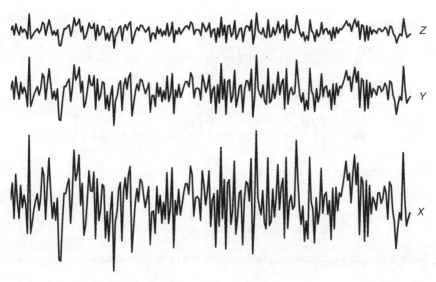

Figure 2.2 White Noise Time Series

variance of the white noise input from σ_a^2 to σ_X^2, σ_Y^2, and σ_Z^2. In a second filter, addition of constants μ_X, μ_Y, and μ_Z transforms the mean from $\mu_a = 0$ to μ_X, μ_Y, and μ_Z. We write this as

$$a_t \times \left(\frac{\sigma_X}{\sigma_a}\right) + \mu_X = X_t$$

$$a_t \times \left(\frac{\sigma_Y}{\sigma_a}\right) + \mu_Y = Y_t$$

$$a_t \times \left(\frac{\sigma_Z}{\sigma_a}\right) + \mu_Z = Z_t$$

Since their means and variances are not identical, X, Y, and Z are different processes. Due to their common serial independence, however, X_t, Y_t, and Z_t are all members of the same white noise family. Serial independence is defined as

$$\gamma_{k>0} = 0$$

It may be "obvious" that X_t, Y_t, and Z_t are serially independent. Demonstrating serial independence is an important procedure in subsequent sections, however, so we take time now to introduce the method.

To demonstrate serial independence for Z_t, begin with the definition of γ_k,

$$\gamma_k = E[(Z_t - \mu_Z)(Z_{t-k} - \mu_Z)]$$

Then, since

$$Z_t = \left(\frac{\sigma_Z}{\sigma_a}\right) a_t + \mu_Z$$

By substitution

$$\gamma_k = E\left[\left(\frac{\sigma_Z}{\sigma_a} a_t + \mu_Z - \mu_Z\right)\left(\frac{\sigma_Z}{\sigma_a} a_{t-k} + \mu_Z - \mu_Z\right)\right]$$

The μ_Z terms cancel, leaving the simpler expression

$$\gamma_k = E\left[\left(\frac{\sigma_Z}{\sigma_a} a_t\right)\left(\frac{\sigma_Z}{\sigma_a} a_{t-k}\right)\right] = E\left[\left(\frac{\sigma_Z}{\sigma_a}\right)^2 (a_t a_{t-k})\right]$$

Since σ_Z/σ_a is a constant, this term factors out of the expectation.

$$\gamma_k = \left(\frac{\sigma_Z}{\sigma_a}\right)^2 E(a_t a_{t-k}) = \frac{\sigma_Z^2}{\sigma_a^2} E(a_t a_{t-k})$$

Now for $k = 0$,

$$\gamma_0 = \frac{\sigma_Z^2}{\sigma_a^2} E(a_t a_t)$$

And since $E(a_t a_t) = \sigma_a^2$ by definition,

$$\gamma_0 = \frac{\sigma_Z^2}{\sigma_a^2} \sigma_a^2 = \sigma_Z^2$$

But for $k > 0$, also by definition, $E(a_t a_{t-k}) = 0$, so

$$\gamma_{k>1} = \frac{\sigma_Z^2}{\sigma_a^2} E(a_t a_{t-k}) = 0$$

Following this same procedure, readers may demonstrate as an exercise that X_t and Y_t are serially independent. In every case, begin with definitions, make appropriate substitutions, and take expected values. Readers who are unfamiliar with expectation algebra are directed to Appendix 2A. This general procedure cannot be used to demonstrate serial independence for a_t, however. Random shocks are serially independent by definition and without this definition, the serial independence of other processes cannot be demonstrated. This emphasizes the importance of the random shock process. Random shocks are the "driving forces" of other processes and, also, the common metric of every time series process.

2.2 *AR*1 AND *MA*1 PROCESSES

Unlike white noise, successive realizations of autoregressive (AR) and moving average (MA) processes are not serially independent. The first-order AR or $AR1$ process,

$$Y_t = a_t + \phi Y_{t-1} \quad \text{where} \quad |\phi| < 1$$

and the first-order MA or $MA1$ process,

$$Y_t = a_t + \theta a_{t-1} \quad \text{where} \quad |\theta| < 1$$

belong to distinct stationary families. It is sometimes said that $AR1$ and $MA1$ processes "remember" their pasts. Although this is a useful analogy, we must explain that what these processes "remember" are past white noise shocks. We should add that their memories are imperfect. As time passes, both processes "forget." What distinguishes $AR1$ and $MA1$ processes is the ways that they "remember."

To explain this difference, we derive covariances, beginning with the $MA1$ process. Following the general procedure, write γ_0 as

$$\gamma_0 = E[(Y_t - \mu_Y)(Y_t - \mu_Y)] = \sigma_Y^2$$

Then for the $MA1$ process,

$$Y_t = a_t - \theta a_{t-1}$$

By substitution,

$$\gamma_0 = E[(a_t - \theta a_{t-1} - \mu_Y)(a_t - \theta a_{t-1} - \mu_Y)]$$

We may assume with no loss of generality that $\mu_Y = 0$, so

$$\begin{aligned}
\gamma_0 &= E[(a_t - \theta a_{t-1})(a_t - \theta a_{t-1})] \\
&= E(a_t^2 - 2\theta a_t a_{t-1} + \theta^2 a_{t-1}^2) \\
&= E(a_t^2) - 2\theta E(a_t a_{t-1}) + \theta^2 E(a_{t-1}^2)
\end{aligned}$$

Now $E(a_t a_{t-1}) = 0$ and $E(a_t^2) = E(a_{t-1}^2) = \sigma_a^2$, so

$$\gamma_0 = \sigma_a^2 - 0 + \theta^2 \sigma_a^2 = \sigma_a^2(1 + \theta^2)$$

We derive γ_1 in more or less the same way. Beginning with the definition

$$\gamma_1 = E(Y_t Y_{t-1})$$

By substitution,

$$\gamma_1 = E[(a_t - \theta a_{t-1})(a_{t-1} - \theta a_{t-2})]$$
$$= E(a_t a_{t-1} - \theta a_t a_{t-2} - \theta a_{t-1}^2 + \theta^2 a_{t-1} a_{t-2})$$
$$= E(a_t a_{t-1}) - \theta E(a_t a_{t-2}) - \theta E(a_{t-1}^2) + \theta^2 E(a_{t-1} a_{t-2})$$

And since a_t, a_{t-1}, and a_{t-2} are all independent, the first, second, and fourth terms are zero.

$$\gamma_1 = -\theta E(a_{t-1}^2) = -\theta \sigma_a^2$$

The same procedure shows that γ_2 is zero.

$$\gamma_2 = E[(a_t - \theta a_{t-1})(a_{t-2} - \theta a_{t-3})]$$
$$= E(a_t a_{t-2} - \theta a_t a_{t-3} - \theta a_{t-1} a_{t-2} + \theta^2 a_{t-1} a_{t-3})$$
$$= E(a_t a_{t-2}) - \theta E(a_t a_{t-3}) - \theta E(a_{t-1} a_{t-2}) + \theta^2 E(a_{t-1} a_{t-3})$$

But a_t, a_{t-1}, a_{t-2}, and a_{t-3} are all independent, so

$$\gamma_2 = 0$$

It should be clear from this derivation that $\gamma_{k>2}$ are also zero.

To derive γ_k for the AR1 process, begin anew with the definition of γ_k. Once again, if $\mu_Y = 0$,

$$\gamma_k = E(Y_t Y_{t-k})$$

Substituting the AR1 identities of Y_t and Y_{t-k},

$$\gamma_k = E(a_t + \phi Y_{t-1})(a_{t-k} + \phi Y_{t-k-1})$$
$$= E(a_t a_{t-k} + \phi a_t Y_{t-k-1} + \phi Y_{t-1} a_{t-k} + \phi^2 Y_{t-1} Y_{t-k-1})$$
$$= E(a_t a_{t-k}) + \phi E(a_t Y_{t-k-1}) + \phi E(Y_{t-1} a_{t-k}) + \phi^2 E(Y_{t-1} Y_{t-k-1})$$

Now since a_t is wholly random, it is independent of all prior shocks and observations, so $E(a_t Y_{t-k-1}) = 0$ for any lag-k. Thus,

$$\gamma_k = E(a_t a_{t-k}) + \phi E(Y_{t-1} a_{t-k}) + \phi^2 E(Y_{t-1} Y_{t-k-1})$$

This expression can be further simplified with the AR1 identity

$$a_{t-k} = Y_{t-k} - \phi Y_{t-k-1}$$

Substituting $Y_{t-k} - \phi Y_{t-k-1}$ for a_{t-k},

$$
\begin{aligned}
\gamma_k &= E[a_t(Y_{t-k} - \phi Y_{t-k-1})] + \phi E[(Y_{t-1})(Y_{t-k} - \phi Y_{t-k-1})] \\
&\quad + \phi^2 E(Y_{t-1} Y_{t-k-1}) \\
&= E(a_t Y_{t-k} - \phi a_t Y_{t-k-1}) + \phi E(Y_{t-1} Y_{t-k} - \phi Y_{t-1} Y_{t-k-1}) \\
&\quad + \phi^2 E(Y_{t-1} Y_{t-k-1}) \\
&= E(a_t Y_{t-k}) - \phi E(a_t Y_{t-k-1}) + \phi E(Y_{t-1} Y_{t-k}) - \phi^2 E(Y_{t-1} Y_{t-k-1}) \\
&\quad + \phi^2 E(Y_{t-1} Y_{t-k-1})
\end{aligned}
$$

The second term of this expression is zero for all k and the last two terms cancel. Thus

$$
\gamma_k = E(a_t Y_{t-k}) + \phi E(Y_{t-1} Y_{t-k})
$$

For $k = 0$, this expression yields

$$
\begin{aligned}
\gamma_0 &= E(a_t a_t) + \phi^2 E(Y_{t-1} Y_{t-1}) \\
&= E(a_t^2) + \phi^2 E(Y_{t-1}^2)
\end{aligned}
$$

Since $E(a_t^2) = \sigma_a^2$ and $E(Y_{t-1}^2) = \sigma_Y^2$,

$$
\gamma_0 = \sigma_a^2 + \phi^2 \sigma_Y^2
$$

Finally, using the identity $\gamma_0 = \sigma_Y^2$,

$$
\begin{aligned}
\gamma_0 &= \sigma_a^2 + \phi^2 \gamma_0 \\
\gamma_0 - \phi^2 \gamma_0 &= \sigma_a^2 \\
\gamma_0(1 - \phi^2) &= \sigma_a^2 \\
\gamma_0 &= \frac{\sigma_a^2}{(1 - \phi^2)}
\end{aligned}
$$

For $k = 1, 2,$ and 3, the γ_k is evaluated as

$$
\begin{aligned}
\gamma_1 &= E(a_t Y_{t-1}) + \phi E(Y_{t-1} Y_{t-1}) = \phi \gamma_0 \\
\gamma_2 &= E(a_t Y_{t-2}) + \phi E(Y_{t-1} Y_{t-2}) = \phi \gamma_1 \\
\gamma_3 &= E(a_t Y_{t-3}) + \phi E(Y_{t-1} Y_{t-3}) = \phi \gamma_2
\end{aligned}
$$

Since $\gamma_2 = \phi \gamma_1$,

$$
\gamma_3 = \phi(\phi \gamma_1) = \phi^2 \gamma_1
$$

Table 2.1. THREE BASIC AUTOCOVARIANCE FUNCTIONS

	γ_0	γ_1	$\gamma_{k \geq 2}$
White Noise	σ_a^2	0	0
MA1	$\sigma_a^2(1+\theta^2)$	$-\theta\sigma_a^2$	0
AR1	$\sigma_a^2/(1-\phi^2)$	$\phi^1\gamma_0$	$\phi^k\gamma_0$

And since $\gamma_1 = \phi\gamma_0$

$$\gamma_3 = \phi^2(\phi\gamma_0) = \phi^3\gamma_0$$

Continuing this procedure, it is simple (though tedious) to show that

$$\gamma_k = \phi^k\gamma_0 \quad \text{for} \quad k = 0, 1, 2, \dots$$

So the covariance function of an AR1 process "decays" with ϕ^k approaching zero as k grows large.

Table 2.1 summarizes the autocovariance functions of white noise, MA1, and AR1 processes. In principle, an unknown generating process can be inferred from the estimated covariance function. If $\gamma_1 \neq 0$, for example, white noise is ruled out. If $\gamma_2 \neq 0$, MA1 is ruled out, and so forth. The unstandardized form of γ_k makes interpretation difficult, however. For this reason, we divide γk by γ_0 to derive a standardized covariance function or, as we call it hereafter, an autocorrelation function (ACF), denoted by ρ_k.

$$\rho_k = \frac{\gamma_k}{\gamma_0} \quad \text{for} \quad k = 0, 1, 2, \dots$$

Unlike γk, ρ_k is standardized. For $k = 0$, $\rho_1 = 1$, which is the variance of the standardized process. For $k > 0$,

$$-1 \leq \rho_k \leq +1$$

For long time series, ρ_k approaches the Pearson product-moment correlation of Y_t and Y_{t-k}. It has the same interpretation—a measure of association—and because it is standardized, the ρ_k are comparable across series.

It should be obvious that the correlation between Y_t and Y_{t+k} is the same as the correlation between Y_{t-k} and Y_t. Thus,

$$\rho_k = \rho_{-k}$$

Since ρ_k is an "even" function, we need only examine its positive lags. Lagged values of a white noise process are independent,

$$E(a_t a_{t \pm k}) = 0 \quad \text{for} \quad k \neq 0$$

So it follows that all nonzero lags of ρ_k are zero.

$$\rho_{k>0} = \gamma_{k>0} = 0$$

For the $MA1$ process,

$$\rho_1 = \frac{\gamma_1}{\gamma_0} = \frac{-\theta}{1+\theta^2}$$

$$\rho_{k>1} = \frac{\gamma_{k>1}}{\gamma_0} = 0$$

Finally, for the $AR1$ process,

$$\rho_1 = \frac{\phi\gamma_0}{\gamma_0} = \phi$$

$$\rho_2 = \frac{\phi^2\gamma_0}{\gamma_0} = \phi^2$$

$$\rho_3 = \frac{\phi^3\gamma_0}{\gamma_0} = \phi^3$$

For $AR1$ processes, then, ρ_k decays geometrically from lag to lag.

Figure 2.3 shows two $MA1$ ACFs. A white noise process (which may be considered an $MA1$ process with $\rho_1 = 0$) has null values for all k. Other than this trivial case, however, $MA1$ processes have $\rho_1 \neq 0$ In every case, ρ_1 is a function of θ. Specifically,

$$\rho_1 = \frac{-\theta}{1+\theta^2}$$

When $\theta = .7$, for example, $\rho_1 = -.47$ and when $\theta = -.7$, $\rho_1 = .47$. In practice, ρ_k is estimated from a finite sample of the process—from a time series. If $\widehat{\rho}_k = 0$ for all $k > 0$, the generating process is white noise. If $\widehat{\rho}_1 \neq 0$ but $\widehat{\rho}_k = 0$ for $k > 1$, on the other hand, as in Figure 2.3, the process is $MA1$. This oversimplifies the

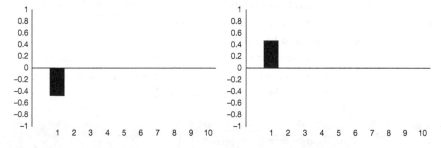

Figure 2.3 Two $MA1$ ACFs

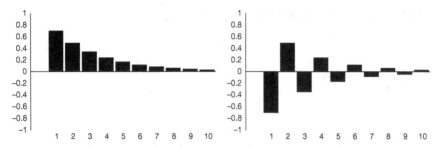

Figure 2.4 Two *AR*1 *ACF*s

empirical task, of course. We address these issues in Chapter 3. For the time being, we note only that, in practice, time series analysis consists largely of comparing estimated and expected *ACF*s to divine the structure of the underlying process. In this sense, *ACF*s are the "workhorse" statistics of time series analysis.

Figure 2.4 shows two *AR*1 *ACF*s. Each decays from lag-1 at a rate determined by the value of ϕ. In all cases, however, *AR*1 *ACF*s "die out" within a few lags. This typical *AR*1 pattern of decay should be compared with the *ACF*s expected of *MA*1 processes (Figure 2.3). In terms of ρ_k, the two processes are so distinct that they could not be confused. This ignores the problem of estimating ρ_k, of course, but that is another matter.

In addition to the *MA*1 and *AR*1 *ACF*s, summarized in Figures 2.3 and 2.4, this section introduces the reader to a general procedure for deriving γ_k. Begin with a definition; simplify the expression by appropriate (but sometimes nonobvious) substitutions; and evaluate the expression. This general procedure will be used again and again. Readers who have difficulty with these derivations are directed to Appendix 2A.

2.3 INPUT-OUTPUT DYNAMICS

Input-output diagrams give another insight into the properties of *AR*1 and *MA*1 processes. For this purpose, think of the process as a "black box" with two registers called MEMORY and HOLDING. If the process operates at discrete times, $T_{-k}, \ldots, T_0, \ldots T_k$, a snapshot taken just before T_1 reveals (future) random shock inputs queued up on the left ready to enter the "black box" and (past) realization outputs stacked up on the right, ready to be analyzed.

$$\ldots a_3, a_2, a_1 \implies \boxed{\begin{array}{c} \text{MEMORY} \\ \hline \text{HOLDING} \end{array}} \implies Y_0, Y_{-1}, Y_{-2}$$

From this point on, *AR* and *MA* processes are distinguished by their MEMORY structures. In the *MA*1 scheme of things, each shock lives for two instants, the first as an input and the second as a memory. As T_0 ends, a portion of the random shock a_0 waits in the HOLDING register. The MEMORY register is empty.

$$\ldots a_3, a_2, a_1 \implies \boxed{\begin{array}{c} \\ \hline -\theta_1 a_0 \end{array}} \implies Y_0, Y_{-1}, Y_{-2}$$

In an eyeblink, a_1 joins $-\theta_1 a_0$ in the HOLDING register as all future shocks move up one position in the queue.

$$\ldots a_4, a_3, a_2 \implies \boxed{\begin{array}{c} \\ \hline a_1 - \theta_1 a_0 \end{array}} \implies Y_0, Y_{-1}, Y_{-2}$$

The newly entered shock is imperfectly reproduced in the MEMORY register as $-\theta_1 a_1$:

$$\ldots a_4, a_3, a_2 \implies \boxed{\begin{array}{c} -\theta_1 a_1 \\ \hline a_1 - \theta_1 a_0 \end{array}} \implies Y_0, Y_{-1}, Y_{-2}$$

As T_1 draws to a close, the contents of the HOLDING register are emptied as Y_1.

$$\ldots a_4, a_3, a_2 \implies \boxed{\begin{array}{c} -\theta_1 a_1 \\ \hline \end{array}} \implies Y_1, Y_0, Y_{-1}$$

And the MEMORY register is emptied into the HOLDING register:

$$\ldots a_4, a_3, a_2 \implies \boxed{\begin{array}{c} \\ \hline -\theta_1 a_1 \end{array}} \implies Y_1, Y_0, Y_{-1}$$

As T_1 comes to an end, a_2 readies itself for input and the process repeats. These diagrams illustrate what we mean when we say that *MA*1 processes have imperfect, finite, memories. By "imperfect," we mean that only a portion of each shock is remembered. By "finite," we mean that the memory of a shock vanishes after one instant in the *MA*1 model.

AR1 systems "remember" past realizations, not past shocks. As T_0 ends, then, a portion of Y_0 waits in the HOLDING register; the MEMORY register is empty.

$$\ldots a_3, a_2, a_1 \implies \boxed{\begin{array}{c} \\ \hline \phi_1 Y_0 \end{array}} \implies Y_0, Y_{-1}, Y_{-2}$$

As T_1 begins, a_1 enters the system to join Y_0 in HOLDING.

$$\dots a_4, a_3, a_2 \implies \boxed{\begin{array}{c} \\ \hline \phi_1 Y_0 + a_1 \end{array}} \implies Y_0, Y_{-1}, Y_{-2}$$

The contents of the HOLDING register are simultaneously copied into MEMORY and emptied as Y_1.

$$\dots a_4, a_3, a_2 \implies \boxed{\begin{array}{c} \phi_1 Y_0 + a_1 \\ \hline \end{array}} \implies Y_1, Y_0, Y_{-1}$$

Then, as T_1 draws to a close, MEMORY is copied imperfectly into HOLDING:

$$\dots a_4, a_3, a_2 \implies \boxed{\begin{array}{c} \\ \hline \phi_1 Y_0 + a_1 \end{array}} \implies Y_1, Y_0, Y_{-1}$$

and the process repeats itself.

Input-out diagrams emphasize the fact that $AR1$ and $MA1$ processes are distinguished by what they remember. $MA1$ processes remember part of a preceding shock, $-\theta_1 a_{t-1}$, while $AR1$ processes remember part of the preceding realization, $\phi_1 Y_{t-1}$. Input-output diagrams obscure an important $AR1$ identity, however. To see this identity, solve the $AR1$ process for a_t,

$$a_t = Y_t - \phi_1 Y_{t-1}$$

Since $Y_{t-1} = a_{t-1} + \phi_1 Y_{t-2}$, by substitution,

$$a_t = Y_t - \phi_1(a_{t-1} + \phi_1 Y_{t-2})$$
$$= Y_t - \phi_1 a_{t-1} - \phi_1^2 Y_{t-2}$$

Adding $\phi_1 a_{t-1}$ to both sides,

$$a_t + \phi_1 a_{t-1} = Y_t - \phi_1^2 Y_{t-2}$$

And because $Y_{t-2} = a_{t-2} + \phi_1 Y_{t-3}$, by substitution,

$$a_t + \phi_1 a_{t-1} = Y_t - \phi_1^2(a_{t-2} + \phi_1 Y_{t-3})$$
$$= Y_t - \phi_1^2 a_{t-2} - \phi_1^3 Y_{t-3}$$

Then adding $\phi_1^2 a_{t-2}$ to both sides,

$$a_t + \phi_1 a_{t-1} + \phi_1^2 a_{t-2} = Y_t - \phi_1^3 Y_{t-3}$$

Continuing this backward substitution indefinitely, we arrive at the identity.

$$Y_t = a_t + \phi_1 a_{t-1} + \phi_1^2 a_{t-2} + \cdots + \phi_1^k a_{t-k} + \cdots = \sum_{k=0}^{\infty} \phi_1^k a_{t-k}$$

AR1 processes may be written identically as an infinite sum of past shocks. Although the AR1 memory is finite in terms of past realizations—only Y_{t-1} is remembered—its memory of past shocks is infinite, though imperfect. The memory of a shock decays as time passes, but no shock is ever completely forgotten.

To emphasize this point, compare MA1 and AR1 processes where $\phi_1 = \theta_1 = .7$. Whereas the MA1 process remembers only one shock:

$$Y_t = a_t - .7 a_{t-1}$$

the AR1 process

$$Y_t = \sum_{k=0}^{\infty} .7^k a_{t-k}$$

remembers all past shocks, weighted by $.7^k$. Tracking a specific shock through both systems reveals this important difference:

t	AR1	MA1
0	1.0	1.0
1	0.7	0.7
2	0.49	
3	0.343	
4	0.2401	
5	0.16807	
:	:	
$k > 5$	$1 - .7^k$	0.0

In the MA1 model, the shock dies abruptly after two instants. In the AR1 model, on the other hand, the shock never really dies but, rather, "fades away" like the Old Soldier. The AR1 system never completely forgets a shock, in other words, but the part remembered decreases geometrically while the part forgotten increases as a unit complement.

Like an elephant, the AR system "never forgets," although, after a few instants, the memory is weak. The relative strength of a memory, moreover, holding elapsed time constant, is a function of the absolute values of the AR and MA parameters. Thus, the *MA*1 process with $\theta_1 = .9$

$$Y_t = a_t - .9a_{t-1}$$

and the *AR*1 process with $\phi_1 = .9$

$$Y_t = a_t - Y_{t-1} = a_t - .9a_{t-1} - .81a_{t-2} - .729a_{t-3} - .6561a_{t-4} - \cdots$$

are very different, at least in terms of past shocks. In contrast, consider the difference between *MA*1 and *AR*1 processes with $\theta_1 = \phi_1 = .1$.

> *MA*1: $Y_t = a_t - .1a_{t-1}$
>
> *AR*1: $Y_t = a_t - .1a_{t-1} - .01a_{t-2} - .001a_{t-3} - .0001a_{t-4} - \cdots$

As a practical matter, short time series generated by *MA*1 and *AR*1 models with $\phi_1 = \theta_1 = .1$ could not be confidently distinguished from each other or from a white noise process. But this empirical issue must wait for the next chapter.

To end this discussion of *MA*1 and *AR*1 input-output dynamics, rewrite the *MA*1 process as

$$a_t = Y_t + \theta_1 a_{t-1}$$

Then, since $a_{t-1} = Y_{t-1} + \theta_1 a_{t-2}$, by backward substitution

$$a_t = Y_t + \theta_1(Y_{t-1} + \theta_1 a_{t-2})$$
$$= Y_t + \theta_1 Y_{t-1} + \theta_1^2 a_{t-2}$$

And since $a_{t-2} = Y_{t-2} + \theta_1 a_{t-3}$,

$$a_t = Y_t + \theta_1 Y_{t-1} + \theta_1^2(Y_{t-2} + \theta_1 a_{t-3}) = Y_t + \theta_1 Y_{t-1} + \theta_1^2 Y_{t-2} + \theta_1^3 a_{t-3}$$

Continuing the backward substitution indefinitely, we discover that *MA*1 processes may be written identically as an infinite sum of past realizations.

$$\sum_{k=0}^{\infty} \theta_1^k Y_{t-k}$$

Note this symmetry. *MA*1 processes may be written in terms of present and past shocks or as a power series of past realizations. *AR*1 processes, similarly, may be written either in terms of a present shock and a past realization or as a power series of past shocks. This result proves quite useful. It allows us to solve *MA*1 and *AR*1 processes for realizations or shocks when the need arises. Virtually all *AR*1 and *MA*1 properties stem from these symmetries. We are now ready to introduce the most important properties.

2.4 HIGHER-ORDER AND MIXED PROCESSES

Now in the general case, qth-order MA and pth-order AR processes consist of a present shock, a_t, and weighted parts of q past shocks and p past realizations respectively.

$$Y_t - \phi_1 Y_{t-1} - \phi_2 Y_{t-2} - \cdots - \phi_p Y_{t-p} + a_t - \theta_1 a_{t-1} - \theta_2 a_{t-2} - \cdots - \theta_q a_{t-q}$$

Of course, the finite, imperfect memories of MA1 and AR1 processes generalize to MAq and ARp processes. In MAq processes, each shock lives for $q+1$ instants, the first as an input and the next q instants as a memory. While shocks never die in ARp processes, they decay geometrically from the first and each successive instant corresponding to nonzero k.

Derivation of MAq and ARp ACFs is made easier by the use of a special notation. Hereafter, $\phi(B)$ and $\theta(B)$ denote MA and AR polynomials of the qth and pth orders:

$$\phi_p(B) = (1 - \phi_1 B - \phi_2 B^2 - \cdots - \phi_p B^p)$$
$$\theta_q(B) = (1 - \theta_1 B - \theta_2 B^2 - \cdots - \theta_q B^q)$$

So long as the parameters of $\phi(B)$ and $\theta(B)$ are constrained to the bounds of stationarity-invertability, both have inverses that allow us to solve for the observation

$$Y_t = \frac{1 - \theta_1 B - \theta_2 B^2 - \cdots - \theta_q B^q}{1 - \phi_1 B - \phi_2 B^2 - \cdots - \phi_q B^q} a_t$$

or for the shock

$$a_t = \frac{1 - \phi_1 B - \phi_2 B^2 - \cdots - \phi_p B^p}{1 - \theta_1 B - \theta_2 B^2 - \cdots - \theta_q B^q} Y_t$$

With this notation understood, to derive an MAq ACF, take the product of Y_t and Y_{t-k}:

$$
\begin{aligned}
Y_t Y_{t-k} &= \theta(B) a_t \theta(B) a_{t-k} \\
&= [a_t - \theta_1 a_{t-1} - \cdots - \theta_q a_{t-q}] \theta(B) a_{t-k} \\
&= a_t \theta(B) a_{t-k} - \theta_1 a_{t-1} \theta(B) a_{t-k} - \cdots - \theta_q a_{t-q} \theta(B) a_{t-k} \\
&= \theta(B)[a_t a_{t-k} - \theta_1 a_{t-1} a_{t-k} - \cdots - \theta_q a_{t-q} a_{t-k}]
\end{aligned}
$$

Then take expected values of both sides.

$$
\begin{aligned}
E(Y_t Y_{t-k}) &= \theta(B) E[a_t a_{t-k} - \theta_1 a_{t-1} a_{t-k} - \cdots - \theta_q a_{t-q} a_{t-k}] \\
\gamma_k &= \theta(B)[E(a_t a_{t-k}) - \theta_1 E(a_{t-1} a_{t-k}) - \cdots - \theta_q E(a_{t-q} a_{t-k})]
\end{aligned}
$$

Since random shocks are independent, each right-hand-side term of this expression has at most one nonzero expected value. Thus, when $k = 0$, the expression reduces to

$$\gamma_{k=0} = \theta(B)[E(a_t a_t) - \theta_1 E(a_{t-1} a_t) - \cdots - \theta_q E(a_{t-q} a_t)]$$
$$= \theta(B)\sigma_a^2$$
$$= (1 - \theta_1 B - \cdots - \theta_q B^q)\sigma_a^2$$

And since σ_a^2 is constant for all t, this expression simplifies to

$$\gamma_0 = (1 - \theta_1 - \cdots - \theta_q)\sigma_a^2$$

which is the MAq variance. For $q \geq 1$,

$$\gamma_{q \geq 1} = -\theta_q(1 - \theta_1 - \cdots - \theta_q)\sigma_a^2$$

This expression gives the ACFs for any MAq process. To illustrate, consider the case of an $MA3$ process where $\theta_1 = .4$, $\theta_2 = -.3$, $\theta_3 = .2$, and $k > 3 = 0$:

$$Y_t = a_t - .4a_{t-1} + .3a_{t-2} - .2a_{t-3}$$

From the formula for γ_k, we have

$$\gamma_0 = (1 - .4 + .3 - .2)\sigma_a^2 = .7\sigma_a^2$$
$$\gamma_1 = -.4(1 - .4 + .3 - .2)\sigma_a^2 = -.28\sigma_a^2$$
$$\gamma_2 = .3(1 - .4 + .3 - .2)\sigma_a^2 = -.21\sigma_a^2$$
$$\gamma_3 = -.2(1 - .4 + .3 - .2)\sigma_a^2 = -.14\sigma_a^2$$
$$\gamma_{q>3} = 0$$

and thus,

$$\rho_1 = \frac{\gamma_1}{\gamma_0} = \frac{-.28\sigma_a^2}{.7\sigma_a^2} = -.4$$

$$\rho_2 = \frac{\gamma_2}{\gamma_0} = \frac{.21\sigma_a^2}{.7\sigma_a^2} = .3$$

$$\rho_3 = \frac{\gamma_3}{\gamma_0} = \frac{-.14\sigma_a^2}{.7\sigma_a^2} = -.2$$

$$\rho_{q>3} = 0$$

This same procedure can be used to derive the ACF of any MAq process.

Figure 2.5 shows two high-order MA ACFs; each has discrete "spikes" corresponding to a nonzero k; after lag-q, the ACF dies abruptly. As these ACFs

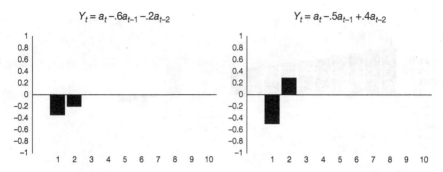

Figure 2.5 Two *MA2 ACFs*

suggest, *MA* processes of different orders are easily distinguished by their *ACFs*. Given certain values of k, however, high-order *MA* processes can be mistaken for low-order *AR* processes.

Although *ARp ACFs* can be derived with the same squaring and expectation procedures used to derive the *AR1 ACF*, the algebra is tedious. A more direct, tractable procedure uses the $Y_{t-k}Y_t$ product:

$$Y_{t-k}Y_t = Y_{t-k}(a_t + \phi_1 Y_{t-1} + \cdots + \phi_p Y_{t-q})$$
$$= Y_{t-k}a_t + \phi_1 Y_{t-k}Y_{t-1} + \cdots + \phi_p Y_{t-k}Y_{t-q}$$

Taking expected values,

$$E(Y_{t-k}Y_t) = E(Y_{t-k}a_t) + \phi_1 E(Y_{t-k}Y_{t-1}) + \cdots + \phi_p E(Y_{t-k}Y_{t-p})$$
$$\gamma_k = \phi_1 \gamma_{k-1} + \cdots + \phi_p \gamma_{k-p} \quad \text{for} \quad k > 1$$

Then dividing by γ_0,

$$\rho_k = \phi_1 \rho_{k-1} + \cdots + \phi_p \rho_{k-p} \quad \text{for} \quad k > 1$$

From this result, $\rho_1, \ldots, \rho_k$ are solved iteratively.

Figure 2.6 shows two *ARp ACFs* that decay in the typical *AR* manner. The salient difference between these *ACFs* and the *AR1 ACFs* shown in Figure 2.4 is that *ARp ACFs* decay from each of the lags corresponding to a nonzero value of k. As these *ACFs* suggest, given certain values of ϕ_1 and ϕ_2, *AR1* and *AR2 ACFs* are nearly indistinguishable; this empirical issue will be addressed at length in the next chapter.

If our experiences are typical, most social science time series are well fit by pure *AR* or *MA* models, but some are best fit by mixed *ARMA* models, which

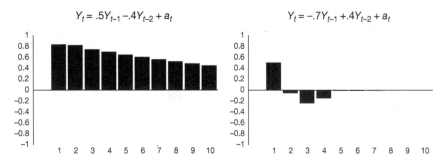

Figure 2.6 Two *AR2 ACFs*

we write as

$$Y_t - \phi_1 Y_{t-1} - \cdots - \phi_p Y_{t-p} = a_t - \theta_1 a_{t-1} - \cdots - \theta_q a_{t-q}$$
$$Y_t(1 - \phi_1 B - \cdots - \phi_p B^p) = a_t(1 - \theta_1 B - \cdots - \theta_q B^q)$$
$$Y_t = \frac{1 - \theta_1 B - \cdots - \theta_q B^q}{1 - \phi_1 B - \cdots - \phi_p B^p} a_t$$

AR models, due to G.U. Yule (1921), and *MA* models, due to E. Slutzky (1937), have longer histories than *ARMA* models and are better understood. It is perhaps for this reason that social scientists have been reluctant to use *ARMA* models. This is unfortunate.

Prior to Box and Jenkins (1970), higher-order *AR* or *MA* models were often used to represent low-order *ARMA* processes. For example, the *ARMA* process

$$(1 - .5B)Y_t = (1 + .4B)a_t$$

is solved for Y_t as

$$\begin{aligned}
Y_t &= (1 - .5B)^{-1}(1 + .4B)a_t \\
&= (1 + .5B + .25B^2 + .125B^3 + .0625B^4 + \cdots)(1 + .4B)a_t \\
&= (1 + .9B + .45B^2 + .225B^3 + .1125B^4 + .05625B^5 + \cdots)a_t
\end{aligned}$$

So the *ARMA* process can be approximated by higher-order *MA* or *AR* models. This requires as many as six parameters, of course, versus the two required for an *ARMA* model.

Using an *MA* identity, any time series process can be approximated by an *AR* model. If a process is *MA*, however, an *MA* model has fewer parameters than its *AR* approximation. Likewise, if a process is *ARMA*, an *ARMA* model has fewer parameters than its *AR* or *MA* approximation. This rule of parsimony cannot be fully appreciated until the practical work of time series analysis begins in

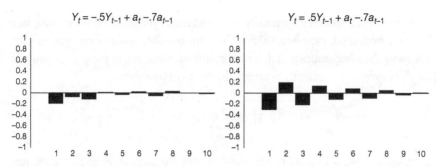

Figure 2.7 Two *ARMA ACFs*

the next chapter. For now, we simply note that "true" models are preferred to approximations. *ARMA* processes deserve *ARMA* models.

A caveat is in order here. While pure *AR* and *MA* models only approximate an *ARMA* process, many *AR* and *MA* processes have exact *ARMA* identities. The simple white noise process, for example, can be written identically as an *ARMA* process:

$$Y_t = a_t = \frac{1 - \theta_1 B - \cdots - \theta_q B^q}{1 - \phi_1 B - \cdots - \phi_p B^p} a_t$$

where $p = q$ and $\phi_j = \theta$. In this case, the numerator and denominator of the model "cancel," leaving a simple white noise model. It follows from this result that we can use any symmetric *ARMA* model to represent a white noise process. When simple *MA* and *AR* processes are modeled identically as complicated *ARMA* models, the resulting parameter redundancies (Box and Jenkins, 1970, 7.3.5) have unpredictable consequences. Sometimes the consequences are merely aesthetic; the model may be less elegant than it could be or too "messy." At the other extreme, parameter redundancies may invalidate an analysis.

Figure 2.7 shows two *ARMA ACFs*, which, not surprisingly, tend to mix discrete *MA* "spikes" and *AR* "decay." Each ρ_k depends on the orders of the *AR* and *MA* structures and values of the ϕs and θs. As these *ACFs* suggest, *ARMA ACFs* are often similar to high-order *AR* and *MA ACFs*, but more specific statements are difficult at this point. If our experience is typical again, high-order *ARMA* processes are rarely encountered in the social sciences while low-order *ARMA* processes are not uncommon.

2.5 INVERTIBILITY AND STATIONARITY

The *MA*1 bounds of invertibility and the *AR*1 bounds of stationarity constrain θ_1 and ϕ_1 to less than unity in absolute value. Although we have stated these bounds, we have not yet defined invertibility or stationarity, even in an heuristic sense, nor have we explained, even heuristically, how invertibility differs from stationarity. We have already demonstrated, by backward substitution, that the $AR1$ process can be expressed identically as an infinite series of past shocks:

$$Y_t = \sum_{k=0}^{\infty} \phi_1^k a_{t-k}$$

$AR1$ stationarity is implied by this power series representation of Y_t. If ϕ_1 is not constrained to the $AR1$ bounds of invertibility, successive terms of the power series grow larger in absolute value and the variance of the $AR1$ process grows infinitely large. Since stationarity requires a finite variance, it follows that the process is stationary only if is smaller than unity in absolute value. To demonstrate this, square both sides of $AR1$ power series representation:

$$Y_t^2 = \left(\sum_{k=0}^{\infty} \phi_1^k a_{t-k} \right) \left(\sum_{k=0}^{\infty} \phi_1^k a_{t-k} \right)$$

Then take expected values:

$$E(Y_t^2) = E\left[\left(\sum_{k=0}^{\infty} \phi_1^k a_{t-k} \right) \left(\sum_{k=0}^{\infty} \phi_1^k a_{t-k} \right) \right]$$

The left-hand side is simply $\gamma_0 = \sigma_Y^2$, the $AR1$ variance. The right-hand side is the expected value of the squared power series, which, while seemingly formidable, reduces to a very simple expression. Since

$$E(a_t a_{t-k}) = 0 \quad \text{for} \quad k > 0$$

the expected values of all cross-product terms in the squared power series are zero. Thus,

$$\begin{aligned}
\gamma_0 &= E(a_t a_t + \phi_1 a_{t-1} \phi_1 a_{t-1} + \cdots + \phi_1^k a_{t-k} \phi_1^k a_{t-k} + \cdots \\
&= E(a_t^2) + \phi_1^2 E(a_{t-1}^2) + \cdots + \phi_1^{2k} E(a_{t-k}^2) + \cdots \\
&= \sigma_a^2 + \phi_1^2 \sigma_a^2 + \cdots + \phi_1^{2k} \sigma_a^2 + \cdots \\
&= \sigma_a^2 (1 + \phi_1^2 + \cdots + \phi_1^{2k} + \cdots) \\
&= \sigma_a^2 \sum_{k=0}^{\infty} \phi_1^{2k}
\end{aligned}$$

Although this series has infinitely many terms, its sum is a finite number so long as ϕ_1 is constrained to the $AR1$ bounds of stationarity. When ϕ_1 lies outside these bounds, the *AR*1 variance approaches infinity and, by definition, the process is nonstationary. An example will clarify this point. When $\phi_1 = .5$, the power series representation of γ_0 gives the *AR*1 variance as

$$\gamma_0 = \sigma_a^2 \sum_{k=0}^{\infty} (.5)^{2k}$$

$$= \sigma_a^2 (.5^0 + .5^2 + .5^4 + .5^6 + \cdots)$$

$$= \sigma_a^2 (1 + .25 + .0625 + .01625 + \cdots)$$

Successive terms of this series grow smaller in absolute value. If we then approximate the value of the infinite series with a finite number of its terms, the approximation converges on a finite number. Using only the first term

$$\widehat{\gamma_0} \approx \sigma_a^2 (1) = \sigma_a^2$$

Using only the first two terms

$$\widehat{\gamma_0} \approx \sigma_a^2 (1 + .25) = 1.25 \sigma_a^2$$

Using only the first three terms

$$\widehat{\gamma_0} \approx \sigma_a^2 (1 + .25 + .0625) = 1.3125 \sigma_a^2$$

Using only the first four terms

$$\widehat{\gamma_0} \approx \sigma_a^2 (1 + .25 + .0625 + .01625) = 1.32813 \sigma_a^2$$

The fifth and subsequent terms of the series are so small that they do not appreciably change the sum. If we were interested only in approximating the variance of the *AR*1 process, we could stop at four terms. There is no need for an approximation, however. It is a simple matter to show that the sum converges to

$$\gamma_0 = \frac{\sigma_a^2}{1 - .5^2} = \frac{4}{3} \sigma_a^2$$

Now consider an *AR*1 process where $\phi_1 = 1.5$. Here the variance is

$$\gamma_0 = \sigma_a^2 \sum_{k=0}^{\infty} (1.5)^{2k}$$

$$= \sigma_a^2 (1.5^0 + 1.5^2 + 1.5^4 + 1.5^6 + \cdots)$$

$$= \sigma_a^2 (1 + 2.25 + 5.0625 + 25.6289 + \cdots)$$

Successive terms of the series now grow larger in absolute value and approximations to the sum do not converge. On the contrary, they explode! Approximating
γ_0 by one, two, three, and four terms,

$$\widehat{\gamma_0} \approx \sigma_a^2(1) = \sigma_a^2$$
$$\widehat{\gamma_0} \approx (1 + 2.25)\sigma_a^2 = 3.25\sigma_a^2$$
$$\widehat{\gamma_0} \approx (1 + 2.25 + 5.0625)\sigma_a^2 = 8.315\sigma_a^2$$
$$\widehat{\gamma_0} \approx (1 + 2.25 + 5.0625 + 25.6289) = 33.9439\sigma_a^2$$

Since successive terms of the series grow larger, we cannot stop here or, for
that matter, at any finite point. Whenever ϕ_1 lies outside the AR1 bounds of
stationarity, the power series fails to converge—successive terms do not grow
smaller in absolute value, that is—and the variance of the AR1 process is
undefined.

This is not generally true of the MA1 process. When θ_1 lies outside the
MA1 bounds of invertibility, the process is still stationary. To demonstrate this,
consider an MA1 process where $\theta_1 = 1.5$. Here the variance is

$$\sigma_Y^2 = E(a_t - 1.5a_{t-1})^2$$
$$= E(a_t^2 - 3a_t a_{t-1} + 2.25a_{t-1}^2)$$
$$= E(a_t^2) - 3E(a_t a_{t-1}) + 2.25E(a_{t-1}^2)$$
$$= \sigma_a^2 + 2.25\sigma_a^2 = 2.25\sigma_a^2$$

which is a finite number.

In sum, when ϕ_1 lies outside the AR1 bounds of stationarity, σ_Y^2 is infinitely
large and, thus, undefined; the process is consequently nonstationary by our
definition. When θ_1 lies outside the MA1 bounds of invertibility, on the other
hand, σ_Y^2 will be a finite number and the process will be stationary. If θ_1 is
not constrained to the bounds of invertibility, however, there is no unique
correspondence between a process and its ACF. To illustrate this problem,
consider MA1 processes X and Y,

$$X_t = a_t - .5a_{t-1} \quad \text{and} \quad Y_t = a_t - 2a_{t-1}$$

Since $X \neq Y$, we expect X and Y to be unique and identifiable—though
"similar"—processes. This is not the case, however. The two processes have
identical ACFs and, therefore, are virtually indistinguishable. Since X and Y are
MA1 processes, their ACFs are determined by γ_0 and γ_1. For X, the variance is

calculated as:

$$\gamma_1(X) = E(X_t X_{t-1})$$
$$= E(a_t - .5a_{t-1})(a_{t-1} - .5a_{t-2})$$
$$= E(a_t a_{t-1}) - .5E(a_t a_{t-2}) - .5E(a_{t-1}^2) + .25E(a_{t-1}a_{t-2})$$
$$= -.5\sigma_a^2$$

And the lag-1 autocovariance is calculated as

$$\gamma_1(X) = E(X_t X_{t-1})$$
$$= E(a_t - .5a_{t-1})(a_{t-1} - .5a_{t-2})$$
$$= E(a_t a_{t-1}) - .5E(a_t a_{t-2}) - .5E(a_{t-1}^2) + .25E(a_{t-1}a_{t-2})$$
$$= -.5\sigma_a^2$$

From these values of $\gamma_0(X)$ and $\gamma_1(X)$, the autocorrelation function is

$$\rho_1(X) = \frac{-.5\sigma_a^2}{1.25\sigma_a^2} = -.4 \text{ and } \rho_{k>1}(X) = 0$$

Following the same steps, the variance of Y is

$$\gamma_0(Y) = E(a_t - 2a_{t-1})^2$$
$$= E(a_t^2) - 4E(a_t a_{t-1}) + 4E(a_{t-1}^2)$$
$$= \sigma_a^2 + 4\sigma_a^2$$
$$= 5\sigma_a^2$$

The lag-1 autocovariance is

$$\gamma_1(Y) = E(Y_t Y_{t-1})$$
$$= E(a_t - 2a_{t-1})(a_{t-1} - 2a_{t-2})$$
$$= E(a_t a_{t-1}) - 2E(a_t a_{t-2}) - 2E(a_{t-1}^2) + 4E(a_{t-1}a_{t-2})$$
$$= -2\sigma_a^2$$

From these values of $\gamma_0(Y)$ and $\gamma_1(Y)$,

$$\rho_1(Y) = \frac{-2\sigma_a^2}{5\sigma_a^2} = -.4 \text{ and } \rho_{k>1}(X) = 0$$

So although X and Y are distinct $MA1$ processes, they have identical ACFs and are indistinguishable. One might argue that X and Y can be distinguished by their variances, of course. But although $\sigma_X^2 \neq \sigma_Y^2$, this difference is illusory. Both variances are stated in the metric of σ_a^2, which, in practice, is unknown. The mere fact that $\sigma_X^2 \neq \sigma_Y^2$ cannot then distinguish one process from the other.

There is a functional relationship between X and Y that, while not obvious, informs this discussion. The values of $\theta_1(X)$ and $\theta_1(Y)$, .5 and 2.0, are inverses. In fact, for every $MA1$ process X with a "legal" θ_1-value,

$$-1 \leq \theta_1(X) \leq +1$$

there is an $MA1$ process Y with the "illegal" θ_1-value,

$$\theta_1(Y) = \frac{1}{\theta_1(X)}, \quad \theta_1(X) \neq 0$$

Since the "legal" X and "illegal" Y have identical $ACFs$, to distinguish these two processes, θ_1 is constrained to the $MA1$ bounds of invertibility.

The parameters of higher-order ARp and MAq processes must be constrained to the bounds of invertibility and stationarity for the same reasons: to ensure the stationarity of AR processes and ensure the uniqueness of MA processes. The bounds required will depend on the integer values of p and q, however. In general, MAq and ARp processes will have $q+1$ and $p+1$ bounds.

Derivation of the MAq and ARp invertibility-stationarity bounds is simplified by the use of a backshift operator, B. As its name implies, the backshift operator "shifts" a time series backwards. That is,

$$BY_t = Y_{t-1}$$

B is also called, sometimes, the lag operator for obvious reasons: Its operation lags the series. The algebra of B obeys the Law of Exponents:

$$B^0 Y_t = Y_t; \text{ i.e., } B^0 = 1$$
$$B^k Y_t = Y_{t-k} \quad \text{and} \quad B^{-k} Y_t = Y_{t+k}$$
$$B^j B^k Y_t = B^{j+k} Y_t = Y_{t-j-k}$$

On the face of it, B introduces a degree of stylistic parsimony. An MAq process may be written explicitly as

$$Y_t = a_t - \theta_1 a_{t-1} - \theta_2 a_{t-2} - \cdots - \theta_q a_{t-q}$$

or identically in terms of the backshift operator as

$$Y_t = a_t - \theta_1 B a_t - \theta_2 B^2 a_t - \cdots - \theta_q B_q a_t$$
$$= (1 - \theta_1 B - \theta_2 B^2 - \cdots - \theta_q B^q) a_t$$
$$= a_t - \sum_{k-1}^{q} B^k \theta_k a_t$$

But the backshift operator has many advantages other than stylistic parsimony. To introduce these advantages and, also, to define the bounds of stationarity for *AR* processes, we solve the *AR*1 process for its random shock:

$$Y_t = a_t + \phi_1 Y_{t-1}$$
$$Y_t - \phi_1 Y_{t-1} = a_t$$
$$(1 - \phi_1 B) Y_t = a_t$$

The first factor on the left-hand side of this *AR*1 process, $(1 - \phi_1 B)$, is commonly called "the *AR*1 operator." The inverse of this *AR*1 operator has the usual inverse property

$$(1 - \phi_1 B)^{-1} (1 - \phi_1 B) = (1 - \phi_1 B)(1 - \phi_1 B)^{-1} = 1$$

Using this property, the *AR*1 process can be solved by multiplying both sides of the model by the inverse operator:

$$(1 - \phi_1 B)^{-1} (1 - \phi_1 B) Y_t = (1 - \phi_1 B)^{-1} a_t$$
$$Y_t = (1 - \phi_1 B)^{-1} a_t$$

if the inverse exists. We demonstrated in Section 2.2, by backward substitution, that an *AR*1 process could be represented identically as

$$Y_t = \sum_{k=0}^{\infty} \phi_1^k a_{t-k}$$

And it follows from this identity that the inverse of the *AR*1 operator is a power series in ϕ_1 and B:

$$(1 - \phi_1 B)^{-1} = \sum_{k=0}^{\infty} \phi_1^k B^k$$

In the same way and for the same reasons, the inverse of the $MA1$ operator is

$$(1 - \theta_1 B)^{-1} = \sum_{k=0}^{\infty} \theta_1^k B^k$$

In general, each AR and MA operator has an inverse that may be used to solve the process for Y_t or a_t.

The AR and MA operators are extremely useful. To derive the bounds of stationarity for an $AR1$ process, for example, we set the $AR1$ operator equal to zero and solve it as a polynomial in B. That is,

$$1 - \phi_1 B = 0, \ \phi_1 \neq 0$$
$$\phi_1 B = 1$$
$$B = \frac{1}{\phi_1}$$

Stationarity requires that all roots of the polynomial be greater than unity in absolute value and this requirement is satisfied by any value

$$-1 < \phi_1 < +1$$

which are the $AR1$ bounds of stationarity.

To derive the bounds of stationarity for an $AR2$ process, we set the $AR2$ operator equal to zero and solve for B:

$$1 - \phi_1 B - \phi_2 B^2 = 0$$
$$B = \frac{-\phi_1 \pm \sqrt{\phi_1 + 4\phi_2}}{-2\phi_2}$$

As with any quadratic equation, there are two solutions and stationarity requires that all roots be greater than unity in absolute value, a condition satisfied only when

$$|\phi_2| < 1 \quad \text{and} \quad \phi_1 + \phi_2 < 1$$

The $MA1$ and $MA2$ bounds of invertibility are derived in the same way: by setting the operators to zero and solving for B. The $MA1$ and $MA2$ invertibility bounds are identical to the $AR1$ and $AR2$ invertibility bounds, of course.

Finally, the bounds of stationarity for an ARp process are derived by setting the ARp operator equal to zero; solving for B; and requiring all roots to be greater than unity in absolute value. ARp and MAq processes have p and q roots respectively, so deriving ARp and MAq bounds is a tedious chore. Fortunately, most modern software packages automatically check estimated models for stationarity and invertibility. In practice, the analyst will be required to understand why the ϕs and θs must be constrained but, given access to an appropriate time series software package, the analyst will never be required to derive the invertibility-stationarity bounds of higher-order processes.

2.6 INTEGRATED PROCESSES

While many social science time series are stationary and adequately modeled as stationary-invertible *ARMA* processes, it may well be that *most* are nonstationary. Many of these nonstationary processes can be modeled as simple variations of the "random walk," which we write as

$$Y_t = Y_{t-1} + a_t$$

Each realization of the random walk is a sum of the preceding realization and a white noise shock. If we think of the random walk as an *AR*1 process with $\phi=1$, then given the *AR*1 stationarity bounds, the random walk is nonstationary by definition. Backward substitution demonstrates an identity of the random walk. For two consecutive realizations of the random walk, Y_{t-1} and Y_t,

$$Y_{t-1} = Y_{t-2} + a_{t-1} \quad \text{and} \quad Y_t = Y_{t-1} + a_t$$

By substitution,

$$Y_t = Y_{t-2} + a_{t-1} + a_t$$

Similarly, substituting for Y_{t-2},

$$Y_t = Y_{t-3} + a_{t-2} + a_{t-1} + a_t$$

Continuing the substitution indefinitely, we discover that Y_t is the sum of all past random shocks.

$$Y_t = a_t + a_{t-1} + a_{t-3} + \cdots = \sum_{k=0}^{\infty} a_{t-k}$$

Since the random walk is an integration or summation of past random shocks, it is commonly called an "integrated" process.

Suppose that a gambler bets on the outcome of a coin flip, winning \$1 for each "head" and losing \$1 for each "tail." Let a_k denote the outcome of the kth flip:

$$a_k = \pm\$1$$

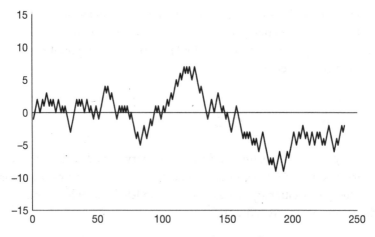

Figure 2.8 $Y_t = a_t + a_{t-1} + \cdots + a_{t-k}$, $E(a_t = 0.00)$

Assuming a "fair" coin,

$$E(a_k) = (.5)(+\$1) + (.5)(-\$1) = 0$$

the expected outcome of any flip is zero. To calculate the net outcome after k flips, we merely sum the a_k. Denoting this sum by Y_k,

$$Y_k = a_t + a_{t-1} + \cdots + a_{t-k} = \sum_{j=0}^{k} a_{t-j}$$

We see that Y_k is a random walk. One could argue that the expected value of Y_k is zero,

$$E(Y_k) = E(a_t + a_{t-1} + \cdots + a_{t-k})$$
$$= E(a_t) + E(a_{t-1}) + \cdots + E(a_{t-k})$$
$$= \sum_{j=0}^{k} E(a_{t-j}) = 0$$

This use of "expected value" is deceiving, of course, because nonstationary processes do not have expected values in the normal sense.

Figures 2.8 and 2.9 show 250 consecutive realizations of two processes generated by summing random coin flips. The time series plotted in Figure 2.8 exhibits the typical stochastic "drift" associated with zero-sum random walks. Because the time series makes wide swings away from the point where it started—$Y_k = 0$, i.e.—if two gamblers start this game with limited funds, one or the other is likely to be bankrupted before Y_k drifts back to zero. This phenomenon is known as

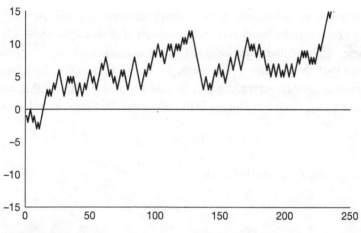

Figure 2.9 $Y_t = a_t + a_{t-1} + \cdots + a_{t-k}, E(a_t = 0.20)$

"gambler's ruin." The time series in Figure 2.9 was generated from nonzero coin flips. When $E(a_k) = \$0.20$, the integration of a_k has a pronounced upward *trend*. Although this process is on a random walk, because the coin flips have a nonzero mean, Y_k moves steadily away from its starting value, $Y_k = 0$. The process *trends*, in other words, and the waiting time for a return to the starting value grows larger as time passes.

The input-output dynamics of a random walk are different from the input-output dynamics of *ARMA* processes in one crucial respect: As time passes, *ARMA* systems "forget" each and every white noise input. Random walks, in contrast, never "forget" an input. The random walk begins at t with future white noise shocks queued up at the entrance to a "black box." The sum of all past random shocks waits inside.

$$\ldots a_{t+2}, a_{t+1}, a_t \quad \Longrightarrow \quad \boxed{\sum_{k=1}^{\infty} a_{t-k}} \quad \Longrightarrow \ldots$$

Upon entering the "black box," a_t is integrated with the sum of past random shocks up to time t.

$$\ldots a_{t+3}, a_{t+2}, a_{t+1} \quad \Longrightarrow \quad \boxed{\sum_{k=0}^{\infty} a_{t-k}} \quad \Longrightarrow \ldots$$

The contents of the "black box" can be written identically as the sum of all past shocks up to time t, as $(Y_{t-1} + a_t)$ or as Y_t. In each of these three identities, the process "memory" is infallible. All prior shocks are "remembered." As the process clock strikes $t + 1$, the "black box" holds the sum of all shocks up to $t + 1$, which, of course, can be written identically as $(Y_{t-1} + a_t)$ or as Y_t.

If the input shocks have a zero mean, Y_t "drifts" aimlessly. Otherwise, if the input shocks have a nonzero mean, Y_t follows a secular trend. In either case, the nonstationary process is stationary in its differences. Writing the random walk as

$$Y_t = Y_{t-1} + \theta_0 + a_t$$

and subtracting Y_{t-1} from both sides,

$$Y_t - Y_{t-1} = \theta_0 + a_t$$

the differenced random walk is equal to a constant, which may be zero, plus white noise. Differenced, in other words, the *nonstationary* random walk is a stationary white noise process.

The algebra of an integrated process meshes neatly with the algebra of stationary processes. Using the backshift operator, differencing can be represented as

$$(1 - B)Y_t = \theta_0 + a_t$$

By convention, we use ∇ to denote $(1 - B)$, the differencing operator.[2]

$$\nabla \equiv (1 - B)$$

The tth realization of the differenced Y_t then is ∇Y_t. The inverse of ∇ is

$$\nabla^{-1} = (1 - B)^{-1} = 1 + B + B^2 + B^3 + \cdots = \sum_{k=0}^{\infty} B^k$$

The series identity of ∇^{-1} can be used to solve the differenced time series for Y_t:

$$\nabla Y_t = \theta_0 + a_t$$
$$\nabla^{-1} \nabla Y_t = \nabla^{-1}(\theta_0 + a_t)$$
$$Y_t = \sum_{k=0}^{\infty} B^k(\theta_0 + a_t)$$
$$Y_t = \sum_{k=0}^{\infty} B^k \theta_0 + \sum_{k=0}^{\infty} B^k a_{t-k}$$

---

2. Readers sometimes confuse ∇ ("nabla") with Δ.

Of course, Y_t need not be white noise but, in general, may be the realization of any stationary *ARMA* process:

$$\nabla Y_t = \phi(B)^{-1}\theta(B)a_t$$

This most general univariate model is an *Auto Regressive Integrated Moving Average (ARIMA)* model.

The mean of a nonstationary integrated process is undefined and, since covariance is defined in terms of the mean,

$$\gamma_k = E(Y_t - \mu_Y)(Y_{t-k} - \mu_Y)$$

covariance is undefined as well. Means and covariances are consequently a function of the specific realization string. The input-output dynamics of a random walk are different from the input-output dynamics of *ARMA* processes in one crucial respect. As time passes, *ARMA* systems "forget" each and every white noise input. Random walks, in contrast, never "forget" an input.

Figure 2.10 plots the sample *ACF*s for the simulated random walks in Figures 2.8 and 2.9. Both of these sample *ACF*s are "typical" of random walks in that they die out slowly from lag to lag. Integrated processes often generate realization strings with *ACF*s where

$$\rho_1 \approx \rho_2 \approx \cdots \approx \rho_k \approx \rho_{k+1} \approx \cdots$$

But since μ_Y and γ_k are undefined, this rule cannot be taken literally.

In principle, a time series can be differenced d times before its differences are stationary. A dth-order random walk

$$\nabla^d Y_t = a_t$$

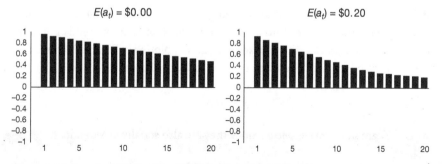

Figure 2.10 Sample *ACF*s for Two Simulated Random Walks

implies a binomial integration. When $d = 2$, for example,

$$\nabla^2 Y_t = a_t$$
$$(1 - B)^2 Y_t = a_t$$
$$(1 - 2B + B^2) Y_t = a_t$$
$$Y_t - 2Y_{t-1} + Y_{t-2} = a_t$$

Solving for Y_t and substituting for Y_{t-1},

$$\begin{aligned} Y_t &= 2Y_{t-1} - Y_{t-2} + a_t \\ &= 2(2Y_{t-2} - Y_{t-3} + a_{t-1}) - Y_{t-2} + a_t \\ &= 3Y_{t-2} - 2Y_{t-3} + 2a_{t-1} + a_t \end{aligned}$$

And substituting for Y_{t-2},

$$\begin{aligned} Y_t &= 3Y_{t-2} - 2Y_{t-3} + 2a_{t-1} + a_t \\ &= 3(2Y_{t-3} - Y_{t-4} + a_{t-2}) - 2Y_{t-3} + 2a_{t-1} + a_t \\ &= 4Y_{t-3} - 3Y_{t-4} + 3a_{t-2} + 2a_{t-1} + a_t \end{aligned}$$

Continuing the backward substitution algorithm, we can see that

$$Y_t = a_t + 2a_{t-1} + 3a_{t-2} + \cdots = \sum_{k=0}^{\infty} k a_{t-k}$$

High-order integrated processes are rarely encountered in the social sciences, however.

2.7 STATIONARITY REVISITED

Although nonstationary processes often generate time series that trend or drift away from the mean, definitions of nonstationarity that focus on trend or drift are incomplete. To illustrate, the time series X_t and Y_t plotted in Figures 2.11 and 2.12 were generated from independent zero-mean Normal processes. Since

$$\mu_X = \mu_Y = 0$$

X_t and Y_t are *stationary-in-mean*. Since they are also serially independent,

$$E(X_t X_{t-k}) = E(Y_t Y_{t-k}) = 0, k > 0$$

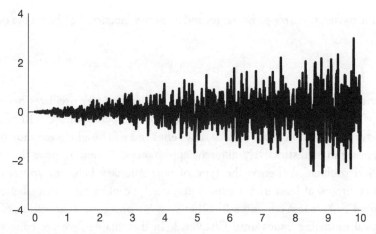

Figure 2.11 X_t: $\mu_X = 0, \sigma_X \propto t$

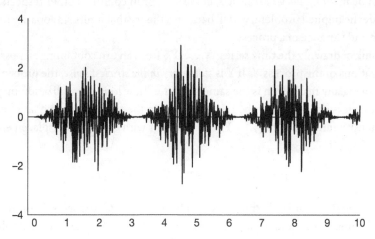

Figure 2.12 Y_t: $\mu_Y = 0, \sigma_Y \propto sin^2 t$

X_t and Y_t have much in common with white noise time series such as those plotted in Figure 2.2. No one would mistake these time series for white noise, however, because unlike white noise, X_t and Y_t are *nonstationary-in-variance*.

When we say that a time series is *not* stationary-in-variance, we mean that its variance changes over time or that its variance is a function of t. For this particular X_t,

$$\sigma_X \propto t$$

As time passes, then, σ_X grows larger and X_t grows "noisier." For Y_t, on the other hand,

$$\sigma_Y \propto \sin^2 t$$

As time passes, σ_Y oscillates between zero and one and Y_t oscillates between "noisy" and "quiet." Both oscillations recur on a fixed period or cycle. Recurring cycles are common in social science time series and will be addressed shortly.

Ignoring their distinctively different appearances, X_t and Y_t pose the same practical problem. Whereas the type of nonstationary behavior apparent in X_t is common, at least in our experience, the type of nonstationary behavior apparent in Y_t is less common. In either case, we postpone a discussion of the practical modeling issues until Chapter 3. In this chapter, we are concerned exclusively with the broader theory of stationarity. If a time series can be *nonstationary-in-mean* and *nonstationary-in-variance*, it follows that a time series might be *nonstationary-in-skewness*, *in-kurtosis*, or in countless other respects. To handle the implied problem, we fall back on a theory that limits stationarity to the mean and variance of a process.

Think of drawing the time series $Y_1, \ldots, Y_N$ from an urn containing all possible realizations of the process Y. If Y is *stationary in the strictest sense*, the probability of drawing any realization is the same no matter how long the realization may be or when it is drawn. Formally, Y is stationary in the strictest sense if and only if the density function $\Pr(Y_1, \ldots, Y_N)$ is invariant with respect to displacement in time. Thus, if

$$\Pr(Y_1, \ldots, Y_N) = \Pr(Y_{1+k}, \ldots, Y_{N+k})$$

for any length-N or lag-k, then Y is stationary in the *strictest sense*. This implies that the mean and variance of Y are constant and that all higher moments about the mean are zero. That is,

$$E(Y_t) = \mu_Y$$
$$E(Y_t - \mu_Y)^2 = \sigma_Y^2 \text{ and}$$
$$E(Y_t - \mu_Y)^j = 0 \text{ for } j > 2$$

Since we cannot empirically verify that all higher moments of Y are zero, strictest-sense stationarity is impractical. If μ_Y and σ_Y^2 are constants, however, Y is stationary in the *widest sense* whether its higher moments are zero or not. The two conditions of *widest-sense* stationarity can always be empirically verified and, if we can assume that Y is Gaussian—which we do throughout this volume—then processes that are stationary in the widest sense are stationary in the strictest sense as well.

Widest-sense stationarity imposes a more realistic set of conditions. Y is stationary in the widest sense (also called *covariance* stationary) if μ_Y and σ_Y^2 are constants, regardless of whether its higher moments about the mean are zero. More important from the practical modeling perspective, widest-sense stationarity can be tested empirically. If Y is Gaussian, moreover, a process that is stationary in the widest sense is stationary in the strictest sense as well. In what follows, then, we assume that Y is a Gaussian process. If the mean and variance of Y_t are constant, we then infer that Y is stationary in the strictest sense. If the mean and variance of Y_t are *not* constant, of course, we can transform and difference Y_t to find a Z_t time series whose mean and variance are constant. Following the same argument, we can infer that the process Z is stationary in the strictest sense.

Although practical modeling issues are not considered until Chapter 3, readers may wonder about the sample *ACF*s of variance nonstationary time series. In most instances, the sample *ACF* of a variance-nonstationary time series will resemble the sample *ACF* of a white noise time series. Sample *ACF*s for X_t and Y_t, plotted in Figure 2.13, are typical in that respect.

If the point is not clear, we need stationarity to draw inferences about the underlying time series process. If the process is stationary, sample realizations of the process—time series—have comparable means, variances, autocovariances, and so on. Given this, we can draw inferences about the generating process from a time series. Stationarity implies that the time series process operated identically in the past as it does in the present and that it will continue to operate identically in the future. Without stationarity, the properties of the time series would vary with the timeframe and no inferences about the underlying process would be possible. Without stationarity, in other words, time series analysis would be impossible.

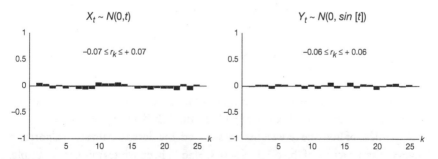

Figure 2.13 Sample *ACF*s for X_t and Y_t

2.8 SEASONAL MODELS

We define seasonality as any cyclical or periodic fluctuation in a time series that recurs or repeats itself at the same phase of the cycle or period. Retail sales normally peak in December when families buy Christmas presents, for example, and unemployment typically peaks in early June when students seek summer jobs. If we knew nothing else about retail sales or unemployment, we could guess when these series would peak. That is the crux of seasonality.

For most purposes, seasonality is "noise" that must be removed or controlled. There are three ways to do this: causal modeling, deseasonalization, and *ARIMA* modeling. Causal modeling is the absolute "best" method of handling seasonality. On this point, we cite Nerlove (1964, p. 263):

> In one sense the whole problem of seasonal adjustment of economic time series is a spurious one. Seasonal variations have causes (for example, variations in the weather), and insofar as these causes are measurable they should be used to explain changes that are normally regarded as seasonal ... Ideally, one should formulate a complete econometric model in which the causes of seasonality are incorporated directly in the equations ... On the practical side the problems include the lack of availability of many relevant series, the non-measurability of key items, and the lack of appropriate statistical methodology ... In addition, the precise structure of the model will very much affect the analysis of seasonal effects ... On the conceptual side, the problem is basically one of continuing structural change, which is essentially the sort of thing which causes seasonality to show up.

Unfortunately, even when the causal mechanism is known, time series observations of the causes are not available.

On the other extreme, deseasonalizing a series prior to analysis is not recommended for most purposes. Virtually all deseasonalization methods create a new series as a weighted average of the old. We write this as

$$Z_t = \omega_1 Y_t + \omega_2 Y_{t-1} + \cdots + \omega_s Y_{t-s}$$

where $\omega_1, \omega_2, \ldots, \omega_s$ are a set of weights and where s is the cycle or period of the data; i.e., $s = 4$ for quarterly data, $s = 12$ for monthly data, and so forth.

Regardless of how the ω-weights are selected, the deseasonalization algorithm changes the structure of the original series. Had Y_t been white noise, for example, the first s lags of the sample *ACF* for Z_t, the deseasonalized time series, would be nonzero. Specifically,

$$E(Z_t Z_{t-1}) = (\omega_1 a_t + \cdots + \omega_s a_{t-s})(\omega_1 a_{t-1} + \cdots + \omega_s a_{t-1-s}) = \omega_1 \omega_2 \sigma_a^2$$
$$E(Z_t Z_{t-2}) = (\omega_1 a_t + \cdots + \omega_s a_{t-s})(\omega_1 a_{t-2} + \cdots + \omega_s a_{t-2-s}) = \omega_1 \omega_3 \sigma_a^2$$

$$\cdots$$

$$\cdots$$

$$E(Z_t Z_{t-k}) = (\omega_1 a_t + \cdots + \omega_s a_{t-s})(\omega_1 a_{t-k} + \cdots + \omega_s a_{t-k-s}) = \omega_1 \omega_{k+1} \sigma_a^2$$

Depending on the values of $\omega_1, \omega_2, \ldots, \omega_s$, this new structure may be nearly impossible to represent as a low-order ARMA model. In our experience, deseasonalization almost always results in a time series that is difficult to model adequately.

The third method of handling seasonality, which is endorsed here, is to model the seasonal variance as an ARMA structure of order s. If we write out M years of a time series in explicit form

$$
\begin{array}{ccccc}
Y_1 & Y_2 & \cdots & Y_{s-1} & Y_s \\
Y_{s+1} & Y_{s+2} & \cdots & Y_{2s-1} & Y_{2s} \\
\cdots & \cdots & \cdots & \cdots \\
\cdots & \cdots & \cdots & \cdots \\
Y_{Ms-s+1} & Y_{Ms-s+2} & \cdots & Y_{Ms-1} & Y_{Ms}
\end{array}
$$

we see that seasonal dependencies between Y_t and Y_{t+s} are expected for the reason that nonseasonal dependencies between Y_t and Y_{t+1} are expected. These seasonal dependencies can be modeled with empirically identified ARMA structures of order s.

A seasonally nonstationary process drifts or trends in annual steps. This behavior figures prominently in agricultural production series (due presumably to the prominence of crop seasons in the process). Seasonal nonstationarity can be modeled with seasonal differencing

$$\nabla^s Y_t = Y_t - Y_{t-s}$$

Stationary seasonal processes can be modeled as seasonal autoregression

$$(1 - \phi_s B^s) Y_t = Y_t - \phi_s Y_{t-s}$$

or as a seasonal moving average

$$(1 - \theta_s B^s) a_t = a_t - \theta_s a_{t-s}$$

In either case, of course, the "best" seasonal model structure is the one that transforms the series to white noise with the fewest number of parameters.

Time series that exhibit both seasonal and nonseasonal behaviors—which are not unusual—introduce another modeling decision. If an *AR* process has both seasonal and nonseasonal structures, for example, the process can be represented as an additive model

$$(1\phi_1 B - \phi_s B^s)Y_t = a_t$$

or as a multiplicative model

$$(1 - \phi_1 B)(1 - \phi_s B^s)Y_t = a_t$$

The two *AR* terms in this multiplicative model are its factors. Expanding the two-factor *AR* model,

$$(1 - \phi_1 B - \phi_s B^s + \phi_1 \phi_s B^{s+1})Y_t = a_t$$

The additive and multiplicative seasonal *AR* models differ by a cross-product term, $\phi_1\phi_s$, which additive models lack. When both ϕ_1 and ϕ_s are small, their product is approximately zero, of course, so there is little difference in that case between additive and multiplicative models. When ϕ_1 and ϕ_s are large, on the other hand, the additive and multiplicative models reflect very different processes.

In practice, we draw no substantive conclusions from the model's form. The fact that an additive or multiplicative model fits a series "best" tells us nothing about the underlying process. An apparent exception to this rule occurs when the series has been differenced both regularly and seasonally. Writing the regular and seasonal difference operators out explicitly,

$$\nabla \nabla^s Y_t = (1 - B)(1 - B^s)Y_t = (1 - B - B^s - B^{1+s})Y_t$$

The use of two differencing operators of orders one and s leads to a cross-product term of order $s + 1$. After regular and seasonal differencing, then, a multiplicative disturbance is expected. But this is due to differencing and has nothing to do with the latent process that generated the series.

2.9 CONCLUSION

This chapter has dealt with theoretical issues—*ARIMA* algebra—to the exclusion of practical issues. We will remedy this shortly. But first, summarizing our theory, a stationary time series can be modeled as the *ARMA* process

$$\phi(B)Y_t = \theta(B)a_t$$

where $\phi(B)$ and $\theta(B)$ are the *AR* and *MA* operators

$$\phi(B) = 1 - \phi_1 B - \phi_2 B^2 - \cdots - \phi_p B^p$$
$$\theta(B) = 1 - \theta_1 B - \theta_2 B^2 - \cdots - \theta_q B^q$$

Constraining the parameters of $\phi(B)$ and $\theta(B)$ to the bounds of stationarity-invertibility, the operators have inverses such that

$$\phi(B)[\phi(B)]^{-1} = [\phi(B)]^{-1}\phi(B) = 1$$
$$\theta(B)[\theta(B)]^{-1} = [\theta(B)]^{-1}\theta(B) = 1$$

These inverses allow us to solve the model for the time series

$$Y_t = [\phi(B)]^{-1}\theta(B)a_t$$

or for the white noise inputs

$$[\theta(B)]^{-1}\phi(B)Y_t = a_t$$

An important class of nonstationary processes are stationary after differencing. In the general *ARIMA* model

$$\phi(B)\nabla Y_t = \theta(B)a_t$$

the differenced time series, ∇Y_t, is the realization of a stationary *ARMA* process. This general *ARIMA* model is solved for Y_t as

$$\nabla Y_t = [\phi(B)]^{-1}\theta(B)a_t$$
$$Y_t = \nabla^{-1}[\phi(B)]^{-1}\theta(B)a_t$$

where ∇^{-1} is the sum of $Y_t, Y_{t-1}, \ldots, Y_1$.

It is often useful for didactic purposes to represent an *ARMA* process in terms of inputs to and outputs from a "black box." A coffee-brewing machine is a useful analogy. To brew a pot of coffee, we feed 12 cups of cold water into one end of the machine and, a few moments later, receive 12 cups of coffee from the other end. If we diagram the brewing process as

$$a_t \implies \boxed{\text{COFFEE MACHINE}} \implies Y_t$$

the analogy is clear. To be precise, of course, we never receive *exactly* 12 cups of coffee. The relationship between the sizes of the outputs and inputs is only approximate. Inputting six cups of cold water, for example, we would be surprised if 12 cups of coffee were delivered at the other end of the machine. On the other hand, we might be equally surprised if exactly six cups of coffee were delivered. Inside the coffee machine, the unobserved brewing process delivers slightly more or slightly fewer cups of coffee than the number of cups of water fed into the machine.

If we were interested in the internal process, we could perform the following experiment: Every 15 minutes, we would input a precisely measured amount of cold water. After a few minutes, we would receive an amount of hot coffee from the machine to be measured precisely. To ensure experimental control, each cold water input would be randomly determined. After many trials—say, 500—we could analyze the Y_t output time series to draw inferences about the brewing process. We would discover that Y_t is determined largely by a_t. The more cold water input, in other words, the more hot coffee output. To a lesser extent, Y_t might also be determined by a_{t-1}, the previous input. This might happen because a small fraction of each input remains inside the machine to be delivered in the next output. The larger the input on one trial, of course, the larger the residual remaining inside the machine to be delivered in the next output. Finally, Y_t might also be determined by Y_{t-1}, the previous output. This could happen if a particularly large output, as a result of a particularly large input, affected the efficiency of the brewing process. For the same reasons, Y_t might be determined by inputs and outputs further removed in time, such as a_{t-2} and Y_{t-2}. But higher-order dependencies would be rare.

The coffee-brewing process is well described by an *ARIMA* model. In general, the size of a pot of coffee is determined by the few immediately preceding outputs and inputs. Inputs and outputs further removed from the present, a_{t-3} and Y_{t-3}, for example, may also play some role in the process, but their influence will be so small that they can be ignored. In practice, the number of inputs and outputs required in the *ARIMA* model will be determined empirically but, in nearly every case, no more than two prior inputs and outputs will have a significant influence on the present output.

The algebraic representation of these input-output models is straightforward. Input-output models have no syntax, strictly speaking. *AR* and *MA* filters may be applied in any order. Since $\phi(B)$ and $\theta(B)$ have inverses, input-output models can be run in reverse with Y_t as the input and a_t as the output. This reversed order suggests a modeling strategy. The stationary Y_t is passed through a series of *AR* and *MA* filters that yield a white noise output. For practical-aesthetic purposes, we want to have no more filters than necessary. In practice, we use the filters only as needed or as suggested by the statistical signature of the time series. Our goal is to find a sequence of filters that reduces Y_t to a_t. The empirically determined sequence of filters is then taken as a model of the process.

APPENDIX 2A EXPECTED VALUES

It will be useful to distinguish between discrete and continuous random variables. An example of the first case is the toss of a single die. Denoting the outcome of the die toss by X, we can write the probability space of X as

$$x_i = \{1, 2, 3, 4, 5, 6\}$$

An example of the second case is the realization of a white noise process. Since the random shock a_t may take on any real value, we write the space as

$$-\infty < a_t < +\infty$$

Although the dice-roll probability space has a finite number of values—this is not necessarily true of all discrete spaces. Likewise, although the white noise probability space includes all of the real numbers, this is not necessarily true of all continuous spaces.

Discrete probability spaces are governed by probability distributions, denoted $\Pr(X)$. In a die-toss experiment, for example, where x_i denotes the ith value of the probability space, $\Pr(X)$ is the probability that the random variable X realizes the value x_i. In the dice-roll example, $\Pr(X = x_i)$ is a uniform one-sixth for each of the six possible values

$$\Pr(1 \leq X \leq 6) = \frac{1}{6}$$

and zero for the values that are not possible.

$$\Pr(X \leq 0) = P(X \geq 7) = 0$$

Continuous probability spaces are governed by *probability density functions*, denoted $f(X)$. The probability that X lies in the closed interval bounded by points a and b is given by the integral

$$\Pr(a < X < b) = \int_a^b f(X)dx$$

To illustrate, the probability that the value of the random shock a_t lies in the interval between discrete points a and b is given by the Gaussian or Normal probability density function

$$\Pr(a < a_t < b) = \frac{1}{\sqrt{2\pi\sigma^2}} \int_a^b e^{-\frac{1}{2\sigma_a}a_t^2}$$

Whereas a discrete probability distribution assigns probabilities to point-values of X, a continuous probility density function assigns probabilities to an interval determined by two point-values, a and b in this example.

Discrete probability distributions have two properties. First, since negative probabilities make no sense, the probability distribution is always nonnegative:

$$\Pr(X = x_i) \geq 0$$

Second, the sum of the probability distribution over all values must be unity:

$$\sum_{-\infty}^{+\infty} \Pr(X = x_i) = 1$$

These properties are easily verified for the die-toss experiment. First, since the probability distribution assigns zero to "out of range" values and one-sixth to "in range" values, the probability distribution is always nonnegative:

$$0 \leq \Pr(X = x_i) \leq \frac{1}{6}$$

Second, the sum of the probabilities across the entire range is unity:

$$\sum_{-\infty}^{+\infty} \Pr(X = x_i) = \sum_{-\infty}^{0} \Pr(X \leq 0) + \sum_{1}^{6} \Pr(1 \leq X \leq 6) + \sum_{7}^{+\infty} \Pr(X \geq 7)$$

$$= 0 + \frac{1}{6} + \frac{1}{6} + \frac{1}{6} + \frac{1}{6} + \frac{1}{6} + \frac{1}{6} + 0 = 1$$

Although continuous probability density functions have analogous properties, the properties are more difficult to verify in specific cases. Using the white noise shock as an illustration, we state those properties here as definitions. First, every probability is nonnegative:

$$\Pr(a < a_t < b) = \frac{1}{\sqrt{2\pi\sigma_a^2}} \int_a^b e^{-\frac{1}{2\sigma_a}a_t^2} \geq 0 \text{ for } a \geq b$$

Second, the continuous probability density function sums to unity:

$$\Pr(-\infty < a_t < +\infty) = \frac{1}{\sqrt{2\pi\sigma_a^2}} \int_a^b e^{-\frac{1}{2\sigma_a}a_t^2} = 1$$

With the random variable, probability space, and probability distribution or density function defined, we are ready to introduce the concept of expected value.

The expected value of a discrete random variable X, denoted $E(X)$, is defined as

$$E(X) = \sum_{-\infty}^{+\infty} P(X = x_i) \times x_i$$

If X is the number realized by rolling a "fair" die, for example, then by definition

$$E(X) = 1 \times \Pr(X = 1) + 2 \times \Pr(X = 2) + \cdots + 6 \times \Pr(X = 6)$$
$$= \left(1 \times \frac{1}{6}\right) + \left(2 \times \frac{1}{6}\right) + \left(3 \times \frac{1}{6}\right) + \cdots + \left(6 \times \frac{1}{6}\right) = 3.5$$

When X is continuous, on the other hand, the expected value is defined as

$$E(a_t) = \frac{1}{\sqrt{2\pi \sigma_a^2}} \int_{-\infty}^{+\infty} e^{-\frac{1}{2\sigma_a} a_t^2} = 0$$

Discrete or continuous, the expected value of a random variable is the product of the variable and its probability integrated over all values.

Several useful results follow from this definition. First, the expected value of a constant is the constant. That is,

$$E(K) = K$$

Second, the expected value of the product of a constant and a variable is the product of the constant and the expected value of the variable. That is,

$$E(KX) = KE(X)$$

And since $E(X) = \mu_X$,

$$E(KX) = K\mu_X$$

$E(X)$ is also called the first moment of X. The second moment of X about the mean

$$E(X - \mu_X)^2 = \sigma_X^2$$

is the variance of X. This result generalizes easily to the product of two random variables. For variables X and Y, covariance is defined as

$$E(X - \mu_X)(Y - \mu_Y)$$

We ordinarily assume that X and Y are standardized to have zero means:

$$E(X) = E(Y) = 0$$

Given this, the covariance of X and Y is

$$E(XY) = \gamma_{XY}$$

which is a more tractable, manageable expression.

Variance and covariance illustrate an important property of the expectation operator. For random variables X and Y, the expected value of the sum is the sum of the expected values:

$$E(X+Y) = E(X) + E(Y)$$

The expectation operator distributes across any linear combination of random variables and constants in this general way:

$$E(X_1 + X_2 + \cdots + X_M) = E(X_1) + E(X_2) + \cdots + E(X_M)$$

But the expected value of the product of X and Y is not generally equal to the product of $E(X)$ and $E(Y)$. That is,

$$E(XY) \neq E(X)E(Y)$$

To illustrate this most important point, consider the $MA1$ process:

$$Y_t = a_t - \theta a_{t-1}$$

The expected value of Y_t is

$$E(Y_t) = E(a_t - \theta a_{t-1}) = E(a_t) - \theta E(a_{t-1}) = 0$$

Table 2.2. Rules and Definitions

$E(X) = \displaystyle\sum_{-\infty}^{+\infty} \Pr(X = x_i) \times x_i$	discrete random variable X
$E(X) = \displaystyle\int_{-\infty}^{+\infty} f(X) dx$	continuous random variable X
$E(k) = k$	constant k
$E(kX) = kE(X)$	random variable X
$E(XY) \neq E(X) \times E(Y)$	random variables X and Y
$E(X+Y) = E(X) + E(Y)$	random variables X and Y
$E(X) = \mu_X$	random variable X
$E(X - \mu_X)^2 = \sigma_X^2$	random variable X
$E(X - \mu_X)(Y - \mu_Y) = \sigma_{XY}$	random variables X and Y

And for the same reason,

$$E(Y_{t-1}) = E(a_{t-1} - \theta a_{t-2}) = E(Y_{t-1}) = E(a_{t-1}) - \theta E(a_{t-2}) = E(Y_{t-1}) = 0$$

But the expected value of the product $Y_t Y_{t-1}$ is not equal to the product $E(Y_t)E(Y_{t-1})$. Instead,

$$E(Y_t Y_{t-1}) = \frac{-\theta}{1+\theta^2} \neq 0$$

The procedures demonstrated here are general. For a linear combination of random variables, the expectation operator is distributed across the combination; the expected value of a linear combination of random variables is the linear combination of each expected value. But the expected value of the product of two or random variables must be taken as a given—covariance, for example—or must be transformed into a linear combination.

APPENDIX 2B SEQUENCES, SERIES, AND LIMITS

Once upon a time, a rich (but foolish) king granted a wish to his grand vizier. The vizier asked that the king put one grain of wheat on the first square of a chessboard, two grains on the second square, four grains on the third square, and so on until all 64 squares were filled. Amused with the vizier's apparent modesty—a few thousand grains of wheat?—the king quickly agreed. Attempting to fulfill the wish, the king soon realized that it would require astronomical quantities of wheat. In fact, the vizier's wish involves the sequence of 64 powers of two,

$$2^0, 2^1, 2^2, \ldots, 2^{63}$$

The first dozen or so numbers of this sequence are large but by no means astronomical. At the third rank of the chessboard, for example, the largest quantity is

$$2^{23} = 8,388,608$$

grains of wheat. In the fourth and subsequent ranks, however, the mind-boggling dimensions of the vizier's request are apparent. The sum of 64 powers of two is

$$\sum_{i=0}^{64} 2^i = 18,446,744,073,709,551,615 \text{ grains}$$

This is approximately the world's wheat production for two thousand years. Calculating this number—and solving a set of related problems—assumes a

Table 2.3. FOUR EXAMPLE SEQUENCES

	Explicit Format	nth Term	Recursion Formula
(a)	$1, 2, 3, \ldots$	$u_n = n$	$u_{n+1} = u_n + 1;\ u_1 = 1$
(b)	$\frac{3}{3}, \frac{5}{3}, \frac{7}{3}, \ldots$	$u_n = \frac{1+2n}{3}$	$u_{n+1} = u_n + \frac{2}{3};\ u_1 = \frac{3}{3}$
(c)	$2^0, 2^1, 2^2, \ldots$	$u_n = 2^{n-1}$	$u_{n+1} = 2u_n;\ u_1 = 2^0$
(d)	$\left(\frac{1}{2}\right)^7, \left(\frac{1}{2}\right)^8, \left(\frac{1}{2}\right)^9, \ldots$	$u_n = \left(\frac{1}{2}\right)^{n+6} \ldots$	$u_{n+1} = \frac{1}{2}u_n;\ u_1 = \left(\frac{1}{2}\right)^7$

knowledge of sequences, series, and limits that begins with definitions of these three concepts.

A sequence is a string of numbers indexed by the positive integers. The sequence can be written explicitly as

$$u_1, u_2, u_3, \ldots, u_n, \ldots$$

Ending the sequence in an ellipsis implies an infinite sequence where n ranges to infinity. Any time series satisfies this definition. A more interesting class of sequences follows a progression.

For purposes of this discussion, Table 2.3 gives four example sequences, (a), (b), (c), and (d), in three formats. The explicit format is a convenient way to write the sequence when its progression can be reliably inferred from the first few terms. When the explicit format will not do, the sequence can be identified by its nth term or by a recursion formula that specifies u_{n+1} in terms of a general value, u_n, and a starting value, u_1. In most instances, the three formats are interchangeable. The choice of one over another is ordinarily determined by taste, style, or pragmatic considerations.

Corresponding to every sequence u_n is a series, denoted S_n, defined as the sum of the sequence. In general

$$S_n = u_1 + u_2 + u_3 + \cdots = \sum_{n=1}^{\infty} u_n$$

and corresponding to example sequences (a), (b), (c), and (d),

$$\text{(a)} \quad S_n = 1 + 2 + 3 + \cdots = \sum_{n=1}^{\infty} n$$

(b) $\quad S_n = \dfrac{3}{3} + \dfrac{5}{3} + \dfrac{7}{3} + \cdots = \displaystyle\sum_{n=1}^{\infty} \dfrac{2n+1}{3}$

(c) $\quad S_n = 2^0 + 2^1 + 2^2 + \cdots = \displaystyle\sum_{n=1}^{\infty} 2^{n-1}$

(d) $\quad \left(\dfrac{1}{2}\right)^7 + \left(\dfrac{1}{2}\right)^8 + \left(\dfrac{1}{2}\right)^9 + \cdots = \displaystyle\sum_{n=1}^{\infty} \left(\dfrac{1}{2}\right)^{n+6}$

To be of any practical value, a series must converge. The convergence of S_n is defined in terms of limits. If the sequence u_n approaches the number U as n approaches infinity, then U is the limit of u_n. This is expressed as

$$\lim_{n\to\infty} u_n = U$$

Considering S_n as a sequence of sums,

$$S_n = S_1, S_2, S_3, \ldots$$

The series converges if and only if

$$\lim_{n\to\infty} S_n = S$$

Otherwise, S_n increases without bound as n approaches infinity. S_n diverges, in other words.

Although the definition of convergence is quite simple, practical application of the definition requires ingenuity and, also, some algebraic rules, which are summarized in Table 2.4. Three important limits are given here by definition:

Rule 1: The limit of n as n approaches infinity is undefined.
Rule 2: The limit of $1/n$ as n approaches infinity is zero.
Rule 3: The limit of a constant as n approaches infinity is the constant.

Table 2.4. RULES FOR EVALUATING SERIES

Rule 1	$\lim_{n\to\infty} n = undefined$
Rule 2	$\lim_{n\to\infty} 1/n = 0$
Rule 3	$\lim_{n\to\infty} k = k$
Rule 4	$\lim_{n\to\infty}(C+D) = \lim_{n\to\infty} C + \lim_{n\to\infty} D$
Rule 5	$\lim_{n\to\infty}(CD) = (\lim_{n\to\infty} C)(\lim_{n\to\infty} D)$
Rule 6	$\lim_{n\to\infty} C \div D = (\lim_{n\to\infty} C) \div (\lim_{n\to\infty} D)$

To these three definitions, we add three algebraic rules:

Rule 4: If the limits exist, the limit of a sum is equal to the sum of the limits.
Rule 5: The limit of a product is equal to the product of the limits.
Rule 6: The limit of a quotient is equal to the quotient of the limits.

Although these definitions and rules may seem trivial, they are the basis for evaluating more complicated limits.

A common, useful method for proving that a sequence converges or diverges consists of showing that the nth term of the sequence is smaller than $1/n$ or larger than n. For example, suppose that we want to evaluate the limit

$$\lim_{n \to \infty} \frac{(1/2)^n}{(1/5)^n}$$

First, rewrite the sequence as

$$\lim_{n \to \infty} \left(\frac{1/2}{1/5} \right)^n = \lim_{n \to \infty} \left(\frac{5}{2} \right)^n$$

Then since

$$\left(\frac{5}{2} \right)^n > n \text{ for } n \geq 0$$

By Rule 1, the limit is undefined. Using the same argument, we can show that

$$\lim_{n \to \infty} \frac{(1/5)^n}{(1/2)^n} = 0$$

Again, rewrite the sequence

$$\lim_{n \to \infty} \frac{(1/5)^n}{(1/2)^n} = \lim_{n \to \infty} \left(\frac{1/5}{1/2} \right)^n = \lim_{n \to \infty} \left(\frac{2}{5} \right)^n$$

Then since

$$\left(\frac{2}{5} \right)^n \leq \frac{1}{n} \text{ or } n \geq 0$$

By Rule 2, the sequence must converge. These demonstrations depend on rewriting the ratio of sequences as a sequence of ratios, of course, which is not always possible.

It follows from Rules 1, 2, and 3 that adding a constant to a sequence changes the limit but not the convergent property of the sequence. For example, to evaluate the limit of

$$\lim_{n\to\infty} \left(1 + \frac{2}{n}\right)$$

we rewrite expression as the sum of three parts,

$$\lim_{n\to\infty} \left(1 + \frac{1}{n} + \frac{1}{n}\right)$$

Then we distribute the limit across the sum,

$$\lim_{n\to\infty}(1) + \lim_{n\to\infty}\left(\frac{1}{n}\right) + \lim_{n\to\infty}\left(\frac{1}{n}\right) = 1$$

Generalizing this result, we can show that any multiple of $1/n$ approaches zero as a limit.

A common problem arises whenever the numerator and denominator of a ratio sequence approach limits independently. To find the limit of

$$\lim_{n\to\infty} \frac{2^n}{1+2^n}$$

divide through numerator and denominator by $2n$,

$$\lim_{n\to\infty} \frac{2^n/2^n}{(1+2^n)/2^n} = \lim_{n\to\infty} \frac{1}{1/2^n + 1}$$

Applying Rules 6 and 3,

$$\lim_{n\to\infty} \frac{1}{1/2^n + 1} = \frac{\lim_{n\to\infty}(1)}{\lim_{n\to\infty}(1/2^n + 1)}$$

$$= \frac{1}{\lim_{n\to\infty}(1/2^n + 1)} \frac{1}{\lim_{n\to\infty}(1/2^n) + \lim_{n\to\infty}(1)}$$

Then, applying Rule 4 to the denominator,

$$\frac{1}{\lim_{n\to\infty}(1/2^n) + \lim_{n\to\infty}(1)} = \frac{1}{\lim_{n\to\infty}(1/2)^n + \lim_{n\to\infty}(1)} = \frac{1}{0+1} = 1$$

This is not the only way to evaluate this limit, of course, but all methods lead to the same conclusion.

Arithmetic and Geometric Series. Time and effort can be saved by studying similarities and differences of the algebraic properties of sequences. With no evaluation, for example, we can tell that sequences (a) and (b) do not converge. Both (a) and (b) are arithmetic sequences that, in general, follow the arithmetic progression

$$u_1, (u_1 + \nabla), (u_1 + 2\nabla), \ldots$$

The nth term of an arithmetic sequence is thus

$$u_n = u_1 + (n-1)\nabla$$

Noting that ∇ is the difference of u_{n+1} and u_n, the arithmetic sequence can be written in terms of the nth recursion:

$$u_{n+1} = u_n + \nabla$$

In particular, sequences (a) and (b) can be written as

$$u_{n+1} = u_n + 1; u_1 = 1 \quad \text{and} \quad u_{n+1} = u_n + \frac{2}{3}; u_1 = \frac{3}{3}$$

When a sequence is specified by its the nth recursion, of course, u_1 must also be specified. The recursion form of these sequences highlights their common algebraic property, however, and hints at the most important property of arithmetic series: *Arithmetic series do not converge.*

An analogy between an arithmetic sequence and the expected path of a trending time series may be useful. In both cases, the first difference is interpreted as the linear change. In both cases, furthermore, the first n terms sum to

$$S_n = \frac{n}{2}[2u_1 + (n-1)\nabla]$$

So for, say, $n = 100$, series (a) and (b) are evaluated as

$$S_{100} = \frac{100}{2}[2(1) + (99)1] = 5050$$

and

$$S_{100} = \frac{100}{2}[2\left(\frac{3}{3}\right) + (99)\frac{2}{3}] = 3400$$

But neither series converges. Instead, both series grow larger and larger as n approaches infinity. More generally, no arithmetic series converges. To prove this, we evaluate the limit of a general arithmetic series:

$$\lim_{n\to\infty} S_n = \lim_{n\to\infty} \frac{n}{2}[2u_1 + (n-1)\nabla]$$

$$\lim_{n\to\infty} S_n = \lim_{n\to\infty} \left(nu_1 + \frac{\nabla}{2}n^2 - \frac{\nabla}{2}n\right)$$

$$\lim_{n\to\infty} S_n = \lim_{n\to\infty} nu_1 + \lim_{n\to\infty} \frac{\nabla}{2}n^2 - \lim_{n\to\infty} \frac{\nabla}{2}n$$

$$\lim_{n\to\infty} S_n = \lim_{n\to\infty} \left(u_1 - \frac{\nabla}{2}\right)\lim_{n\to\infty} n + \left(\frac{\nabla}{2}\right)\lim_{n\to\infty} n^2$$

Since both limits are undefined, their sum is undefined. S_n diverges and, so, as claimed, no arithmetic series converges. Needless to say, this limits the usefulness of arithmetic series.

Sequences (c) and (d) present another case. These sequences follow the geometric progression

$$u_1, u_1 \nabla, u_1 \nabla^2, \ldots$$

The nth term of the geometric sequence is thus

$$u_n = u_1 \nabla^{n-1}$$

Here ∇ is the ratio of u_{n+1} and u_n, which leads to the geometric recursion formula

$$u_{n+1} = \nabla u_n$$

For sequence (c)

$$u_{n+1} = 2u_n; \quad u_1 = 2^0 = 1$$

And for sequence (d)

$$u_{n+1} = \frac{1}{2} u_n; \quad u_1 = \left(\frac{1}{2}\right)^7 = \frac{1}{128}$$

Again, the recursion form highlights the common algebraic property of these sequences and hints at a property of geometric series. It can be shown that the first n terms of a geometric sequence sum to

$$S_n = u_1 \frac{1 - \nabla^n}{1 - \nabla}$$

For $n = 100$, then, series (c) is evaluated as

$$S_{100} = (1)\frac{1 - 2^{100}}{1 - 2} = 2^{100} - 1$$

This is an *extremely* large number, so one might guess that (c) does not converge. In fact, it *explodes*. For series (d), on the other hand

$$S_{100} = \left(\frac{1}{2}\right)^7 \frac{1 - (\frac{1}{2})^{100}}{1 - \frac{1}{2}}$$

$$= \left(\frac{1}{2}\right)^6 \left[1 - \left(\frac{1}{2}\right)^{100}\right]$$

$$= \left(\frac{1}{2}\right)^6 - \left(\frac{1}{2}\right)^{106} \approx \frac{1}{64}$$

In this case, one might guess that (d) converges. *In general, a geometric series converges only when ∇ is less than one in absolute value.* To prove this, we evaluate the limit of S_n. Taking limits on both sides of the formula for S_n

$$\lim_{n \to \infty} S_n = \lim_{n \to \infty} u_1 \frac{1 - \nabla^n}{1 - \nabla}$$

We can then factor the constant terms out of the left-hand side:

$$\lim_{n \to \infty} S_n = \frac{u_1}{1 - \nabla} \lim_{n \to \infty} (1 - \nabla^n)$$

Then, distributing the limit,

$$\lim_{n \to \infty} S_n = \frac{u_1}{1 - \nabla} \lim_{n \to \infty} 1 - \frac{u_1}{1 - \nabla} \lim_{n \to \infty} \nabla^n$$

This simplifies to

$$\lim_{n \to \infty} S_n = \frac{u_1}{1 - \nabla} - \frac{u_1}{1 - \nabla} \lim_{n \to \infty} \nabla^n$$

When $\nabla < 1$, the second term of this limit vanishes and

$$\lim_{n \to \infty} S_n = \frac{u_1}{1 - \nabla}$$

On the other hand, when $\nabla > 1$, the second term "explodes," and

$$\lim_{n \to \infty} S_n = \infty$$

which is to say that the limit is undefined. Finally, when $\nabla = 1$, this expression involves division by zero and the limit must be evaluated by other means. However, we state by definition that the limit is undefined for $\nabla = 1$.

Based on this result, we see that for (c), where $\nabla = 2$, the series is undefined. For (d), in contrast, where $\nabla = 1/2$, the series approaches the limit

$$S_n = \frac{1 - \left(\frac{1}{2}\right)^7}{1 - \frac{1}{2}} = \frac{-\frac{127}{128}}{-\frac{64}{128}} = \frac{127}{64} \approx 1.98$$

In general, geometric series converge whenever ∇ is less than one in absolute value. That is,

$$\lim_{n \to \infty} S_n = \frac{u_1}{1 - \nabla} \quad \text{if and only if} \quad -1 < \nabla < 1$$

And because geometric series do converge under these conditions—that is, S_n converges whenever ∇ is smaller than unity in absolute value—power series are a valuable analytic tool. A few examples will demonstrate this point.

In Chapter 2.2, the $AR1$ process was written in its series form by backward substitution. In Chapter 2.4, the series form was used to show that the variance of an $AR1$ process was given by the series

$$\sigma_Y^2 = \frac{\sigma_a^2}{1 + \phi^2 + \phi^6 + \cdots + \phi^{2k}} = \sum_{k=1}^{\infty} \phi^{2(k-1)} \sigma_a^2$$

We can now use the convergence property of geometric series to evaluate σ_Y^2. First, to show that σ_Y^2 is a geometric series, find the ratio of u_{n+1} and u_n:

$$\frac{u_{n+1}}{u_n} = \frac{\phi^{2n}}{\phi^{2(n-1)}} = \phi^{2n-2(n-1)} = \phi^2$$

So the series is based on the sequence

$$u_{n+1} = \phi^2 u_n; \; u_1 = \sigma_a^2$$

which is a geometric series. Now, having shown that the series representation of σ_Y^2 is a geometric series, we know that

$$\sigma_Y^2 = \sum_{k=1}^{\infty} \phi^{2(k-1)} \sigma_a^2 = \frac{\sigma_a^2}{1 - \phi^2} \text{ if and only if } -1 < \phi < 1$$

In other words, as we claimed in Chapter 2.4, the $AR1$ stationarity bounds guarantee the existence of σ_Y^2.

In Chapter 2.4, we derived the reciprocal of the $AR1$ operator by backward substitution. Since the $AR1$ process can be written as a geometric series, however—that is, since

$$Y_t = a_t(1 + \phi B + \phi^2 B^2 + \cdots + \phi^k B^k + \cdots) = \sum_{k=0}^{\infty} \phi^k a_{t-k}$$

the reciprocal can be derived directly from the geometric expansion. For that purpose, note that

$$S_n = \sum_{k=0}^{\infty} \phi^k a_{t-k} = \frac{1}{1 - \phi B}$$

which is what was claimed.

Tests of Convergence. We have already demonstrated, first, that no arithmetic series converges; and second, that geometric series converge if and only if

$$\frac{-1 < u_{n+1}}{u_n < +1} \quad \text{or} \quad -1 < \nabla < +1$$

In other cases, unfortunately, the convergence properties of each series must be established case by case. For this purpose, we develop a set of empirical convergence tests.

Necessary Condition Test. One might think that S_n converges whenever u_n approaches a finite limit. But, in fact, if u_n has a nonzero limit

$$\lim_{n \to \infty} u_n = U, \; U \neq 0$$

then S_n cannot converge. This is the basis of a necessary condition test for convergence. Put simply, if

$$\lim_{n \to \infty} u_n \neq 0$$

then S_n must diverge. Otherwise, S_n may or may not converge. To illustrate, the sequence of natural numbers, $u_n = n$, clearly diverges, so the associated series must diverge. If this were not obvious, we could apply the necessary condition test. Since $u_n = n$, we have by definition

$$\lim_{n \to \infty} n = \infty$$

So the associated series diverges. In contrast, the reciprocal sequence, 1, 1/2, 1/3, . . .,1/n, approaches zero as a limit:

$$\lim_{n \to \infty} \frac{1}{n} = 0$$

This does not imply that the associated series converges, however, because this is only a *necessary* condition. The series still need not converge and, in fact, this series diverges.

Ratio Test for Positive Terms. When a sequence has only positive terms, the ratio of u_{n+1} to u_n can be used to test convergence. If

$$\lim_{n \to \infty} \frac{u_{n+1}}{u_n} < 1$$

then S_n always converges. If

$$\lim_{n \to \infty} \frac{u_{n+1}}{u_n} > 1$$

then S_n always diverges. Finally, when

$$\lim_{n \to \infty} \frac{u_{n+1}}{u_n} = 1$$

the test is inconclusive. To illustrate, consider a ratio whose numerator and denominator are arithmetic and geometric sequences respectively—say,

$$\left(\frac{1}{2}\right)^1, \left(\frac{2}{2}\right)^2, \left(\frac{3}{2}\right)^3, \dots, \left(\frac{n}{2}\right)^n$$

Does S_n converge? The ratio of successive terms of this sequence is

$$\frac{u_{n+1}}{u_n} = \frac{\frac{n+1}{2^{n+1}}}{\frac{n}{2^n}} = \left(\frac{n+1}{2^{n+1}}\right)\left(\frac{2^n}{n}\right)$$

A little algebraic manipulation simplifies this ratio

$$\frac{u_{n+1}}{u_n} = \frac{n+1}{2^{n+1}} \times \frac{2^n}{n} = \frac{n+1}{2n} = \frac{n}{2n} + \frac{1}{n} = \frac{1}{2} + \frac{1}{n}$$

Taking the limit of this expression,

$$\lim_{n \to \infty} \frac{u_{n+1}}{u_n} = \lim_{n \to \infty} \left(\frac{1}{2} + \frac{1}{n}\right) = \lim_{n \to \infty} \left(\frac{1}{2}\right) + \lim_{n \to \infty} \left(\frac{1}{n}\right) = \frac{1}{2}$$

Since this limit is less than unity, S_n must converge.

Although the reciprocal integer sequence satisfies the necessary condition test, the series does not converge. Since $u_n = \frac{1}{n}$ is always positive, we can use the ratio test. The ratio of u_{n+1} to u_n is

$$\frac{u_{n+1}}{u_n} = \frac{n+1}{n} = \frac{n}{n} + \frac{1}{n} = 1 + \frac{1}{n}$$

The limit of the ratio is

$$\lim_{n \to \infty} \frac{u_{n+1}}{u_n} = \lim_{n \to \infty} \left(1 + \frac{1}{n}\right) = \lim_{n \to \infty} (1) + \lim_{n \to \infty} \left(\frac{1}{n}\right) = 1$$

This test too is inconclusive.

Comparison Tests. A series of positive terms must converge if its nth term is smaller than the nth term of a series that is known to converge. If v_n converges, in other words, and if u_n is smaller than v_n, then u_n must also converge. The converse is also true: If v_n diverges and if u_n is larger than v_n, then u_n cannot converge. Although the truth of these claims should be intuitively obvious, their utility may not be apparent. In fact, comparison tests are often the most generally useful convergence tests. Consider the series of reciprocal powers of the natural numbers:

$$S_n = \frac{1}{1^p} + \frac{1}{2^p} + \frac{1}{3^p} + \cdots = \sum_{n=0}^{\infty} \frac{1}{n^p}$$

For $p > 1$, S_n must converge, but for $p \leq 1$, on the other hand, S_n cannot converge.

3

Noise Modeling

All models are wrong [but] some models are useful.

—Box (1979)

For any time series, there are literally thousands of statistically *adequate ARIMA* models. Each transforms the series into white noise. But no more than a half-dozen of these adequate models are *useful* in the sense implied by Box. Differences among the six-or-so useful models might be so small that choosing a specific model from the six would be practically inconsequential. Nevertheless, by convention, the "best" *ARIMA* model is the one of the six-or-so that is *most* useful. As Box's aphorism implies, this "best" *ARIMA* model is categorically *wrong* because even the "best" model is, after all, *only* a model. But to the extent that it serves its intended purpose, the model is *practically* useful.

In the preceding chapter, working in the realm of algebra, we ignored practicalities. We assumed our way around practical obstacles and sometimes used semantic tricks to prove outrageous statements. In practice, on the other hand, we deal with short time series and discover that what is true and obvious in expectation, whether true or not in realization, is seldom obvious. We must now pay somewhat more attention to practicalities, offering a more balanced view of time series modeling.

To motivate this topic, think of modeling as a game where an analyst is given a finite realization string—a time series—and is asked to guess the generating process. To make the game interesting, the analyst pays $1 for the privilege of guessing and wins $2 for each correct guess. Can the analyst win this game? Never. As the "house," we would undoubtedly start with the shortest possible time series, say a single rounded number like 2.782. Infinitely many *ARIMA* processes could generate this number, so the analyst has no chance of winning.

The analyst would undoubtedly demand a refund, arguing that 2.782 is not a time series, but we would argue that 2.782 is indeed a time series, albeit a short one. The argument is moot, however, because we could give the analyst 100 or even 1000 observations without losing our advantage. No matter how different two *ARIMA* processes might be in theory, in practice, they can—and will—generate identical time series.

To stand any chance at all, the analyst must demand credit for reasonably correct guesses. If the integer order of the *AR* and *MA* structures is correctly identified, for example, the guess is 90 percent correct; if the *AR* and *MA* parameter values are guessed within two standard errors, the guess is 95 percent correct, and so forth. With these rules, two very different processes, say,

$$\nabla Y_t = a_t \quad \text{and} \quad (1 - .5B)Y_t = (1 - .8B)a_t$$

can still generate identical realization strings. But the probability that this will happen grows smaller as the realization string grows longer.

Under the new set of rules, the analyst no longer bets that the guess is absolutely correct but that the guess is relatively correct—90, 95, or even 99 percent correct, depending on the time series. The advantage now belongs to the analyst. Finally, if the analyst varies the size of the bet from guess to guess, the game approaches a "sure thing." The wise analyst bets large sums on long, well-behaved series, small sums on short series regardless of how well behaved they may be, and, from time to time, makes no bet at all.

Continuing the gaming analogy, all games of chance require a strategy to maximize the chances of winning and to minimize losses. Time series modeling is no exception. A strategy for finding the "best" *ARIMA* model of a time series is depicted as a flowchart in Figure 3.1. Although in practice this algorithm is nearly

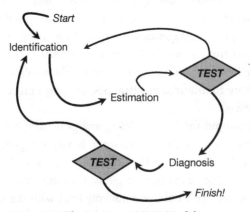

Figure 3.1 The Iterative *ARIMA* Modeling Strategy

optimal for modeling common time series, it is not a substitute for common sense. Nor is it meant to be interpreted literally. Before executing the algorithm, for example, the prudent analyst will inspect the plotted time series, searching for features of the data that might guide the analysis—outliers, nonstationary behavior, and so forth. After the algorithm is finished, the prudent analyst will inspect a plot of a model's residuals to search for anomalous patterns that might suggest misspecification. Within these broad guidelines, however, the algorithm ensures that the model selected is the most parsimonious, statistically adequate model for the time series. Given the salience of the algorithm, we discuss its operations in detail.

Identification. A first approximation to $N(a_t)$ is identified by comparing the sample ACF with the $ACFs$ expected of various $ARIMA$ processes. This involves deciding whether the time series must be differenced and what ARp and/or MAq structures are required to adequately represent the underlying generating process. In theory, each process has a unique ACF. In practice, of course, sample $ACFs$ sometimes bear little resemblance to the parent process. For the stationary series Y_t with sample mean and variance,

$$\overline{Y} = \frac{1}{N}\sum_{t=1}^{N} Y_t \quad \text{and} \quad s^2 = \frac{1}{N}\sum_{t=1}^{N}(Y_t - \overline{Y})^2$$

the lag-k sample ACF is estimated as

$$r_k = \frac{\dfrac{1}{N-k}\sum_{t=1}^{N-k}(Y_t - \overline{Y})(Y_{t-k} - \overline{Y})}{s^2}$$

For an insight into the nature of this formula, lag Y_t backward in time

$$
\begin{array}{ccccc}
Y_1 & Y_2 & \cdots & Y_{N-1} & Y_N \\
 & Y_1 & Y_2 & \cdots & Y_{N-1} & Y_N \\
 & & Y_1 & Y_2 & \cdots & Y_{N-1} & Y_N
\end{array}
$$

and so forth. This array emphasizes the fact that r_1 is the correlation of Y_t and its first lag, Y_{t-1}; r_2 is the correlation of Y_t and its second lag, Y_{t-2}; r_3 is the correlation of Y_t and its third lag, Y_{t-3}; and in general, r_k is the correlation of Y_t and its kth lag, Y_{t-k}. Note further that one pair of observations is lost from the numerator of r_k with successive lags; the numerator of r_1 has $N - 1$ observations, the numerator of r_2 has $N - 2$ observations, and so forth. Since its denominator is always based on $N - k$ observations, r_k is not strictly speaking a Pearson product-moment correlation coefficient. But since r_k approximates

Pearson's correlation for large N, we have no quarrel with that straightforward interpretation.

Since the sample ACF is itself a random variable, the value of r_k varies from realization to realization. The sample variance of r_k is given by

$$s_r^2 = \frac{1 + 2\sum_{t=1}^{k} r_k^2}{N}$$

The null hypothesis that $r_k = 0$ may be tested by comparing r_k to its standard error. For $r_k = 0$, 95 percent of the sample distribution lies in the interval

$$-1.96 s_r < r_k < +1.96 s_r$$

With 95 percent confidence, then, the null hypothesis that $r_k = 0$ is rejected whenever r_k lies outside this interval. Questions about the significance of r_k typically arise when two alternative models are distinguished by a specific lag of the ACF. White noise and $MA1$ models differ only by the value of r_1, for example, and this implies the null hypothesis

$$H_0: \quad r_1 = 0; \text{ White Noise}$$

If r_1 lies in the closed interval $\pm 1.96 s_r$, H_0 is accepted. Otherwise, H_0 is rejected with 95 percent confidence and the alternative hypothesis

$$H_A: \quad r_1 \neq 0; MA1$$

is accepted. All commonsense rules of hypothesis testing apply, of course. If a series is unusually short, say, $N < 50$, large r_k may be insignificant; and if a series is unusually long, say, $N > 250$, small r_k may be significant. Otherwise, values of r_k in the closed interval of $\pm 1.96 s_r$ are ignored for most identification tasks.

Estimation. With a tentative model identified, parameters are estimated. To pass this step, the algorithm requires that all parameters be statistically significant and that AR and MA parameters be stationary-invertible. Failing the first criterion need not force a return to the identification step. Instead, by dropping insignificant parameters, a more parsimonious version of the original model is re-estimated. The second criterion is not so forgiving. A nonstationary or noninvertible parameter estimate often rules out an entire class of tentative models, so dropping a problematic parameter may not solve the problem. In either case, however, failing the estimation step provides valuable information to be used in subsequent iterations of the algorithm.

Diagnosis. Passing both estimation tests, the algorithm proceeds to the diagnostic step where the model residuals are compared to white noise. The residuals are said to be "not different than white noise" if they have a Normal distribution

$$a_t \backsim \text{Normal}(0, \sigma_a^2)$$

and if they are independent

$$E(a_t a_{t-k}) = 0$$

Although Normality can be tested by any goodness-of-fit statistic, we prefer the Kolmogorov-Smirnov (KS) statistic. Whatever statistic is used, the Normality of a model's residuals must be tested and confirmed prior to any further consideration.

When the Normality criterion is satisfied, the independence criterion is tested with a residual ACF. For that purpose, the independence H_0 is reformulated as

$$H_0: r_1 = r_2 = \cdots = r_k = 0; \; a_t \backsim \text{iid Normal}(0, \sigma_a^2)$$

The Q-statistic (or the "portmanteau statistic") is the most popular test of this null hypothesis. An early version of the Q-statistic, due to Box and Pierce (1970), is given by

$$Q_k = N \sum_{i=1}^{k} r_k^2$$

where k is the number of lags of the ACF tested under H_0. Under H_0, the Box-Pierce Q-statistic is distributed approximately as χ_k^2. Simulation experiments found the Box-Pierce Q-statistic departed from the χ^2 distribution in even moderately long time series, however. To remedy this problem, Ljung and Box (1978) proposed a corrected Q-statistic,

$$Q_k = N(N+2) \sum_{i=1}^{k} (N-k)^{-1} r_k^2$$

Like the Box-Pierce Q-statistic, the Ljung-Box Q-statistic is approximately distributed as χ_k^2 and is now the preferred version of the test.

One potential problem in using the Q-statistic is choosing k, the number of lags to include in testing the independence H_0. The power of the test decreases as the lag increases, making it desirable to select a relatively small number of lags. Other than that, the choice is ultimately arbitrary. When seasonality is a possibility, as with monthly data, one rule is to select k to be twice the length of the cycle (that is, 24 observations with monthly data). Another strategy is to use a mechanical rule, such as $k = N/4$, where N is the length of the time series (Wei, 2006, p. 109). Based on simulation experiments, Tsay (2002, p. 25) argues that tests based on

$k = ln(N)$ are more powerful. Tsay's approach selects a very small number of lags even with long series, however, and we have not found it to be useful.

The choice of a specific k is less important if the test rejects or fails to reject H_0 over a wide range of possible values. Most *ARIMA* software packages will display the value of the Q-statistic for each lag to some upper limit, and often all reasonable values lead to the same inference.

Applied to the residuals of an estimated model, the degrees of freedom for the test decrease with the number of coefficients. Specifically, using model residuals, Q has a χ^2 distribution with degrees of freedom equal to k minus the number of coefficients (including the constant if one appears in the estimates). Nevertheless, a common practice is to report results using k degrees of freedom regardless of the model estimates.

If the model residuals satisfy both the Normality and independence criteria, the model is said to be "statistically adequate" and the algorithm stops. If the residuals fail either criterion, on the other hand, the tentative model is rejected and the algorithm returns to an earlier step.

Remaining questions about the modeling algorithm are best answered by a few in-depth example analyses. The time series analyzed in this chapter and in Chapter 5 were selected to illustrate the most common practical problems that analysts are likely to encounter. The time series can be found through the publisher's web portal. Readers are encouraged to replicate our analyses, checking (or challenging) our results.[1]

3.1 WHITE NOISE

Figure 3.2 shows a time series of β-particle hits on a Geiger-Mueller tube (Topsoe and Stillwell, 1990). Since radioactive decay processes typically have "random" (i.e., Poisson) outcomes, we suspect that a white noise model will fit the β-particle time series. A full analysis is required to confirm this suspicion, of course.

In the social sciences, on the other hand, white noise processes are thought to be rare; in our experience, they are. Figure 3.3 shows a rare exception. These data are monthly homicides in South Carolina for 1950 through 1963. King (1978) argues that these data reveal the "brutalization" effect of capital punishment: Homicides rise following an execution. Indeed, since there were 182 homicides in the 10 months immediately following an execution but only 162 in the 10 months immediately preceding an execution, King's argument seems to be supported. But is this difference statistically significant? Plugging the means and standard

---

1. *ARIMA* parameters reported in this and subsequent chapters were estimated with the SCA Statistical System (Liu and Hudak, 1983) and were replicated with SAS and Stata.

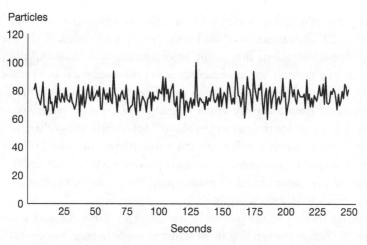

Figure 3.2 β-Particles

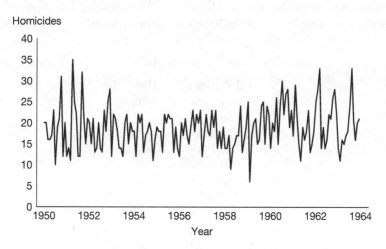

Figure 3.3 South Carolina Homicides (King, 1978)

deviations for the pre- and post-execution months into the familar formula for the difference-of-means *t*-test,

$$t_{After-Before} = \frac{16.2 - 18.2}{\sqrt{\frac{3.71}{10} + \frac{2.86}{10}}} = 2.47$$

So homicides do indeed rise in the month following an execution, as King claims, and if we can trust a simple difference-of-means *t*-test, the difference is significant. Nearly all tests of significance assume white noise, of course, and in our experience, white noise processes are rare in the social sciences. A valid test of the null hypothesis must therefore wait on a formal analysis of this time series.

Analysis begins with a visual inspection of the raw time series. Both time series have the "flat" appearance associated with stationary processes. While each has one or two observations that might be characterized as "outliers," the values are neither so extreme nor so numerous as to pose an obstacle to identification of $N(a_t)$. Although experienced analysts believe that they can identify a white noise process from a cursory visual inspection of the time series, we remain skeptical. Even novice analysts will be able to spot problematic outliers, however, and distinguish between stationary and nonstationary processes. These goals motivate the preliminary visual inspection of a raw time series. Satisfied that both processes are stationary and that neither time series has flagrant outliers, we move on to a formal time series analysis.

Identification. The sample *ACF*s are listed in Table 3.1 and plotted in Figure 3.4. Before interpreting these statistics, we anticipate two general questions. First, how long should a sample *ACF* be? Shorter or longer *ACF*s would identify the same models for these time series. Since roughly 1 in 20 r_k are statistically significant by chance, $k=20$ lags might be preferred for interpretability.

Table 3.1. SAMPLE *ACF*s

	β-Particles		Homicides	
k	r_k	s_r	r_k	s_r
1	.01	.06	.11	.08
2	−.05	.06	−.00	.08
3	.01	.06	.07	.08
4	.06	.06	.03	.08
5	.05	.06	−.06	.08
6	.10	.06	.03	.08
7	−.06	.06	−.04	.08
8	.07	.06	.12	.08
9	.02	.06	.02	.08
10	.05	.06	−.07	.08

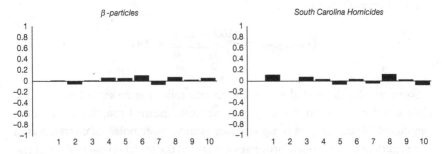

Figure 3.4 Sample *ACF*s, β-Particles and South Carolina Homicides

Table 3.2. ESTIMATION AND DIAGNOSIS

		Estimate	SE	t	
β-particles	$\hat{\theta}_0$	75.51	0.42	179.77	$RSE = 6.64$
					$Q_{20} = 19.8$
					$Z_{KS} = 0.09$
Homicides	$\hat{\theta}_0$	18.77	0.39	−.28	$RSE = 5.06$
					$Q_{20} = 20.5$
					$Z_{KS} = 0.10$

Because these time series are stationary and nonseasonal, however, 10 lags should be sufficient. We revisit this question at a later point. Second question, what are the relative advantages of reporting a sample ACF as a tabulation (Table 3.1) or as a "correlogram" (Figure 3.4)? The reporting format is a matter of taste. Some prefer tabulations; some prefer ACF plots. We present both in this chapter.

In either reporting format, the sample ACFs clearly identify white noise models for both series. Not one r_k is significantly different than zero. This rules out all models except white noise.

Estimation. Parameter estimates for the two white noise models, along with basic model statistics, are presented in Table 3.2. There is little to say about these estimates and, hopefully, their origins are no mystery. For white noise, the single model parameter is estimated as the arithmetic mean. For the $β$-particle and homicide series respectively,

$$\hat{\theta}_0 = \frac{1}{249} \sum_{t=1}^{249} Y_t = 75.51 \text{ and } \hat{\theta}_0 = \frac{1}{168} \sum_{t=1}^{168} Y_t = 18.77$$

We would ordinarily check for stationarity-invertibility and significance. Strict adherence to the iterative model-building strategy (Figure 3.1) makes little sense when a white noise model is identified, however.

Diagnosis. A model is said to be "statistically adequate" or "adequate" if its residuals are not different than white noise. This implies two distinct tests. The model residuals must be (1) Normal and (2) independent. We discuss the Normality test in detail in the next section. For now, we note that Normal distributions fit the residuals of both models quite well. Independence can be tested with a Q-statistic estimated from the residual ACF. For white noise, the raw series and the model residuals differ by a constant (θ_0), so the time series ACF (Table 3.1) and the residual ACF are identical. For a white noise null hypothesis, with 20 degrees of freedom, 95 percent of the χ^2 distribution lies between zero and 31.41. Since the values of $Q_{20} = 19.8$ and $Q_{20} = 20.5$ are smaller than the

95th percentile, the white noise null hypothesis cannot be rejected. Accordingly, we conclude that these series are white noise.

3.2 THE NORMALITY ASSUMPTION: A DIGRESSION

Normality is often taken for granted or assumed without question, and this can be a grave error. At the first model-building stage, violation of the Normality assumption can distort a sample *ACF*, making identification hopelessly difficult. At the second stage, violation of the Normality assumption can lead to biased parameter estimates and invalid inferences. At the third stage, non-Normal residuals can result in a model being accepted when, in fact, it should be rejected. In sum, violations of the Normality assumption can and do affect every stage of the model-building strategy. The consequences can be so serious, moreover, that the analyst is advised to make a formal test of the Normality assumption prior to any attempt at modeling.

Cumulative frequencies of the β-particle and homicide time series are plotted in Figure 3.5; cumulative Normal distributions are superimposed. The slight discrepancies to the left of the modes indicate that both time series are skewed slightly to the left. Otherwise, both distributions appear approximately Normal. Formal goodness-of-fit tests, which are recommended in all cases, require cumulative distributions such as these.

The best-known and (probably) most widely used goodness-of-fit test is based on the Pearson (1900) goodness-of-fit statistic:

$$X^2 = \sum_{i=1}^{N} \frac{(O_i - E_i)^2}{E_i}$$

where O_i and E_i are the ith observed and expected cumulative frequencies. Values of O_i and E_i are listed in Table 3.3 for the two time series, along with

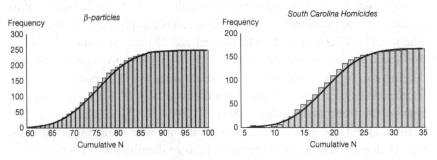

Figure 3.5 Cumulative Normal Distributions

the values of the X^2 statistic. Under the null hypothesis of identical Normality, X^2 is distributed as χ^2 with $n - 1$ degrees of freedom. In this case, we have $n - 1 = 31$ and $n - 1 = 26$ degrees of freedom for the β-particle and homicide series. Consulting a table of the χ^2, the 95th percentiles for 31 and 26 degrees of freedom are 45.51 and 38.88, so

$$H_0: X^2 < 45.51 \quad \text{and} \quad H_0: X^2 < 38.88$$

From Table 3.3, however, we calculate $X^2 = 11.46$ and $X^2 = 20.42$. Since neither χ^2 statistic is large enough to reject H_0, the Normality assumption is warranted for both residual time series.

Under some circumstances, the X^2 goodness-of-fit test has serious limitations. While the β-particle and homicide time series fall neatly into 32 and 27 discrete categories, for example, continuous values of Y_t must be forced into an arbitrary number of categories. This practical consideration aside, the X^2 goodness-of-fit statistic has a notoriously quirky power curve that too often supports false conclusions. The KS goodness-of-fit test has a more acceptable power curve and requires no arbitrary categorization.

The KS test statistic is the absolute difference of standardized observed and expected frequencies. For data arrayed as in Table 3.3, that is

$$D_{max} = max \left| \frac{O - E}{N} \right|$$

Unlike χ^2, D_{max} can be computed directly from the series values (vs. category totals). For the β-particle and homicide residuaals,

$$D_{max} = .0604 \quad \text{and} \quad D_{max} = .0708$$

For a one-tailed hypothesis test, the 95th percentile of D_{max} is

$$D_{.05} = \frac{1.36}{\sqrt{N}}$$

For $N = 249$ and $N = 168$ observations, then, Normality is rejected if

$$D_{max} > \frac{1.36}{\sqrt{249}} \approx .086 \quad \text{and} \quad D_{max} > \frac{1.36}{\sqrt{168}} \approx 0.105$$

Since D_{max} is less than $D_{.05}$ in both cases, however, the Normality assumption holds for both series.

Every analysis should begin with a visual inspection of the plotted time series to search for outliers, to judge whether the series is nonstationary or seasonal in appearance, and to search for other features that might inform the analysis.

Table 3.3. GOODNESS-OF-FIT STATISTICS FOR β-PARTICLES AND SOUTH CAROLINA HOMICIDES

	β-Particles					Homicides			
Y_t	O	E	X^2	D	Y_t	O	E	X^2	D
60	3	2.43	.13	.0023	6	1	.97	.00	.0002
61	4	3.60	.04	.0016	9	2	4.48	1.37	.0148
62	5	5.23	.01	.0009	10	3	6.96	2.25	.0236
63	9	7.43	.33	.0063	11	7	10.46	1.14	.0206
64	11	10.36	.04	.0026	12	16	15.18	.04	.0049
65	15	14.15	.05	.0034	13	23	21.34	.13	.0099
66	19	18.96	.00	.0002	14	38	29.04	2.76	.0533
67	25	24.93	.00	.0003	15	49	38.32	2.98	.0636
68	34	32.17	.10	.0073	16	58	49.06	1.63	.0532
69	45	40.74	.45	.0171	17	70	61.04	1.32	.0533
70	53	50.68	.11	.0093	18	85	73.86	1.68	.0663
71	64	61.93	.07	.0083	19	95	87.07	.72	.0472
72	81	74.40	.59	.0265	20	110	100.17	.96	.0585
73	94	87.89	.42	.0245	21	123	112.65	.95	.0616
74	113	102.16	1.15	.0435	22	136	124.09	1.14	*.0708
75	132	116.94	1.94	*.0605	23	144	134.18	.72	.0584
76	146	131.88	1.51	.0567	24	149	142.73	.28	.0373
77	160	146.66	1.21	.0536	25	154	149.71	.12	.0255
78	176	160.95	1.41	.0604	26	156	155.18	.00	.0049
79	186	174.45	.76	.0464	27	157	159.30	.03	.0092
80	194	186.92	.27	.0284	28	161	162.30	.01	.0077
81	204	198.19	.17	.0233	29	162	164.39	.03	.0142
82	215	208.14	.23	.0276	30	163	165.79	.05	.0166
83	224	216.74	.24	.0292	31	164	166.69	.04	.0160
84	229	223.99	.22	.0201	32	165	167.25	.03	.0133
85	234	229.97	.07	.0162	33	167	167.59	.00	.0035
86	237	234.80	.02	.0088	35	168	167.89	.00	.0006
88	240	241.54	.02	.0062					
89	242	243.75	.02	.0070					
90	245	245.38	.00	.0015					
94	248	248.33	.00	.0013					
100	249	248.97	.00	.0001					

A formal test of the Normality assumption should be conducted prior to each analysis. If a formal test rejects Normality, the time series must be made Normal prior to analysis. The procedures for making a time series Normal range from removing a few outliers—"Winsorizing"—to a transformation. We revisit this topic throughout this chapter and in Chapter 6 when we develop statistical conclusion validity.

3.3 *AR*1 AND *MA*1 TIME SERIES

In our experience, *AR*1 and *MA*1 processes are relatively common. *MA*1 processes are often vestigial artifacts of statistical adjustment or norming. The arithmetic procedures that are used to transform counts into population rates, for example, often create *MA*1 errors. *AR*1 processes are relatively more common, arising from natural processes.

3.3.1 Canadian Inflation

Figure 3.6 shows an annual time series of Canadian inflation rates for 1956 through 2008. $N = 53$ years is a relatively short time series, especially for one as volatile as this one. After a period of relative stability in the late 1950s and early 1960s, the time series level rises abruptly in the early 1970s. The level then dips just as abruptly and climbs steadily to peak in the early 1980s. After pausing in the late 1980s, the series level falls to a low point in the early 1990s, where it remains for more than a decade. Based on a visual inspection, we suspect that this time series will be difficult to model.

Ten lags of the sample *ACF* for $Infltn_t$ are plotted in the left-hand panel of Figure 3.7. Although the values of $r_{k>3}$ are large, they are not statistically significant by a $\pm 2s_r$ criterion. Otherwise, the pattern of decay in the first three lags is consistent with an *AR*1 process. Recall that for an *AR*1 process, we expect

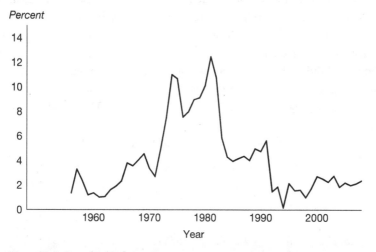

Figure 3.6 Canadian Inflation Rate

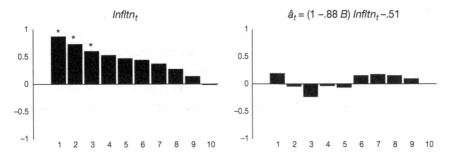

Figure 3.7 Sample ACFs, Canadian Inflation Rate

$r_2 = r_1^2$ and $r_3 = r_1^3$. Given the observed value of $r_1 = 0.87$,

$$r_1^2 = (0.87)^2 = 0.7$$
$$r_1^3 = (0.87)^3 = 0.66$$

Since the values of r_1^2 and r_1^3 are not much different than the observed values of $r_2 = 0.73$ and $r_3 = 0.60$, the sample ACF identifies the AR1 model

$$(1 - \phi_1 B)Infltn_t = \theta_0 + a_t$$

Parameter estimates for this AR1 model are reported as Model 1 in Table 3.4. The value of $\hat{\phi}_1 = 0.8799$ is statistically significant and lies within the AR1 stationarity bounds. The value of $\hat{\theta}_0 = 0.5113$ is not statistically significant, but we will ignore that problem for the moment. With that exception, Model 1 passes our estimation criteria, so we move on to model diagnosis.

The diagnostic test of statistical adequacy has two criteria: Residuals must be both Normal *and* independent. Under the Normality hypothesis, the value of $Z_{KS} = 0.72$ for the residuals of Model 1 occurs with probability $p < 0.67$, so Normality is not rejected.

Ten lags of the ACF for the residuals of Model 1 are plotted in the right-hand panel of Figure 3.7. Under the independence hypothesis, the value of $Q_{10} = 11.4$ for the residuals occurs with probability $p < 0.33$, so independence is

Table 3.4. ESTIMATION AND DIAGNOSIS, *Infltn_t*

		Estimate	SE	t	Diagnosis
Model 1	$\hat{\theta}_0$	.5113	.3296	1.55	$RSE = 1.4207$
	$\hat{\phi}_1$	.8799	.0645	13.64	$Q_{10} = 11.4$
					$Z_{KS} = 0.72$
Model 2	$\hat{\mu}$	4.2580	.6635	2.56	$RSE = 1.4207$
	$\hat{\phi}_1$	.8799	.0645	13.64	$Q_{10} = 11.4$
					$Z_{KS} = 0.72$

not rejected. Since its residuals are not different than white noise, Model 1 is statistically adequate.

We can now return to the problem of the statistically insignificant value of $\hat{\theta}_0$. Rounding to two decimal places, we evaluate Model 1 as

$$(1 - 0.88B)Infltn_t = 0.51 + a_t$$

Solving for $Infltn_t$,

$$Infltn_t = \frac{0.51 + a_t}{1 - 0.88B}$$

Using the infinite series identity for an inverse $AR1$ operator,

$$\frac{1}{1 - 0.88B} \equiv (1 - 0.88B)^{-1} \equiv \sum_{k=0}^{\infty} 0.88^k B^k$$

We can write Model 1 as

$$
\begin{aligned}
Infltn_t &= \sum_{k=0}^{\infty} 0.88^k B^k (0.51 + a_t) \\
&= 0.51 \sum_{k=0}^{\infty} 0.88^k B^k + \sum_{k=0}^{\infty} 0.88^k B^k a_t \\
&= \frac{0.51}{1 - 0.88} + \sum_{k=0}^{\infty} 0.88^k B^k a_t \\
&= 4.25 + \sum_{k=0}^{\infty} 0.88^k B^k a_t
\end{aligned}
$$

The first term on the right-hand-side is the mean of $Infltn_t$. Subtracting this mean from both sides,

$$Infltn_t - 4.25 = \sum_{k=0}^{\infty} 0.88B^k a_t$$

Recognizing the infinite series as an identity of the inverse $AR1$ operator,

$$Infltn_t - 4.25 = \frac{a_t}{1 - 0.88B}$$

Then, solving for a_t

$$(1 - 0.88B)(Infltn_t - 4.25) = a_t$$

The point of this algebraic manipulation is that there are two ways to incorporate a constant in an *AR* model.

The first way was used to specify Model 1:

$$(1 - \phi_1 B)Infltn_t = \theta_0 + a_t$$

The second way is to subtract the mean from the time series:

$$(1 - \phi_1 B)(Infltn_t - \mu) = a_t$$

Parameter estimates for this specification are reported as Model 2 in Table 3.4. The parameter estimates for Model 2 are identical to the estimates for Model 1 with one exception. Whereas $\hat{\theta}_0 = 0.5113$ is *not* statistically significant, $\hat{\mu} = 4.2580$ *is* statistically significant. This apparent contradiction is due to the manner in which the two models are estimated. We address this technical issue in Appendix 3A. But for the practical purpose of interpreting the constant in an *AR* model, readers need to understand that there *are* two ways to specify the constant parameter. When the constant appears in the numerator on the right-hand side of the equation,

$$Y_t = \frac{\theta_0 + a_t}{1 - \phi_1 B}$$

by convention, we denote it as θ_0. But when the constant appears on the left-hand side of the equation,

$$(1 - \phi_1 B)(Y_t - \mu) = a_t$$

we denote it as μ.[2] Since the estimated constants are related by

$$\hat{\mu} \approx \frac{\hat{\theta}_0}{1 - \hat{\phi}_1}$$

even though they have different values, they have the same interpretive implications. The decision to specify the constant as θ_0 or as μ is ordinarily determined by practical considerations such as, in this instance, statistical significance.

Another comment concerns our interpretation of the visual evidence. Some experienced analysts might question our identification of an *AR* model because the plotted time series (Figure 3.6) lacks the "flat" appearance associated with stationary processes. A large exogenous shock and nonstationary "drift" are

---

2. Because not all software packages recognize this convention, it behooves the reader to know whether the estimated constant printed out by a software package is $\hat{\mu}$ or $\hat{\theta}_0$. If $\hat{\mu}$ is subtracted from each Y_t, of course, $\hat{\mu} = \hat{\theta}_0 = 0$.

difficult to distinguish in a short time series. We will revisit this issue when we introduce unit-root statistical tests for homogeneous nonstationarity. Until then, we note that, although visual evidence should never be ignored, it should not be given more weight than any other type of evidence.

3.3.2 U.K. GDP Growth

Figure 3.8 shows an annual time series of growth in the real Gross Domestic Product (GDP) for the United Kingdom, beginning in 1831 and ending in 2010. This is a relatively long time series and, at least compared to the Canadian inflation time series, relatively well behaved. Other than the years of the two world wars, the time series fluctuates around its mean level. The "flat" appearance of this time series is typical of what we expect from a stationary process. The visual evidence suggests that there will be no need for differencing or transforming this time series. As always, of course, our decision will be informed by the sample ACFs.

The construction of this time series provides an insight into the underlying process. Because annual change in GDP is defined as:

$$UKGDP_t = \frac{\text{GDP in year } t - \text{ GDP in year } t - 1}{\text{GDP in year } t - 1}$$

the value of $UKGDP_t$ depends on the value of $UKGDP_{t-1}$. As a definitional consequence, the effect of a large exogenous shock persists for exactly one year, thereby generating an $MA1$ disturbance. In our experience, MA processes are rare

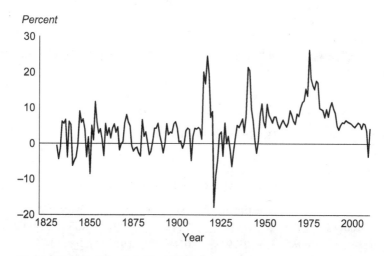

Figure 3.8 U.K. Growth in Real GDP

in social science time series. The exceptions ordinarily involve, as in this instance, a generating mechanism that uses the preceding time series observation to adjust or correct the current observation.

The first 10 lags of the sample ACF for $UKGDP_t$, plotted in the left-hand panel of Figure 3.9, confirm our speculation about MA processes. The value of $r_1 = 0.23$ is significant; the values of $r_{k>1}$ are smaller and insignificant. This sample ACF identifies the $MA1$ model:

$$UKGDP_t = \theta_0 + (1 - \theta_1 B)a_t$$

Parameter estimates for this model are reported as Model 1 in Table 3.5. All of the estimates are statistically significant and the value of $\hat{\theta}_1 = -.2179$ lies inside the $MA1$ invertibility bounds. The model residuals satisfy both diagnostic criteria. Under the Normality hypothesis, a value of $Z_{KS} = 1.03$ occurs with probability $p < 0.24$. A sample ACF for the residuals of Model 1 is plotted in the right-hand panel of Figure 3.9. Under the independence hypothesis, the value of $Q_{10} = 14.5$ for this sample ACF occurs with probability $p < 0.15$. These residuals are not different than white noise.

It will be instructive to compare our analysis of $UKGDP_t$ to our analysis of the Canadian inflation time series. First, unlike the $AR1$ model that we fit to $Infltn_t$, there is only one way to incorporate a constant into this $MA1$ model. Whether the constant appears on the left-hand side or right-hand side of the equation, it is

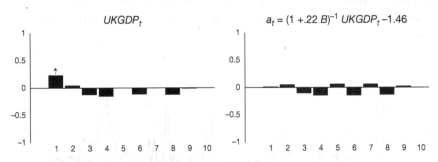

Figure 3.9 Sample ACFs, U.K. Growth in Real GDP

Table 3.5. ESTIMATION AND DIAGNOSIS, $UKGDP_t$

		Estimate	SE	t	Diagnosis
Model 1	$\hat{\theta}_0$	1.4644	.2446	5.99	$RSE = 2.7451$
	$\hat{\theta}_1$	−.2179	.0749	2.91	$Q_{10} = 14.5$
					$Z_{KS} = 1.03$

interpreted as the mean of $UKGDP_t$. Second, although in this instance the plotted time series (Figure 3.8) has the "flat" appearance that we associate with stationary processes, the visual evidence of shorter segments—say, 1910 to 1950—would be ambiguous on this point.

Finally, we have not yet commented on the Residual Standard Errors (*RSEs*) reported in the far-right columns of Tables 3.4 and 3.5. These statistics should be reported for any estimated model. In principle, *RSEs* can be standardized as R^2 statistics. *ARIMA* model R^2 statistics are often quite large, however, near unity, and do not necessarily have straightforward "variance explained" interpretations. We do not recommend reporting R^2 statistics and urge extreme caution in their use and interpretion. On the other hand, *RSE* statistics play invaluable roles in *ARIMA* modeling. We discuss the role of *RSEs* in parameter estimation model selection later in this chapter. Other important roles of *RSEs* will be developed in great detail in Chapters 6 and 7.

3.3.3 Pediatric Trauma Admissions

Figure 3.10 shows a weekly time series of pediatric patients with assault-related injuries at the Children's Hospital of Philadelphia, a level-one trauma center.[3] The weekly time series has a volatile appearance but seems stationary.

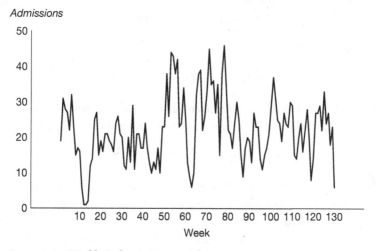

Figure 3.10 Weekly Pediatric Trauma Admissions

3. This time series was given to us by colleague Joel Fein, MD, MPH, of the Violence Intervention Project at the Children's Hospital of Philadelphia.

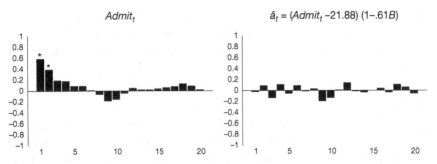

Figure 3.11 Sample *ACF*, Weekly Pediatric Trauma Admissions

Table 3.6. ESTIMATION AND DIAGNOSIS, *Admit$_t$*

		Estimate	SE	t	Diagnosis
Model 1	$\hat{\mu}$	21.8761	1.6678	13.12	$RSE = 7.4632$
	$\hat{\phi}_1$	.6059	.0713	8.50	$Q_{20} = 20.1$
					$Z_{KS} = 0.72$
Model 2	$\hat{\mu}$	21.8081	1.2860	16.96	$RSE = 7.4273$
	$\hat{\theta}_1$	−.5967	.0822	−7.26	$Q_{20} = 17.4$
	$\hat{\theta}_2$	−.3648	.0823	−4.43	$Z_{KS} = 0.77$

Twenty lags of the sample *ACF* for *Admit$_t$* are plotted in Figure 3.11. The large, statistically significant values of r_1 and r_2 identify either an *AR*1 model,

$$(1 - \phi_1 B)(Admit_t - \mu) = a_t$$

or possibly an *MA*2 model

$$(Admit_t - \mu) = (1 - \theta_1 B - \theta_2 B^2)a_t$$

*AR*1 models are ordinarily preferred on grounds of parsimony. In this instance, moreover, the sample *ACF* exhibits the typical *AR*1 pattern of decay:

$$r_1^2 = (0.59)^2 = 0.3481 \approx r_2 = 0.39$$

To demonstrate a practical point, however, we will consider both models.

Parameter estimates for the *AR*1 model are reported as Model 1 in Table 3.6. Both parameter estimates are statistically significant and the value of $\hat{\phi}_1 = 0.6059$ lies inside the *AR*1 stationarity bounds. The values of $Z_{KS} = 0.72$ and $Q_{20} = 20.1$ for the model residuals are too small to reject a white noise hypothesis, so Model 1 is statistically adequate. But is it the "best" model?

Parameter estimates for the *MA*2 model are reported as Model 2 in Table 3.6. All three parameter estimates are statistically significant and the values of

$\hat{\theta}_1 = -.5967$ and $\hat{\theta}_2 = -.3648$ lie inside the *MA2* invertibility bounds. The values of $Z_{KS} = 0.77$ and $Q_{20} = 17.4$ for the model residuals are too small to reject the white noise hypothesis, so Model 2 is statistically adequate.

With a smaller *RSE* statistic—7.4273 vs. 7.4632—Model 2 is the better-fitting model. But since it has one more parameter than Model 1, we expect it to fit better. Is the slight reduction in *RSE* worth the cost of an additional parameter? We address this question in detail at a later point. So as not to keep the reader in suspense, Model 1 is the "best" model for this time series.

3.4 HIGHER-ORDER *ARMA* PROCESSES

Short time series—say, $N < 100$ observations—are often adequately fit by *AR1* or *MA1* models. Our analysis of the annual Canadian inflation time series, $Infltn_t$, was typical in that respect. Due in part to the problem of the demands of statistical significance, higher-order *ARMA* models are unusual for time series as short as this one. Our analysis of the annual U.K. GDP time series, $UKGDP_t$, was atypical in the same respect. Stationary *ARMA* models are seldom statistically adequate for time series of $N = 180$ observations. On the contrary, long time series—say, $N > 200$ observations—are almost always *non*stationary in mean or variance. After differencing and/or a variance-stabilizing transformation, moreover, these longer time series often require higher-order *ARMA* or *ARIMA* models. This fact complicates model identification and diagnosis and requires new procedures, statistics, and tests. Our introduction to these complications begins with long time series that are stationary in mean.

3.4.1 Beveridge's Wheat Price Time Series

Figure 3.12 shows an annual time series of inflation-adjusted European wheat prices from 1500 to 1869 compiled by Sir William Beveridge (1922). This time series is longer than most of the time series that readers will encounter. Long time series often pose special problems, and this one is not unusual in that respect. A visual inspection of the time series suggests that it is stationary in mean. Due only to inflation, economic time series often have strong secular trends. Although Beveridge's inflation adjustment appears to have detrended this time series, making it stationary in mean, the series variance is uneven. Five or six years of relatively small price changes are punctuated by large spikes.

With more than a dozen large outliers in $N = 370$ years, we would be surprised if this time series satisfied the Normality assumption. A histogram of the time series, shown in Figure 3.13, reinforces our suspicion. The time series is skewed

**Inflation-adjusted
Price in Pounds**

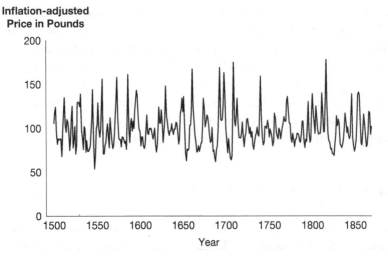

Figure 3.12 Beveridge's Wheat Price Time Series

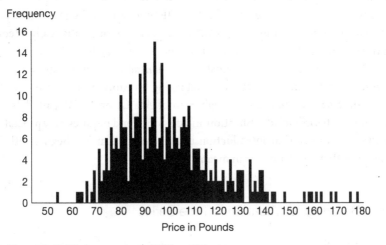

Figure 3.13 Histogram, Annual Wheat Prices

to the right. A *KS* test $(Z_{KS} = 1.63)$ rejects Normality. If the time series must be transformed prior to analysis, we must decide which transformation to use. In the context of a time series analysis, such questions are addressed by the Box-Cox (1964) transformation function. For the time series $Wheat_t$, the Box-Cox function is

$$Wheat_t^{(\lambda)} = \frac{Wheat_t^{\lambda} - 1}{\lambda} \quad \text{for} \quad \lambda \neq 0; \qquad = Ln(Wheat_t) \quad \text{for} \quad \lambda = 0$$

For the limited purpose of transforming $Wheat_t$ to stabilize its variance, the reader will need to know how to *evaluate* the Box-Cox function for $Wheat_t$ and then how to *apply* the results of the evaluation to the transformation task. Beyond this limited purpose, the technical details of the Box-Cox transformation function and its proper application are found in Appendix 3B.

To evaluate the Box-Cox function for a time series, $Wheat_t$ in this instance, we make sure that all of the observations are positive. The plotted time series (Figure 3.12) and histogram (Figure 3.13) show that $Wheat_t > 0$ for all $N = 370$ years. We next divide the time series observations by the geometric mean of the time series. In this instance,

$$\mu_{geometric}(Wheat_t) = \left(\prod_{t=1}^{N=370} Wheat_t \right)^{\frac{1}{370}} \approx 97.43$$

so

$$wheat_t = \frac{Wheat_t}{97.43}; \qquad Wheat_t = 97.43 \times wheat_t$$

Finally, we plot the variance of $wheat_t^{(\lambda)}$ for a range of λ-values. Figure 3.14 plots the variance of $wheat_t^{(\lambda)}$ for $-3.5 < \lambda < 2.5$. The minimum variance in this range of λ-values occurs when $\lambda \approx -0.57$, so we take that value as the "best" Box-Cox transformation.

Readers who did not follow our abridged description of how the variance function in Figure 3.14 was constructed should not be discouraged. A more detailed description of these procedures is found in Appendix 3B. With that material and a little practice, any reader can generate the variance function of a time series. Since most time series software packages generate these functions

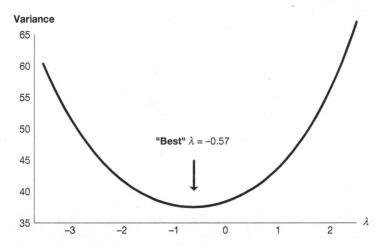

Figure 3.14 Variance for $-3.5 < \lambda < +2.5$

automatically, few readers would want to expend the effort to acquire this skill. The effort is better spent learning how to interpret and use the variance function.

Since the "best" Box-Cox transformation of $Wheat_t$ occurs when $\lambda = -0.57$, it might make sense to model $wheat_t^{(\lambda=-0.57)}$. Although $wheat_t^{(\lambda=-0.57)}$ has ideal statistical properties, however, this might be lost on skeptical journal referees. Few social scientists—and even fewer referees—understand the principles of variance-stabilizing transformations, much less Box-Cox transformation functions. Fortunately, we can almost always find a transformation whose statistical properties are *nearly* ideal but whose structure is better understood and more easily explained.

The first simplification is to transform $Wheat_t$ instead of $wheat_t$. We divided $Wheat_t$ by its geometric mean in order to generate the variance function plotted in Figure 3.14. But since division by a constant does not affect the inflection points of the variance function, $wheat_t^{(\lambda)}$ and $Wheat_t^{(\lambda)}$ have the same variance-stabilizing properties. The second simplification involves finding a λ-value that is not statistically different than the "best" value but that has a more meaningful interpretation. Although it is not the "best" transformation, $Wheat_t^{(\lambda=-0.5)}$ is a "very, very good" transformation, not significantly different than the "best" transformation.

Combining these two simplifications, then, on practical and aesthetic grounds, we choose the reciprocal square-root transformation to stabilize the variance of our time series. The transformed time series, $Wheat_t^{-0.5}$ or $Wheat_t^{-1/2}$, is plotted in Figure 3.15. The transformed time series has no extreme outliers and has a

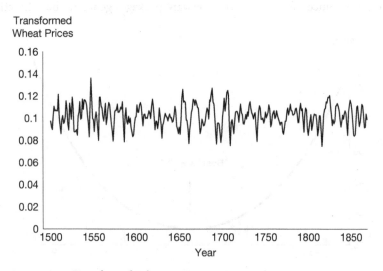

Figure 3.15 Transformed Wheat Price Time Series

Table 3.7. IDENTIFICATION, $Wheat_t^{-1/2}$

k	$Wheat_t^{-1/2}$				$\hat{a}_t$	
	r_k	Q_k	r_{kk}	s_r	r_k	Q_k
1	.61	138.	.61	.05	.02	0.2
2	.15	146.	−.35	.05	−.06	1.7
3	−.05	147.	.07	.05	.06	3.0
4	−.10	151.	−.07	.05	−.01	3.1
5	−.11	155.	−.03	.05	−.01	3.1
6	−.15	164.	−.14	.05	−.07	5.2
7	−.22	183.	−.11	.05	−.07	6.8
8	−.27	210.	−.13	.05	−.18	18.6
9	−.19	224.	.03	.05	−.10	22.2
10	−.07	226.	−.04	.05	−.00	22.2
11	−.02	227.	−.05	.05	.01	22.2
12	−.03	227.	−.07	.05	−.03	22.7
13	−.01	227.	.01	.05	−.04	23.2
14	.06	228.	.03	.05	.05	24.0
15	.12	234.	.02	.05	.03	24.2
16	.16	244.	.05	.05	.10	27.8
17	.12	250.	−.04	.05	.07	29.8
18	.02	250.	−.04	.05	.00	29.8
19	−.05	251.	−.03	.05	−.05	30.6
20	−.04	252.	.02	.05	−.04	31.4

smoother, more homogeneous appearance. The value of $Z_{KS} = 0.59$ for this distribution is too small to reject Normality

Satisfied with this transformation, we proceed to identify an *ARIMA* model for $Wheat_t^{-1/2}$. Table 3.7 reports the first 20 lags of the sample *ACF* for $Wheat_t^{-1/2}$ along with the corresponding Q-statistics. We have already used the Q-statistic to test the independence hypothesis for a set of model residuals. Under the null hypothesis

$$H_0: r_1 = \cdots = r_k = 0$$

Q_k is distributed as χ^2 with k degrees of freedom. Q-statistics can also be used to test the significance of a single r_k. Under the null hypothesis

$$H_0: r_k = 0$$

the difference of Q_k and Q_{k-1} is distributed as χ^2 with one degree of freedom. Compared to the ratio of r_k to its standard error, the Q-statistic provides a more powerful test of significance. Q-statistics are more difficult to display graphically, however, and must be reported in a table.

At the conventional 95 percent confidence level, the sample ACF for $Wheat_t^{-1/2}$ has a large, significant spike at r_1 and smaller significant spikes at r_6, r_7, r_8, and r_9. Though statistically significant, the values of r_6, r_7, r_8, and r_9 are small enough to be ignored at this early stage. For a time series as long as $Wheat_t^{-1/2}$, relatively small but significant r_k are a nuisance. Analysts are advised to view the sample ACF critically in the initial stages. Ignoring the r_6, r_7, r_8, and r_9, this sample ACF might identify a simple $MA1$ model:

$$Wheat_t^{-1/2} = \theta_0 + (1 - \theta_1 B)a_t$$

But since values of $r_1 > 0.5$ imply non-invertible values of θ_1, the sample ACF argues against this identification. Ruling out an $MA1$ model, a mixed $ARMA$ model or, perhaps, a simple AR model is possible. An $AR1$ model seems unlikely, given the sample ACF. An $AR1$ ACF is expected to decay exponentially. For $r_1 = 0.61$, that is, we expect

$$r_2 = .61^2 \approx .37$$
$$r_3 = .61^3 \approx .23$$

But the values of r_2 and r_3 are much smaller than what we would expect of an $AR1$ process. If $Wheat_t^{-1/2}$ is driven by an AR process, it is likely to be a higher-order process, perhaps $AR2$ or even $AR3$.

There are several ways to identify the order of an ARp process. Some analysts claim to be able to divine the likely order of the process from its sample ACF. Other analysts fit successively higher ARp models to the time series, stopping when the residuals of a model are not different than white noise. While these methods often "work" to some extent, neither is recommended. The first method involves guesswork and is at least inefficient. The second method often leads to a non-parsimonious, over-fitted ARp model.

The most reliable and efficient method of identifying the order of an ARp process relies on the sample Partial AutoCorrelation Function ($PACF$). The sample $PACF$ for $Wheat_t^{-1/2}$ is reported in the middle columns of Table 3.7 along with its standard error. As its name suggests, the lag-k $PACF$, denoted r_{kk}, is the correlation of Y_t and Y_{t-k} with the effects of all intermediate-lag correlations "partialled" out.

The $PACF$ is estimated from an equation system due to Yule (1927) and Walker (1931). The Yule-Walker equations equate the value of r_k with the sum of the lagged values of the ACF weighted by the ARp parameters:

$$r_1 = \phi_1 r_0 + \phi_2 r_1 + \cdots + \phi_{p-1} r_{p-2} + \phi_p r_{p-1}$$
$$r_2 = \phi_1 r_1 + \phi_2 r_2 + \cdots + \phi_{p-1} r_{p-3} + \phi_p r_{p-2}$$
$$\cdots$$
$$r_p = \phi_1 r_{p-1} + \phi_2 r_{p-2} + \cdots + \phi_{p-1} r_1 + \phi_p r_0$$

Box and Jenkins (1970, pp. 65-66) use an iterative algorithm to solve the Yule-Walker equations for the first three lags of the sample PACF:

$$r_{11} = r_1$$
$$r_{22} = \frac{r_2 - r_1^2}{1 - r_1^2}$$
$$r_{33} = \frac{r_3 + r_1 r_2^2 + r_1^3 - 2r_1 r_2 - r_1^2 r_3}{1 + 2r_1^2 r_2 - 2r_2^2 - r_1^2}$$

Comparing these solutions to the analogous Pearson partial correlation coefficients reinforces the idea that the PACF is a measure of partial *auto*correlation.

The PACF of an ARp process has a "spike" for each significant ϕ_p parameter. By that rule, the sample PACF reported in Table 3.7 identifies an AR2 process:

$$(1 - \phi_1 B - \phi_2 B^2) Wheat_t^{-1/2} = \theta_0 + a_t$$

This identification follows from the large values of r_{11} and r_{22}. Asymptotic standard errors of r_{kk} are given by

$$s_r = \frac{1}{\sqrt{N}}$$

By the $\pm 2s_r$ criterion, r_{11} and r_{22} are statistically significant, identifying strong first- and second-order AR components. The values of $r_{66}, r_{77},$ and r_{88} are also statistically significant, of course, but we choose to ignore $r_{66}, r_{77},$ and r_{88} at this early stage. This AR2 identification is not ideal but it is the most plausible model for now. So we accept it and hope that subsequent evidence will better inform the identification.

Parameter estimates for the AR2 model are reported as Model 1 in Table 3.8. The values of $\hat{\phi}_1 = .8193$ and $\hat{\phi}_2 = -.3490$ are stationary and statistically significant. Although the value of $Z_{KS} = 0.91$ is too small to reject Normality for the Model 1 residuals, the Q-statistic is larger than what we would like to see. Under the independence hypothesis, the value of $Q_{20} = 31.4$ occurs with probability $p <$ 0.049, so we reject the white noise hypothesis for these residuals—though just barely.

Table 3.8. ESTIMATION AND DIAGNOSIS, $Wheat_t^{-1/2}$

		Estimate	SE	t	Diagnosis
Model 1	$\hat{\theta}_0$	.1018	.0007	142.13	$RSE = .0073$
	$\hat{\phi}_1$	.8193	.0488	16.79	$Q_{20} = 31.4$
	$\hat{\phi}_2$	−.3490	.0488	−7.15	$Z_{KS} = 0.91$
Model 2	$\hat{\theta}_0$	.1018	.0006	177.48	$RSE = .0072$
	$\hat{\phi}_1$	.8015	.0489	16.40	$Q_{20} = 19.7$
	$\hat{\phi}_2$	−.3513	.0488	−7.19	$Z_{KS} = 0.67$
	$\hat{\theta}_8$	.1584	.0518	3.06	

To identify a better model, we consult the sample *ACF* for the Model 1 residuals. The sample *ACF* for $\hat{a}_t$, reported in Table 3.7, shows that the *AR2* parameters fit the low-order lags adequately but leave a small, statistically significant value of r_8. This isolated spike can be fit by an *MA8* component:

$$(1 - \phi_1 B - \phi_2 B^2)Wheat_t^{-0.5} = \theta_0 + (1 - \theta_8 B^8)a_t$$

Parameter estimates for this model are reported as Model 2 in Table 3.8. Estimates of $\hat{\theta}_8$=.1584, $\hat{\phi}_1$=.8015, and $\hat{\phi}_2$=−.3513 are invertible-stationary and statistically significant. The values of Q_{20}=19.7 and Z_{KS}=0.67 for the Model 2 residuals are too small to reject a white noise hypothesis, so Model 2 is a statistically adequate representation of the generating process or, in plain words, Model 2 fits $Wheat_t^{-0.5}$.

We leave three questions unanswered. First, what can our analysis of $Wheat_t^{-0.5}$ tell us about $Wheat_t$? Second, although Model 2 is the "better" of the two models, is it that much better than Model 1? Third, what is the substantive meaning of the isolated spike at r_8 of the residual *ACF*? We postpone our discussion about interpreting transformed effects and models until Chapter 5. Likewise, we postpone our discussion of model selection until a later point in this chapter. That leaves the unexplained spike at r_8 of the residual *ACF*. The answer is that this spike has no substantive meaning. We have always suspected that it is an artifact of the "smoothing" algorithm employed by Sir William Beveridge to deflate this time series. But that amounts to speculation. Regardless of its origin, in this instance, the spike at lag-8 of the residual *ACF* had to be modeled.

In closing our analysis of $Wheat_t$, we return to the the Box-Cox transformation function. We discuss the consequences of *not* transforming a time series that is nonstationary in variance in Chapter 6 as a threat to statistical conclusion validity. *The consequences are dire.* Because transformations involve dense mathematics, however, and because the threats to statistical conclusion validity are not well known or understood, variance-stabilizing transformations are not widely used in time series experiments. We hope to change this dismal state of affairs. Table 3.9

Table 3.9. The Box-Cox Transformation Function

$\lambda > 1$	$Y_t^{(\lambda)} \propto Y_t^{\lambda}$	**Power**
$\lambda = 1$	$Y_t^{(\lambda)} \propto Y_t$	**No transformation**
$0 < \lambda < 1$	$Y_t^{(\lambda)} \propto \sqrt[\lambda]{Y_t}$	**Root**
$\lambda = 0$	$Y_t^{(\lambda)} = Ln\,(Y_t)$	**Natural log**
$0 > \lambda > -1$	$Y_t^{(\lambda)} \propto \dfrac{1}{\sqrt[\lambda]{Y_t}}$	**Reciprocal root**
$\lambda = -1$	$Y_t^{(\lambda)} \propto \dfrac{1}{Y_t}$	**Reciprocal**
$\lambda < -1$	$Y_t^{(\lambda)} \propto \dfrac{1}{Y_t^{\lambda}}$	**Reciprocal power**

lists the λ-values corresponding to the power, root, logarithm, reciprocal root, and reciprocal power transformations. The "best" of these variance-stabilizing transformations is the one nearest the λ-value that minimizes the variance function of a time series.

3.4.2 Zurich Sunspot Numbers

Figure 3.16 plots another long annual time series, the Zurich relative sunspot numbers (Yule, 1921). This long annual time series presents many of the same practical problems encountered in our analysis of Beveridge's wheat price time series. Like the wheat price time series, this sunspot time series must be transformed prior to analysis. The need for transformation is more obvious in this instance. For more than three decades, beginning in the 1890s, year-to-year fluctuations in the time series are smaller than the years before or after. The appropriate transformation will yield a smoother, more homogeneous time series.

Figure 3.17 plots the variance function for $sunspot_t^{(\lambda)}$ where $sunspot_t$ is defined as

$$sunspot_t = \frac{Sunspot_t + 0.1}{29.13}, \mu_{geometric}(Sunspot_t + 0.1) = 29.13$$

for $-2 < \lambda < 4$. Because $Sunspot_t = 0$, we added the constant 0.1 to each observation. It is instructive to compare this variance function to the function for Beveridge's wheat time series (Figure 3.14). Whereas that function has an aesthetically satisfying parabolic shape with a noticeable inflection point at the "best" value of λ, this function runs parallel to the horizontal axis between the values of $\lambda = -1$ and $\lambda = 2$. Although the function turns at the "best" value

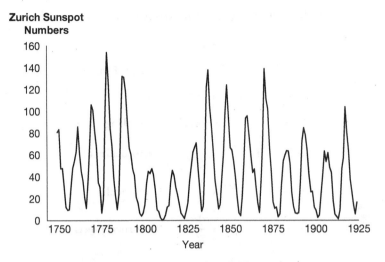

Figure 3.16 Annual Zurich Sunspot Numbers (Yule, 1921)

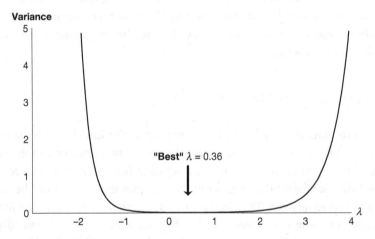

Figure 3.17 Variance, $-2 < \lambda < +4$

of $\lambda = .36$, detecting the minimum by crude "eyeballing" taxes the imagination. Given the flat shape of this function, instead of using the "best" value of $\lambda = .36$, we will use the more practical value of $\lambda = .5$, which corresponds to the square-root transformation.

The transformed time series, $Sunspot_t^{1/2}$, is plotted in Figure 3.18. Although the 1790-to-1820 period has a noticeably lower mean level, the variance of the time series is now homogeneous. The transformation seems to have accomplished its goal.

The sample *ACF* and *PACF* for $Sunspot_t^{1/2}$ are reported in Table 3.10. The *PACF* is again used to identify the order of an *ARp* process. Exponential decay in the first

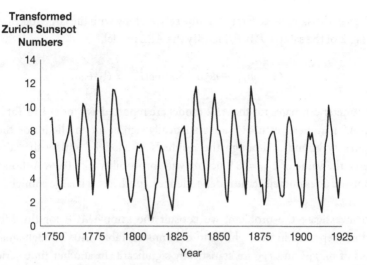

Figure 3.18 Transformed Annual Zurich Sunspot Numbers

Table 3.10. IDENTIFICATION, $Sunspot_t^{1/2}$

	$Sunspot_t^{-1/2}$				$\hat{a}_t$	
k	r_k	Q_k	r_{kk}	s_r	r_k	Q_k
1	.82	120.	.82	.08	.01	0.0
2	.45	157.	−.65	.08	−.04	0.1
3	.06	158.	−.11	.08	.05	0.3
4	−.25	169.	−.02	.08	.11	1.2
5	−.41	200.	−.05	.08	.07	1.5
6	−.41	230.	.12	.08	−.13	2.5
7	−.24	241.	.16	.08	.02	2.6
8	.03	241.	.14	.08	.01	2.6
9	.30	258.	.17	.08	.29	8.8
10	.50	306.	.05	.08	.09	9.4
11	.56	366.	.06	.08	−.04	9.6
12	.47	409.	.01	.08	−.01	9.6
13	.27	423.	−.02	.08	.05	9.8
14	.04	423.	.11	.08	−.03	9.9
15	−.15	427.	.01	.08	.05	10.1
16	−.27	441.	−.15	.08	−.04	10.3
17	−.30	459.	−.05	.08	.02	10.3
18	−.27	473.	−.17	.08	−.11	11.4
19	−.16	478.	−.02	.08	.02	11.4
20	−.02	478.	−.03	.08	−.01	11.5

few lags of the sample ACF for this time series, along with the large spikes at lag-1 and lag-2 of the sample PACF, identify the AR2 model,

$$(1 - \phi_1 B - \phi_2 B^2) Sunspot_t^{1/2} = \theta_0 + a_t$$

Parameter estimates for the AR2 model are reported as Model 1 in Table 3.11. Both AR parameter estimates are statistically significant and lie inside the AR2 stationarity bounds. Although the residuals of Model 1 satisfy the adequacy criteria, the value of $Q_{20}=28.9$ occurs with probability $p > 0.09$. Although this Q-statistic does not reject the independence hypothesis, it is large enough to raise concerns.

To investigate the problem, we consult the sample ACF for the Model 1 residuals reported in the right-hand columns of Table 3.10. Though small, the values of r_9, r_{11}, and r_{12} are statistically significant. In another time series, we might ignore these small autocorrelations. Because sunspot activity waxes and wanes in a cycle of approximately 11 years (Izenman, 1983), however, these autocorrelations are expected. We add MA9, MA11, and MA12 parameters to accommodate the significant values of r_9, r_{11}, and r_{12}.

$$(1 - \phi_1 B - \phi_2 B^2) Sunspot_t^{1/2} = \theta_0 + \left(1 - \theta_9 B^9 - \theta_{10} B^{10} - \theta_{11} B^{11}\right) a_t$$
$$Sunspot_t^{1/2} = \frac{\theta_0 + \left(1 - \theta_9 B^9 - \theta_{10} B^{10} - \theta_{11} B^{11}\right) a_t}{(1 - \phi_1 B - \phi_2 B^2)}$$

Parameter estimates for Model 2, reported in Table 3.11, are statistically significant and stationary-invertible. The values of $Q_{20}=16.2$ and $Z_{KS}=0.59$ for the Model 2 residuals are too small to reject the white noise null hypothesis. Model 2 is statistically adequate.

Table 3.11. ESTIMATION AND DIAGNOSIS, $Sunspot_t^{1/2}$

		Estimate	SE	t	Diagnosis
Model 1	$\hat{\theta}_0$	6.0982	.2936	20.77	RSE = 1.1606
	$\hat{\phi}_1$	1.3632	.0569	23.95	Q_{20} = 28.9
	$\hat{\phi}_2$	−.6630	.0571	−11.62	Z_{KS} = 0.88
Model 2	$\hat{\theta}_0$	6.0240	.4103	14.68	RSE = 1.0922
	$\hat{\phi}_1$	1.2705	.0622	20.43	Q_{20} = 16.2
	$\hat{\phi}_2$	−.5872	.0619	−9.49	Z_{KS} = 0.59
	$\hat{\theta}_9$	−.2810	.0745	−3.77	
	$\hat{\theta}_{11}$	−.1696	.0758	−2.24	
	$\hat{\theta}_{12}$	−.2032	.0753	−2.70	

3.5 INTEGRATED MODELS

The salient contributions of Box and Jenkins (1970) included unifying the existing *AR* and *MA* models into a larger *ARMA* model and devising a practical, reliable modeling strategy (Figure 3.1) for fitting *ARMA* models to stationary time series. To extend their modeling strategy to nonstationary time series, Box and Jenkin proposed difference equations:

> Many empirical time series (for example, stock prices) behave as if they had no fixed mean. Even so, they exhibit homogeneity in the sense that, apart from local level, or perhaps local level and trend, one part of the series behaves much like any other part. Models which describe such homogeneous nonstationary behavior can be obtained by supposing some suitable difference of the process to be stationary. (Box and Jenkins, 1970, p. 85)

Since many if not most social science time series are nonstationary in the homogeneous sense, the routine use of difference equations is the most important contribution of Box and Jenkins. From a practical modeling perspective, then, an *ARIMA* model is nothing more than an *ARMA* model that adequately fits a differenced time series. Finding no reasonable *ARMA* model that fits the time series, we difference the time series and try again.

3.5.1 Kroeber's Skirt-Width Time Series

Difference-and-try-again works well in simple, obvious cases such as Kroeber's skirt-width time series, which we introduced in Chapter 1. The time series, $Skirt_t$, and its first-difference, $\nabla Skirt_t$, are plotted in Figure 3.19. Kroeber's (1969; Richardson and Kroeber, 1940) theory of "cultural unsettlement" held that fashions changed only gradually during periods of peace and prosperity but then changed rapidly during periods of war and depression. Kroeber interpreted the 1860 peak in $Skirt_t$ as corroboration for his theory. When the time series is differenced, however, the 1860s are unremarkable. Although fluctuations in $\nabla Skirt_t$ coinciding roughly with the Napoleonic wars (1802–1803) and World War I (1918) seem to corroborate Kroeber's theory, correlational time series designs are difficult to interpret. Differencing serves another purpose, of course. Whereas $Skirt_t$ drifts aimlessly, $\nabla Skirt_t$ fluctuates about a well-defined, visually apparent mean. It is *stationary* in mean.

Though $\nabla Skirt_t$ appears to be stationary in mean, however, it does not appear to be stationary in variance. The extreme "outliers" in 1802–1803 and 1918 suggest that $\nabla Skirt_t$ may not be Normal. In a time series as long as this one, appearances can be deceiving. Preliminary statistical analyses, not reported here, do not reject the Normality assumption. $\nabla Skirt_t$ can be modeled as a stationary process.

Skirt Widths

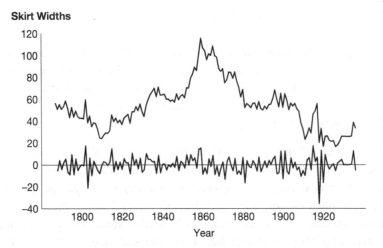

Figure 3.19 Kroeber's Skirt-Width Time Series and its First Difference

Table 3.12. IDENTIFICATION, $Skirt_t$

	$Skirt_t$		$\nabla Skirt_t$				$\hat{a}_t$	
k	r_k	Q_k	r_k	Q_k	r_{kk}	s_r	r_k	Q_k
1	.94	134.	−.38	21.6	−.38	.08	.01	0.0
2	.92	265.	.23	29.9	.11	.08	−.04	0.1
3	.87	383.	−.13	32.4	−.01	.08	.05	0.3
4	.84	494.	.03	32.6	−.04	.08	.11	1.2
5	.80	595.	−.05	33.0	−.04	.08	.07	1.5
6	.77	689.	.05	33.3	.03	.	−.13	2.5
7	.74	776.	.03	33.5	.08	.08	.02	2.6
8	.69	853.	−.06	34.0	−.05	.08	.01	2.6
9	.66	923.	.09	35.3	.05	.08	.29	8.8
10	.61	985.	−.08	36.4	−.01	.08	.09	9.4
11	.57	1039.	.14	39.7	.11	.08	−.04	9.6
12	.52	1084.	−.17	44.1	−.08	.08	−.01	9.6
13	.49	1123.	.11	46.1	−.01	.08	.05	9.8
14	.44	1156.	−.09	47.4	−.00	.08	−.03	9.9
15	.41	1184.	.04	47.6	−.01	.08	.05	10.1
16	.37	1206.	−.02	47.7	−.00	.08	−.04	10.3
17	.33	1225.	−.11	49.8	−.16	.08	.02	10.3
18	.30	1241.	.08	50.8	−.00	.08	−.11	11.4
19	.27	1253.	−.09	52.1	−.01	.08	.02	11.4
20	.26	1265.	.11	54.0	.04	.08	−.01	11.5

Sample *ACFs* and *PACFs* for $Skirt_t$ are reported in Table 3.12. The sample *ACF* confirms the obvious: $Skirt_t$ must be differenced. If this identification is unclear, note that the value of $r_1=.94$ lies well outside the invertibility bounds of any legal MA model. Low-order AR models are ruled out by the absence of lag-to-lag decay. The values of r_1 through r_{11} are all large and statistically significant. With low-order $ARMA$ models ruled out, by a strict process of elimination, the sample ACF identifies an integrated model. This process of elimination is typical of model identification. Even when a sample ACF does not point to a particular model, the sample ACF rules out a set of models. This particular sample ACF has all of the characteristics of a nonstationary process: The value of r_1 is greater than, say, 0.8; the ACF decays slowly from lag to lag; and $r_k > 0$ for large k. This sample ACF screams: Difference this series.

The sample ACF for $\nabla Skirt_t$ identifies either of two models: an $AR1$ model,

$$(1 - \phi_1 B)\nabla Skirt_t = \theta_0 + a_t$$
$$Skirt_t = \frac{\theta_0 + a_t}{(1 - \phi_1 B)\nabla}$$

or an $MA2$ model:

$$\nabla Skirt_t = \theta_0 + (1 - \theta_1 B - \theta_2 B^2)a_t$$
$$Skirt_t = \frac{\theta_0 + (1 - \theta_1 B - \theta_2 B^2)a_t}{\nabla}$$

These identifications follow from the large, statistically significant values of $r_1 = -.38$ and $r_2 = +.23$ and from the small, insignificant values of $r_k \geq 3$. It is difficult at this early stage to choose between the two models. On the one hand, the sample ACF seems to decay exponentially with alternating signs, suggesting an $AR1$ process with $\phi_1 < 0$. On the other hand, what appears to be exponential decay might be two discrete spikes, suggesting an $MA2$ process. We consider both models.

Parameter estimates for the two tentative models are reported in Table.3.13. The estimate of θ_0 is not statistically significant in either model and can be dropped. Estimates of ϕ_1, θ_1, and θ_2 are statistically significant and lie within the bounds of stationarity-invertibility. Both models are acceptable at this stage.

Table 3.13. ESTIMATION AND DIAGNOSIS, $Skirt_t$

		Estimate	SE	t	Diagnosis
Model 1	$\hat{\theta}_0$	−.1175	.4123	−0.28	$RSE = 6.8886$
	$\hat{\phi}_1$	−.3780	.0761	−4.97	$Q_{20} = 13.6$
					$Z_{KS} = 0.64$
Model 2	$\hat{\theta}_0$	−.1294	.4835	−0.27	$RSE = 6.8837$
	$\hat{\theta}_1$	.3145	.0806	3.90	$Q_{20} = 15.2$
	$\hat{\theta}_2$	−.1862	.0816	−2.28	$Z_{KS} = 0.55$

Values of Q_{20} are too small to reject white noise hypotheses for either model. Both models are statistically adequate. The $AR1$ model is the "better" on the criterion of parsimony but, otherwise, the two models are practically indistinguishable. At this point, we postpone discussion of this topic.

3.5.2 Annual U.S. Tuberculosis Cases

The time series plotted in Figure 3.20 illustrates another common type of non-stationarity, *secular trend*. Aside from a "blip" in the 1940s, the annual incidence of tuberculosis diminishes steadily from 1930 to 1998. The trend continues after 1980 but at a diminishing rate, approaching the natural floor of zero cases. When a time series approaches its natural floor, as in this instance, a log-transformation is often recommended. A decision on the most appropriate transformation awaits the results of a more complete analysis, of course.

Meanwhile, a plot of the differenced time series in Figure 3.21 demonstrates an implication of the natural floor. As $Tubrc_t$ approaches its floor, the range of $\nabla Tubrc_t$ grows smaller and smaller. The visual evidence convinces us that $Tubrc_t$ is nonstationary in mean and in variance. A more complete Box-Cox analysis will be needed.

To find an appropriate transformation, we create the time series $tubrc_t^{(\lambda)}$ defined as

$$tubrc_t = \frac{Tubrc_t}{28.52}, \qquad \mu_{geometric}(Tubrc_t) = 28.52$$

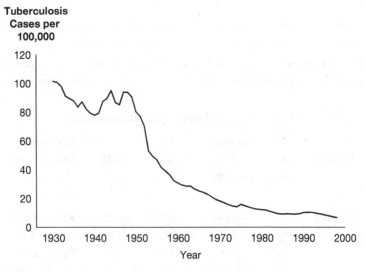

Figure 3.20 Differenced Annual Tuberculosis Cases per 100,000

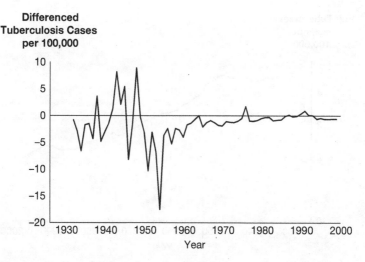

Figure 3.21 Annual Tuberculosis Cases per 100,000

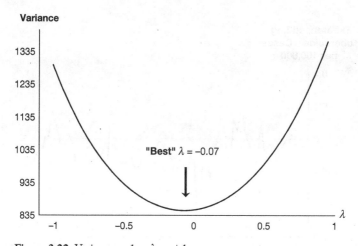

Figure 3.22 Variance, $-1 < \lambda < +1$

We then calculate the variance of $tubrc_t^{(\lambda)}$ for a range of λ-values. Figure 3.22 plots the variance function for $-1 < \lambda < 1$. The variance function confirms our experience with time series of this sort. The "best" estimate of $\lambda = -0.07$ is not far from $\lambda = 0$, the value corresponding to the natural logarithm. On practical and aesthetic grounds, we choose to model $Ln(Tuberc_t)$.

The log-transformed time series, $Ln(Tuberc_t)$, and its first difference, $\nabla Ln(Tuberc_t)$, are plotted in Figures 3.23 and 3.24. In the natural log metric, the secular trend in the time series is approximately linear and, thus, well represented by a difference equation model. A visual inspection of $\nabla Ln(Tuberc_t)$ confirms the choice. In the natural log metric, the annual differences are homogenous

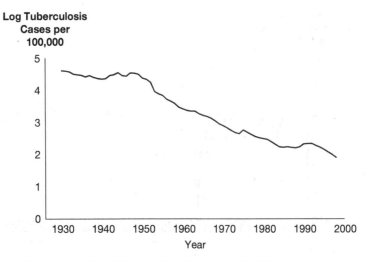

Figure 3.23 Log Annual Tuberculosis Cases per 100,000

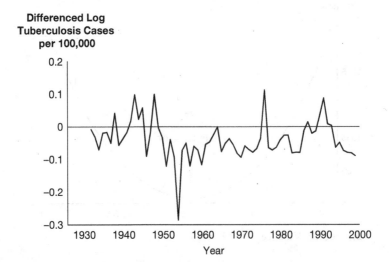

Figure 3.24 Differenced Log Annual Tuberculosis Cases per 100,000

across the 1932-to-2000 period. A large negative shock in 1955 survives the
transformation but poses no insurmountable obstacle to a statistically adequate
model.[4] Satisfied with this transformation, we proceed to the identification stage.

4. Shocks of this sort are often due to changes in the definitions of diseases. The International
Classification of Diseases was revised in 1955. See Mausner and Kramer (1985, p. 76) for another
example and a discussion of the general problems of interpreting historical disease time series. We
return to this topic in Chapter 7.

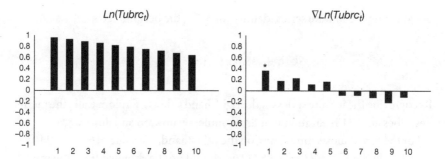

Figure 3.25 Sample ACFs, Log Annual Tuberculosis Cases per 100,000

Table 3.14. ESTIMATION AND DIAGNOSIS, $Ln(Tubrc_t)$

		Estimate	**SE**	**t**	**Diagnosis**
Model 1	$\hat{\theta}_0$	−.0409	.0107	−3.83	$RSE = 0.0556$
	$\hat{\phi}_1$	.3613	.1154	3.13	$Q_{10} = 9.0$
					$Z_{KS} = 0.88$

Sample ACFs for $Ln(Tubrc_t)$ and $\nabla Ln(Tubrc_t)$ are plotted in Figure 3.25. The sample ACF for the undifferenced time series confirms the visual evidence: $Ln(Tubrc_t)$ must be differenced. The sample ACF for the differenced time series, $\nabla Ln(Tubrc_t)$, identifies the AR1 model:

$$(1 - \phi_1 B)\nabla Ln(Tubrc_t) = \theta_0 + a_t$$
$$Ln(Tubrc_t) = \frac{\theta_0 + a_t}{(1 - \phi_1 B)\nabla}$$

Parameter estimates for this model are reported in Table 3.14 as Model 1. Both parameter estimates are statistically significant and $\hat{\phi}_1 = .3613$ lies within the bounds of stationarity. The values $Q_{10} = 9.0$ and $Z_{KS} = 0.88$ are too small to reject a white noise hypothesis for the model residuals, so the AR1 model is statistically adequate. We accept Model 1.

The estimates of θ_0 for the tuberculosis and skirt-width time series reveal the crucial difference between trend and drift. For Kroeber's skirt-width time series, the value of $\hat{\theta}_0 = -.1175$ for the differenced time series is not statistically significant ($t = -0.28$). Invoking the rule of parsimony, we let $\theta_0 = 0$ and accept as the "best" model,

$$(1 + .38B)\nabla Skirt_t = a_t$$

This "best" model is solved for $Skirt_t$ as

$$Skirt_t + .38Skirt_{t-1} = \nabla^{-1}a_t$$

Substituting the infinite series identity for ∇^{-1}, the best model is

$$Skirt_t + .38Skirt_{t-1} = \sum_{k=1}^{\infty} a_{t-k}$$

Recognizing the infinite series on the right-hand side as a random walk, the model describes an $AR1$ realization that drifts aimlessly upward and downward.

For the tuberculosis time series, on the other hand, the value of $\hat{\theta}_0 = -.0409$ is statistically significant ($t = -3.83$) and should not be dropped from the model. In that case, the "best" model is

$$(1 - .36B)\nabla Ln(Tubrc_t) = -.0409 + a_t$$

which is solved for $Ln(Tubrc_t)$ as

$$Ln(Tubrc_t) - .36Ln(Tubrc_{t-1}) = \nabla^{-1}(-.0409 + a_t) = -.0409k + \sum_{k=1}^{\infty} a_t$$

Although this model also describes the random walk of an $AR1$ realization, the level of the $AR1$ realization drops by the constant $\hat{\theta}_0 = -.041$ with each passing year. Instead of being centered on a constant level, this random walk is centered on a level that moves downward in a secular trend. The $AR1$ realization on the left-hand side is a logarithm, of course, which implies a nonlinear trend. Exponentiating both sides of the model transforms the left-hand side into the ratio of $Tubrc_t$ to $Tubrc_{t-1}$.

Ratio models are particularly useful whenever, as in this case, the level of a time series is constrained by a natural floor or ceiling. Otherwise, interpreting the model parameters of a transformed time series introduces complications. We address this topic in detail when the need arises, but that does not happen until Chapter 5.

3.6 SEASONAL MODELS

Seasonality is a cyclical or periodic fluctuation in a time series that recurs or repeats itself at the same phase of the period. If the period s is a calendar year, then $s = 4$ for quarterly data, $s = 12$ for monthly data, and so forth. Seasonal modeling requires a little bit of theory and much pragmatism. On the theoretical side, we agree with Nerlove (1964, p. 263) that "Seasonal variations have causes." We would be surprised if the β-particle time series (Figure 3.2) had a strong seasonal pattern, for example, because physical theory leads us to expect a wholly random time series. On the pragmatic side, because criminological theories emphasize risk factors that peak in the summer months (McDowall and Curtis, 2015), we were surprised to discover that the South Carolina homicide time series (Figure 3.3) does *not* have a strong seasonal pattern. Modeling the weak seasonal pattern would have required a much longer time series or, perhaps, different data. We will address the issue of unmodeled seasonality as a threat to construct validity in Chapter 8. For present purposes, in this chapter, we deal with the practical considerations of representing seasonality in the *ARIMA* noise model.

3.6.1 Anchorage Monthly Precipitation

Though dominated by purely practical considerations, the seasonal modeling strategy requires some reason to *expect* a seasonal process The time series plotted in the left-hand panel of Figure 3.26 consists of 684 monthly average precipitation readings for Anchorage, Alaska. Throughout its long history, from January 1952 through December 2008, the time series, which we call $Prcp_t$, maintains the "flat" appearance of a process that is stationary in mean. As time passes, however, monthly fluctuations grow larger, suggesting that $Prcp_t$ is nonstationary in variance. The visual evidence is unambiguous on that point. Like the annual tuberculosis time series, $Prcp_t$ has a natural floor—zero inches of precipitation—that constrains its variance by season. Monthly fluctuations are relatively large during the wet season but relatively small during the dry season. An appropriate transformation will solve this problem.

To select an appropriate transformation, we create the time series $prcp_t$ defined as

$$prcp_t = \frac{Prcp_t + 0.01}{0.89}, \mu_{geometric}(Prcp_t + 0.01) = 0.89$$

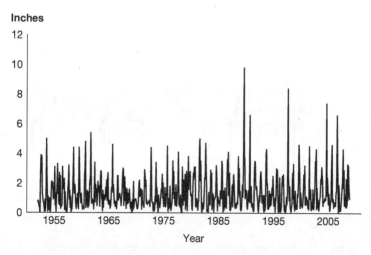

Figure 3.26 Average Monthly Precipitation, Anchorage

Two of the $N=684$ observations are zeroes, so we add the constant 0.01 to $Prcp_t$. The variance of $prcp_t^{(\lambda)}$ for $-1 < \lambda < 2$ is plotted in Figure 3.27.

The minimum variance coincides with the "best" value of $\lambda = 0.26$. Unlike the annual tuberculosis time series, $Prcp_t$ has no secular trend, so there is no reason to prefer a natural log transformation. Bowing to practical and aesthetic demands, we choose the quarter-root transformation. The transformed time series, $Prcp_t^{1/4}$, is plotted in Figure 3.28. The quarter-root transformation appears to have done the trick. The monthly fluctuations in $Prcp_t^{1/4}$ are homogeneous across the seasons. Satisfied, we move on to the identification stage.

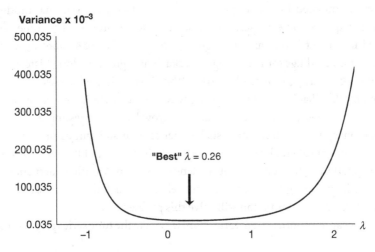

Figure 3.27 Variance, $-1 < \lambda < +2$

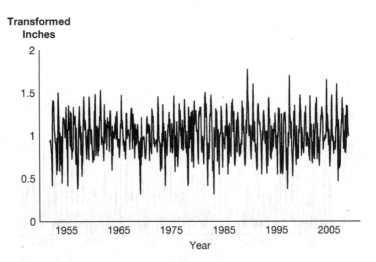

Figure 3.28 Transformed Average Monthly Precipitation, Anchorage

Table 3.15. IDENTIFICATION, $Prcp_t^{1/4}$

	$Prcp_{t^{1/4}}$		$\nabla Prcp_t^{1/4}$		$\nabla^{12} Prcp_t^{1/4}$		$\nabla\nabla^{12} Prcp_t^{1/4}$	
k	r_k	Q_k	r_k	Q_k	r_{kk}	s_r	r_k	Q_k
1	.36	87.8	−.34	80.8	.06	2.2	−.46	142.
2	.16	105.	−.01	80.8	−.02	2.4	−.06	145.
3	−.04	106.	−.05	82.4	.02	2.6	−.01	145.
4	−.17	126.	−.02	82.6	.07	5.8	.04	146.
5	−.28	179.	−.07	85.7	.05	7.5	.01	146.
6	−.30	241.	−.01	85.8	.00	7.5	.00	146.
7	−.31	306.	−.11	93.8	−.04	8.8	−.07	149.
8	−.17	327.	−.01	93.8	.04	10.2	.08	153.
9	−.03	328.	−.05	95.6	−.01	10.3	−.05	155.
10	.17	348.	.05	97.6	.03	10.9	.08	151.
11	.31	415.	−.00	97.6	−.08	15.3	.12	169.
12	.45	553.	.19	123.	−.41	133.	−.40	280.
13	.34	632.	.06	125.	.01	133.	.20	308.
14	.15	649.	.03	126.	.06	135.	.07	312.
15	−.06	652.	−.04	127.	−.03	136.	−.03	312.
16	−.23	687.	−.07	130.	−.07	139.	−.02	312.
17	−.30	751.	−.06	133.	−.07	142.	−.03	313.
18	−.30	812.	−.01	133.	−.01	142.	.02	313.
19	−.28	867.	−.03	134.	−.00	142.	.07	317.
20	−.23	904.	−.13	145.	−.12	152.	−.14	330.
21	−.01	904.	.05	147.	.03	153.	.11	338.
22	.15	919.	−.03	148.	−.03	154.	−.06	341.
23	.34	1003.	.15	164.	.02	154.	.09	347.
24	.35	1008.	.04	165.	−.10	160.	−.11	355.

Sample ACFs for $Prcp_t^{1/4}$, $\nabla Prcp_t^{1/4}$, $\nabla^{12} Prcp_t^{1/4}$, and $\nabla\nabla^{12} Prcp_t^{1/4}$ are reported in Table 3.15 and plotted in Figure 3.29. Seasonal models can be identified from $2S$ lags of the sample ACF. For monthly data, this works out to the $2S = 24$ lags reported in Table 3.15. To illustrate the distinctive signature of a seasonally nonstationary process, 125 lags of the sample ACFs are plotted in Figure 3.29. The visual signature of a seasonally nonstationary process is striking. Nonstationary seasonality is identified by nonzero values of $r_S, r_{2S}, \ldots, r_{kS}$. The values of $r_{24} = 0.35$, $r_{36} = 0.36$, $r_{48} = 0.37$, and $r_{60} = 0.32$ are not particularly large but they are approximately equal. It is this *persistence* of the sample ACF at multiples of lag-S that identifies a seasonally nonstationary process.

Although the sample ACF of $Prcp_t^{1/4}$ identifies a seasonally nonstationary process, it does not identify the exact differences needed to make $Prcp_t^{1/4}$ stationary. For this identification, we compare the sample ACFs for $\nabla Prcp_t^{1/4}$,

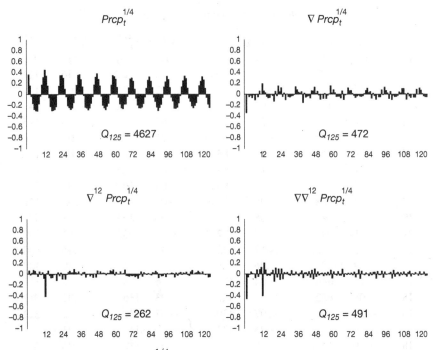

Figure 3.29 Sample ACFs $Prcp_t^{1/4}$

$\nabla^{12}Prcp_t^{1/4}$, and $\nabla\nabla^{12}Prcp_t^{1/4}$. Based on the Q-statistics, $\nabla^{12}Prcp_t^{1/4}$ is the most promising of the three differences. The first-differenced time series, $\nabla Prcp_t^{1/4}$, does surprisingly well. If $Prcp_t^{1/4}$ were a shorter time series, we might reconsider $\nabla Prcp_t^{1/4}$. But given the extraordinary length of this time series—$N=684$ observations—losing 12 observations to seasonal differencing is a trivial cost. Finally, based on the same Q-statistic criterion, $\nabla\nabla^{12}Prcp_t^{1/4}$ is over-differenced.

The sample ACF for $\nabla^{12}P_t^{1/4}$ reported in Table 3.15 has two statistically significant values in the first 12 lags, $r_{11} = 0.08$ and $r_{12} = -.41$. We ignore r_{11} at this early stage: It is relatively small, after all, and *barely* significant. Dismissing r_{11} as an artifact of the large N, the sample ACF identifies the 12th-order IMA model:

$$\nabla^{12}Prcp_t^{1/4} = \theta_0 + (1 - \theta_{12}B^{12})a_t$$

or

$$Prcp_t^{1/4} = \frac{\theta_0 + (1 - \theta_{12}B^{12})a_t}{\nabla^{12}}$$

Parameter estimates for this model are reported as Model 1 in Table 3.16. The value of $\hat{\theta}_{12} = 0.8597$ is invertible and significant. The values $Z_{KS} = 0.78$ and

Table 3.16. ESTIMATION AND DIAGNOSIS, $Prcp_t^{1/4}$

		Estimate	SE	t	Diagnosis
Model 1	$\hat{\theta}_0$	.0002	.0012	0.18	$RSE = 0.1929$
	$\hat{\theta}_{12}$	.8597	.0201	42.81	$Q_{24} = 28.9$
					$Z_{KS} = 0.78$

$Q = 28.9$ are too small to reject a white noise hypothesis for the model's residuals, so Model 1 is accepted.

Because the value of $\hat{\theta}_0 = 0.0002$ is not statistically significant, strictly speaking, the model should be re-estimated without this parameter. When this parameter is dropped from the model, however, the statistics reported in Table 3.16 do not change. Without the constant, the "best" model of $Prcp_t^{1/4}$ is

$$Prcp_t^{1/4} = \frac{a_t - 0.86a_{t-12}}{\nabla^{12}} = \sum_{k=13}^{\infty} (a_t - 0.86a_{t-12})$$

The transformed time series drifts aimlessly, upward and downward, in annual increments.

3.6.2 Monthly Atmospheric CO_2

An important lesson learned from the Anchorage monthly precipitation time series is that—unlike trend, drift, and outliers—seasonality is not always visually obvious. This is particularly true when a time series is extraordinarily long and its underlying process is unusually complex. If the Anchorage monthly precipitation time series (Figure 3.26) illustrates the worst-case scenario, the time series plotted in Figure 3.30 illustrates the best case.

These data are monthly atmospheric parts per million of CO_2 measured from the Mauna Kea Observatory (Keeling et al., 1989). Two properties of this time series are apparent. First, due to the steadily rising use of fossil fuels and incessant deforestation, atmospheric CO_2 levels rise steadily from year to year. Few secular trends are as obviously linear as this one. Second, due to the spring fixation and autumn release of CO_2 by vegetation in the northern hemisphere, within each year, atmospheric CO_2 levels wax and wane predictably. Few annual cycles are as obvious as this one. Knowing nothing about the underlying physical and biological processes, and without consulting any identification statistics, we can be sure that this series is nonstationary from month to month and from year to year. The highly predictable behavior of the time series suggests, further, that there is no need for a transformation. Subsequent analyses confirm this visual impression.

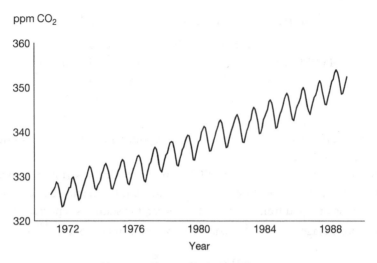

ppm CO_2

Figure 3.30 Monthly Atmospheric CO_2

Although we do not recommend it, some analysts could identify the "best" model for this time series—which we call $CO2_t$—from a visual inspection of the plotted series. Wiser, more prudent analysts would want to rely instead on the sample *ACFs* reported in Table 3.17. As in the Anchorage precipitation time series (Table 3.15), our identification compares the sample *ACFs* for undifferenced time series, $CO2_t$, the first-order differenced time series, $\nabla CO2_t$, the 12th-order differenced time series, $\nabla^{12}CO2_t$, and the first- *and* 12th-order differenced time series, $\nabla\nabla^{12}CO2_t$. This collection of sample *ACFs* will be the standard collection for every monthly seasonal time series identification. Sample *ACFs* for monthly seasonal time series identifications will include the first 24 lags In our experience, shorter *ACFs* miss too much information and longer *ACFs* are confusing.

Based on Q-statistics, the "best" *ARIMA* model will use the first- and 12th-order differenced time series. If this identification is unclear, note first that all 24 lags of the sample *ACF* for $CO2_t$ reported in Table 3.17 are large and statistically significant. The time series *must* be differenced. Given the decision to difference, we compare the values Q_{24} for $\nabla CO2_t$, $\nabla^{12}CO2_t$, and $\nabla\nabla^{12}CO2_t$. The value of $Q_{24} = 70.0$ for $\nabla\nabla^{12}CO2_t$ is lower than the statistic for either $\nabla CO2_t$ ($Q_{24} = 1423$) or $\nabla^{12}CO2_t$ ($Q_{24} = 559$), so it is the "best" difference of the three that we would consider.

Given this decision, large, statistically significant spikes at the first and 12th lags of the sample *ACF* for $\nabla\nabla^{12}CO2_t$ identify the model with *MA1* and *MA12* parameters. These parameters can be incorporated in either of two models: an

Table 3.17. IDENTIFICATION, $CO2_t$

k	$CO2_t$		$\nabla CO2_t$		$\nabla^{12}CO2_t$		$\nabla\nabla^{12}CO2_t$	
	r_k	Q_k	r_k	Q_k	r_{kk}	s_r	r_k	Q_k
1	.97	209.	.71	110.	.81	138.	−.28	15.8
2	.93	401.	.25	124.	.73	249.	.01	15.8
3	.89	576.	−.19	132.	.63	334.	−.06	16.6
4	.85	737.	−.46	180.	.58	404.	.09	18.3
5	.82	889.	−.54	246.	.48	452.	−.04	18.7
6	.81	1035.	−.53	308.	.39	484.	.02	18.8
7	.80	1179.	−.52	369.	.28	501.	−.04	19.2
8	.80	1325.	−.43	411.	.20	509.	−.00	19.2
9	.81	1474.	−.16	416.	.12	513.	.04	19.5
10	.82	1630.	.25	430.	.04	513.	−.04	19.9
11	.83	1790.	.69	541.	−.03	513.	.16	25.2
12	.83	1949.	.90	730.	−.17	519.	−.39	58.3
13	.80	2099.	.68	837.	−.15	524.	.08	59.6
14	.76	2236.	.24	850.	−.16	530.	.01	59.6
15	.72	2359.	−.19	858.	−.16	535.	−.04	60.0
16	.69	2470.	−.44	904.	−.16	541.	−.05	60.5
17	.66	2573.	−.51	966.	−.12	544.	.08	62.1
18	.65	2673.	−.50	1026.	−.12	547.	−.01	62.2
19	.64	2771.	−.48	1082.	−.10	549.	.09	64.1
20	.64	2870.	−.41	1122.	−.12	553.	−.15	69.0
21	.65	2972.	−.15	1128.	−.09	555.	.04	69.5
22	.66	3080.	.23	1141.	−.08	556.	.02	69.5
23	.67	3191.	.65	1245.	−.08	557.	−.04	69.9
24	.67	3302.	.85	1423.	−.07	559.	.03	70.0

additive model,

$$\nabla\nabla^{12}CO2_t = \theta_0 + (1 - \theta_1 B - \theta_{12} B^{12})a_t$$
$$CO2_t = \frac{\theta_0 + (1 - \theta_1 B - \theta_{12} B^{12})a_t}{\nabla\nabla^{12}}$$

or a multiplicative model,

$$\nabla\nabla^{12}CO2_t = \theta_0 + (1 - \theta_1 B)(1 - \theta_{12} B^{12})a_t$$
$$COP2_t = \frac{\theta_0 + (1 - \theta_1 B)(1 - \theta_{12} B^{12})a_t}{\nabla\nabla^{12}}$$

The sample ACF does not distinguish between these two candidate models. Accordingly, we estimate and diagnose both.

Table 3.18. ESTIMATION AND DIAGNOSIS, $CO2_t$

		Estimate	SE	t	Diagnosis
Model 1	$\hat{\theta}_0$	.0058	.0041	1.43	$RSE = 0.3050$
	$\hat{\theta}_1$	.2917	.0524	5.57	$Q_{24} = 14.5$
	$\hat{\theta}_{12}$	.5330	.0532	10.02	$Z_{KS} = 0.88$
Model 2	$\hat{\theta}_0$	.0062	.0061	1.02	$RSE = 0.3016$
	$\hat{\theta}_1$	.3228	.0666	4.85	$Q_{24} = 14.9$
	$\hat{\theta}_{12}$	.6324	.0575	10.99	$Z_{KS} = 0.86$

Parameter estimates for the additive and multiplicative models are reported in Table 3.18 as Model 1 and Model 2 respectively.[5] The estimates of θ_1 and θ_{12} are statistically significant and invertible in both models. The estimates of θ_0 are not statistically significant in either model. We would ordinarily re-estimate the models without the insignificant parameters. The secular trend in this time series is so regular and steady, however, that we feel justified in leaving the models alone. Since the values of Q_{24} and Z_{KS} are too small to reject the white noise hypothesis for either model, both models are statistically adequate. But which model is better? The multiplicative Model 2 has a lower RSE and, thus, is the "best" model. The difference between the two models is trivially small, however, and might be ignored if Model 1 were to prove more useful.

3.6.3 Australian Traffic Fatalities

Except for the complication of choosing between the additive and multiplicative structures, modeling the monthly CO_2 time series was a relatively simple, straightforward exercise. Judging from the visual evidence, modeling the time series plotted in Figure 3.31 will be more challenging. These data are quarterly Australian traffic fatalities (Bhattacharyya and Layton, 1979).

In our experience, quarterly time series are more difficult to model than other seasonal time series. But this *particular* quarterly time series, which we call $AuFtl_t$, has several features that complicate the modeling task. Although traffic fatalities are subject to strong seasonal forces, for example, there is no visually obvious quarterly cycle in the plotted time series. And although $AuFtl_t$ is obviously

---

5. The multiplicative Model 2 is sometimes called the "airline model" because Box and Jenkins (1970, p. 304) used it for their monthly international airline passengers time series. Box and Jenkins paid little attention to additive models. In their experience, multiplicative models produced more accurate forecasts for *most* seasonal time series. Our experience is consistent with theirs. Nevertheless, additive and multiplicative models should be estimated and compared for all time series.

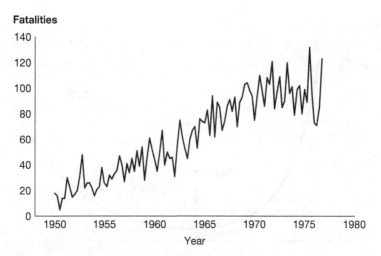

Figure 3.31 Quarterly Australian Traffic Fatalities

nonstationary in mean, its secular trend is ragged. Finally, as time passes, the quarterly fluctuations grow larger, suggesting that $AuFtl_t$ is also nonstationary in variance.

Fatality time series are often well represented as Poisson sequences and $AuFtl_t$ is no exception. If the mean of a Poisson sequence is large, as it is in this time series, the ratio of the mean to its square root is approximately Normal. This Poisson property argues for a square root transformation. Ignoring this theoretical preference, we begin the search for a transformation by creating the time series $AuFtl_t$ defined as

$$auftl_t = \frac{AuFtl_t}{52.84}, \qquad \mu_{geometric}(AuFtl_t) = 52.84$$

Figure 3.32 plots the variance of $auftl_t^{(\lambda)}$ over the interval $-1 < \lambda < 3$. The "best" transformation occurs at $\lambda = 0.66$. Since $\lambda = 0.5$ is not significantly different than this "best" λ-value, we will use the square-root transformation. The square-root time series, plotted in Figure 3.33, fluctuates regularly about a nonstationary mean, so the transformation seems to have done the trick.

Sample ACFs for $AuFtl_t^{1/2}$, $\nabla AuFtl_t^{1/2}$, $\nabla^4 AuFtl_t^{1/2}$, and $\nabla\nabla^4 AuFtl_t^{1/2}$ are reported in Table 3.19. The sample ACF for $AuFtl_t^{1/2}$ leaves no doubt that the time series must be differenced. Based on Q-statistics, the "best" difference is either $\nabla AuFtl_t^{1/2}$ ($Q_8 = 28.5$) or, perhaps, $\nabla^4 AuFtl_t^{1/2}$ ($Q_8 = 32.2$). In addition to a slightly smaller Q-statistic ($Q_8 = 28.5$ vs. 32.2), $\nabla AuFtl_t^{1/2}$ has three more observations (107 vs. 104). This is a relatively minor advantage, however, so after we have finished modeling $\nabla AuFtl_t^{1/2}$, we will explore models for $\nabla^4 AuFtl_t^{1/2}$.

Variance x 10⁻³

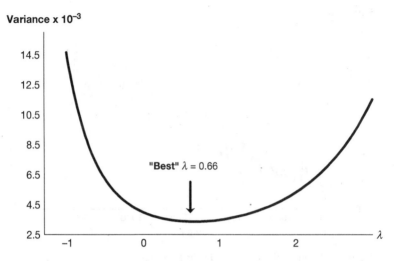

Figure 3.32 Variance, $-1 < \lambda < +3$

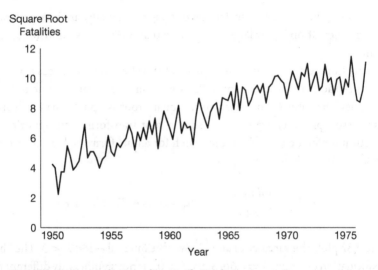

Figure 3.33 Quarterly Australian Traffic Fatalities, Square Roots

After several iterations, an $MA4$ model is identified for $\nabla AuFtl_t^{1/2}$:

$$\nabla AuFtl_t^{1/2} = \theta_0 + (1 - \theta_1 B - \theta_3 B^3 - \theta_4 B^4) a_t$$

Identification of an $MA4$ model from the sample ACF reported in Table 3.19 is not obvious. The insignificant value of $r_4 = 0.06$ argues against an $MA4$ identification, in fact, while the significant value of $r_3 = -0.20$ argues for an $MA3$ model. We could find no reasonable $MA3$ model that fit $\nabla AuFtl_t^{1/2}$ adequately, however—we ask the reader to verify this as an exercise—nor could we find any

Table 3.19. IDENTIFICATION, $AuFtl_t^{1/2}$

	$AuFtl_{t\cdot1/2}$		$\nabla AuFtl_t^{1/2}$		$\nabla^4 AuFtl_t^{1/2}$		$\nabla\nabla^4 AuFtl_t^{1/2}$	
k	r_k	Q_k	r_k	Q_k	r_{kk}	s_r	r_k	Q_k
1	86	82.4	−.40	17.5	.05	0.2	−.45	21.3
2	.82	159.	−.02	17.5	−.01	0.2	.07	21.8
3	.79	228.	−.20	22.0	−.19	4.3	.01	21.8
4	.80	301.	.06	22.3	−.42	23.4	−.46	45.2
5	.79	374.	.17	25.5	.21	28.5	.39	62.1
6	.74	438.	−.14	27.7	.09	29.5	−.08	62.8
7	.74	502.	.04	27.8	.15	32.0	.09	63.8
8	.71	562.	.07	28.5	.03	32.2	.00	63.8

Table 3.20. ESTIMATION AND DIAGNOSIS, $AuFtl_t^{1/2}$

		Estimate	SE	t	Diagnosis
Model 1	$\hat{\theta}_0$	.0550	.0146	3.76	$RSE = 0.7602$
	$\hat{\theta}_1$	.8274	.0717	11.54	$Q_8 = 4.1$
	$\hat{\theta}_3$	.2911	.1033	2.82	$Z_{KS} = 0.68$
	$\hat{\theta}_4$	−.3175	.0944	−3.36	
Model 2	$\hat{\theta}_0$	.2257	.0539	4.18	$RSE = 0.8082$
	$\hat{\theta}_4$	.6300	.0744	8,47	$Q_8 = 9.5$
	$\hat{\theta}_5$	−.2915	.0757	−3.85	$Z_{KS} = 0.40$

statistically adequate model that did not include an $MA4$ term. The discrepancy between the sample ACF and the "best" model should sensitize the reader to the fact that sample $ACFs$ are biased, making the identification of seasonal models particularly difficult.

Parameter estimates for the $MA4$ model are reported as Model 1 in Table 3.20. All of the parameter estimates are statistically significant and invertible. The values of $Z_{KS} = 0.68$ and $Q_8 = 4.1$ are too small to reject the white noise hypothesis for the residuals, so Model 1 is statistically adequate. Rounding to two decimal places, we write Model 1 as

$$AuFtl_t^{1/2} - AuFtl_{t-1}^{1/2} = 0.06 + a_t - .83a_{t-1} - .29a_{t-3} + .32a_{t-4}$$

Successive observations of $AuFtl_t^{1/2}$ rise by $\hat{\theta}_0 = 0.06$ units. Since the secular trend is linear, this amounts to $4\hat{\theta}_0 = 0.24$ units per year.

Although Model 1 is a "good" model, it is not necessarily the "best" model of $AuFtl_t^{1/2}$. From the sample ACF, an $MA5$ model of the fourth-differenced time series is plausible:

$$\nabla^4 AuFtl_t^{1/2} = \theta_0 + (1 - \theta_4 B^4 - \theta_5 B^5)a_t$$

This identification also requires an explanation. Significant values of r_3, r_4, and r_5 in the sample ACF for $\nabla^4 AuFtl_t^{1/2}$ (Table 3.19) identify a model with MA parameters θ_3, θ_4, and θ_5. Whenever we included θ_3 in a model, however, the parameter estimate was not statistically significant. All of the statistically adequate models that we estimated included parameters θ_4 and θ_5. Again, we invite the reader to replicate our analysis as an exercise.

Parameter estimates for the $MA5$ model are reported as Model 2 in Table 3.20. All parameter estimates are statistically significant and invertible again and the residuals are not different than white noise. To two decimal places, we can write Model 2 as

$$AuFtl_t^{1/2} - AuFtl_{t-4}^{1/2} = 0.23 + a_t - 0.63a_{t-4} + 0.29a_{t-5}$$

In Model 2, $AuFtl_t^{1/2}$ rises in annual increments of $\hat{\theta}_0 = 0.23$ units. This is remarkably close to the annual change in level. Although Model 2 is an acceptable model of $AuFtl_t^{1/2}$, based on RSE statistics, Model 1 is the "better" model of $AuFtl_t^{1/2}$. It is now time to address the problem of model selection in greater detail.

3.7 AUXILIARY MODELING PROCEDURES

The Box-Jenkins iterative modeling algorithm diagrammed in Figure 3.1 nearly always leads to the "best" $ARIMA$ model. When the algorithm stalls, a little educated guesswork often serves to nudge it back on track This educated guess-work can include the results of two auxiliary identification procedures. Neither procedure is part of the traditional modeling strategy and, in some respects, both are incompatible with the traditional strategy. Nevertheless, used in conjunction with the iterative algorithm, these auxiliary procedures can shed light on the structure of an underlying time series process.

Information criteria were developed originally to solve a problem posed by extremely long time series. As N grows long, statistical tests of significance and fit become useless. Small high-order AR and MA terms achieve statistical significance and models become needlessly complicated. To solve this statistical problem, Akaike (1974) proposed a measure of fit based on entropy. Although information criteria like Akaike's are not subject to the statistical problems posed by extremely long N, they do not support statistical tests of model fit or adequacy. They can be useful nevertheless.

Unit root tests were developed for the explicit purpose of distinguishing between stationary and nonstationary models. In Chapter 2.6, we noted that the nonstationary random walk model is a special case of the stationary $AR1$ model where $\phi_1 = 1$. When $\hat{\phi}_1$ is approximately equal to one, then, it becomes difficult to choose between the competing $AR1$ and random walk models. Common sense and our experience with significance tests suggest that the choice could be based on the null hypothesis:

$$H_0: \phi_1 = 1$$

Rejecting H_0 chooses the stationary $AR1$ model; failing to reject H_0 chooses the nonstationary random walk model. Common sense and experience fail at this point, unfortunately. The Student's t-distribution that we use to test the statistical significance of $\hat{\phi}_1$ gives a biased test of this particular H_0. Dickey and Fuller (1979) derive the correct distribution. In our experience, Dickey-Fuller unit root tests are less useful for $ARIMA$ models. We will expand on this statement shortly.

3.7.1 Information Criteria

The iterative $ARIMA$ modeling algorithm often leads to two or three statistically adequate models that differ by small degrees. When the difference between the "best" model and a "very good" competing model is small—and that happens often—the analyst must look outside the iterative modeling strategy for advice. Although the model with the smallest RSE is defined as the "best" model, selecting a model on the RSE criterion alone has theoretical and practical shortcomings.

First, since model fit can always be improved by adding parameters, the model with the smallest RSE may be more complicated than necessary. The "best" model may *over*-fit the data, in other words. Although fit is a desirable model property, so is parsimony. When the "best" model and its "very good" competitors belong to the same $ARIMA$ class, the iterative strategy is rational and efficient. When the "best" model and a "very good" competitor belong to different $ARIMA$ classes, on the other hand—say, stationary versus nonstationary—it becomes difficult to weigh model fit against parsimony.

Second, compared to a "very good" competitor, the "best" model may fail to account for troublesome autocorrelations or trend; or it may not perform as well in some application. If a "very good" competing model is a more accurate reflection of theory, common sense, or reality, or if it gives better forecasts or

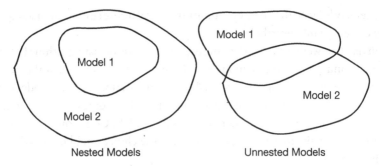

Figure 3.34 Nested vs. Unnested Models

supports a more powerful hypothesis test, there should be some way to justify its selection in lieu of the "best" model.

Both shortcomings point to the need for an *RSE metric* to tell us whether the difference in the *RSEs* of competing models is small enough to be ignored. Unfortunately, no *RSE* metric can be applied to the widest range of models. Instead, there is one strong metric that applies only to *nested* models and a weaker metric that can be applied to *unnested* models

The χ^2 distribution provides a natural metric for competing models that are *nested*. Under a null hypothesis of model equivalence,

$$H_0\text{: } Model1 \cong Model2$$

the weighted difference in *RSEs* between two competing models is distributed as a χ^2 statistic with degrees of freedom determined by the difference in the number of parameters in the two models. Suppose that Model 1 has M parameters, for example, and that Model 2 was created by adding m additional parameters. If the weighted difference in *RSEs* for the two nested models exceeds the 95th percentile of χ^2_m, H_0 is rejected. The incremental fit purchased at the expense of adding m parameters to Model 1 is justified. But if the weighted difference in *RSEs* is smaller than the 95th percentile of χ^2_m, H_0 is rejected. The incremental fit of Model 2 does not justify the loss in parsimony associated with its m additional parameters.

The argument assumes that Model 1 is nested within Model 2, of course, which happens whenever parameters are added to a statistically adequate model. Sample *ACFs* for the Zurich sunspot time series, for example, identified Model 1, which was estimated as:

$$Sunspot_t^{1/2} = \frac{6.10 + a_t}{1 - 1.36B + 0.66B^2}$$

Although Model 1 was statistically adequate, its residual *ACF* revealed an 11-year cycle. The cycle might have been ignored in any other time series, but there are

Table 3.21. MODEL SELECTION CRITERIA

	Model	N	−2LL	df	AIC	BIC
$Sunspot_t^{1/2}$	1	176	553.48	4	561.48	574.16
	2	176	532.44	7	546.44	568.63
$Admit_t$	1	130	891.06	3	897.06	905.66
	2	130	890.56	4	898.56	910.02
$\nabla Skirt_t$	1	149	1001.18	3	1007.17	1016.18
	2	149	1001.64	4	1009.63	1021.65
$\nabla\nabla^{12} CO2_t$	1	204	87.48	4	95.47	108.74
	2	204	79.86	4	87.85	101.12
$\nabla AuFtl_t^{1/2}$	1	107	244.76	5	254.77	268.13
$\nabla^4 AuFtl_t^{1/2}$	2	104	247.18	4	255.17	265.75
$Wheat_t^{-1/2}$	1	370	−2590.58	4	−2582.58	−2566.92
	2	370	−2601.72	5	−2591.72	−2572.16

theoretical grounds for an 11-year sunspot cycle. So Model 2 was identified and estimated as:

$$Sunspot_t^{1/2} = \frac{6.02 + (1 + 0.28B^9 + 0.17B^{11} + 0.20B^{12})a_t}{1 - 1.27B + 0.59B^2}$$

The three added *MA* parameters reduce the *RSE* from 1.1606 in Model 1 to 1.0922 in Model 2. Is this *RSE* reduction large enough to justify the three extra parameters in Model 2?

Since Model 1 is nested within Model 2, we can test H_0 by comparing the difference in their weighted *RSEs* to the distribution of χ_3^2. To demonstrate a point, we write H_0 as:

$$H_0: \text{Model 1} \cong \text{Model 2}; \theta_9 = \theta_{11} = \theta_{12} = 0$$

Nesting equates model equivalence with the *joint* significance of three additional parameters in Model 2. Based on *t*-statistics, $\hat{\theta}_9$, $\hat{\theta}_{11}$, and $\hat{\theta}_{12}$ are each *individually* significant. But this does not guarantee their *joint* significance. Ignoring the issue raised by conducting three sequential *t*-tests, a valid test of H_0 must account for the *correlation* between $\hat{\theta}_9$, $\hat{\theta}_{11}$, and $\hat{\theta}_{12}$. For that, we test the *joint* significance of $\hat{\theta}_9$, $\hat{\theta}_{11}$, and $\hat{\theta}_{12}$—and hence the *equivalence* of Model 1 and Model 2—with a deviance statistic defined as

$$D = [-2LL(\text{Model 2})] - [-2LL(\text{Model 1})]$$

Substituting the values of $-2LL$ for Model 1 and Model 2 reported in Table 3.21:[6]

$$D = 87.48 - 79.86 = 7.62$$

Under H_0, D is distributed as χ_3^2. Since values of $\chi_3^2 \geq 7.62$ occur with probability $p < 0.054$, the difference between Model 1 and Model 2 is *not* statistically significant, so we cannot reject H_0. This test result is tantalizingly close to the critical value, however. Others might reject H_0 on theoretical grounds. We leave that decision to the reader.

When competing models are *not* nested, the weighted difference in *RSEs* is not distributed as χ^2 under H_0. If the weighted *RSEs* are adjusted for their different numbers of parameters, however, they can be interpreted in a relative information metric. One of the most widely used *information criteria* is the Akaike Information Criterion (*AIC*; Akaike, 1973, 1974), defined as

$$AIC(\text{Model}) = -2LL + 2df$$

where *df* is the number of parameters in the Model, including the *RSE*. The *AIC* quantifies the Kullback-Leibler index, a measure of the information lost by using a model to represent reality. Because the underlying reality is unknown, the *AIC* has no *absolute* meaning. Because the biased representation of reality is constant across models of the same reality, however, the *AICs* for competing models can be interpreted as the *relative* information lost by each. Models with smaller information losses and lower *AICs* are preferred.

In computing the *AIC*, the *2df* component acts as a penalty term for model complexity. As a model adds parameters, and so grows more complex, the value of the *AIC* will increase as well. Only if the improvement in fit is larger than the penalty term will the *AIC* select a more complex model over a simpler one. The *AIC* therefore assumes a preference for parsimonious models over complex ones.

To illustrate the *AIC*, consider our analysis of the weekly pediatric trauma admissions time series, $Admit_t$. The sample *ACF* identified Model 1, which was estimated as:

$$Admit_t - 21.88 = \frac{a_t}{1 - .61B}$$

Depending on the value of r_1, AR1 processes can be fit by MA2 models. In this instance, the sample *ACF* identified a Model 2, which was estimated as:

$$Admit_t - 21.81 = (1 + 0.60B + 0.36B^2)a_t$$

---

6. The log likelihood function is developed in Appendix 3A. $-2LL = N \times Ln(RSE^2)$.

By virtue of its smaller *RSE*, Model 2 is the "better" of the two models. Its smaller *RSE* comes at the expense of an extra parameter, however, a difference that the *AIC*s reported in Table 3.21 take into account. Based on its smaller *AIC*— 897.06 vs. 898.56—Model 1 is the "better" of the two models. Since the difference in their *AIC*s is small, one might think that the *relative* difference between Model 1 and Model 2 is small. This would be a fallacy, however.

We encountered the same *AR1-MA2* dilemma in our analysis of Kroeber's skirt-width time series. Model 1 was estimated as

$$\nabla Skirt_t = \frac{a_t - 0.12}{1 + 0.38B}$$

and Model 2 was estimated as

$$\nabla Skirt_t = (1 - 0.31B + 0.19)a_t - 0.12$$

The *AIC*s reported in Table 3.21 are computed from $\nabla Skirt_t$, not from $Skirt_t$. This convention is not motivated by mere aesthetics. We will have more to say about this shortly. For the present, based on *AIC*s, the *AR1* model is "better" than the *MA2* model:

$$AIC(\text{Model 1}) = 1007.17 < AIC(\text{Model 2}) = 1009.63$$

Once again, the magnitude of the difference in *AIC*s says nothing about the difference between the two models. On the contrary, in our experience, *AR1* models are invariably "better" than the competing *MA2* models.

A variation on the *AIC*, the Bayesian Information Criterion (*BIC*, Schwarz, 1978) charges a larger penalty for additional parameters. The *BIC* is defined as:

$$BIC(\text{Model}) = -2LL + df \times Ln(N)$$

Unlike the *AIC*, the *BIC* has a basis in probability theory.[7] Under some conditions, it approximates the Bayes factor, which measures the relative strength of the evidence in favor of a particular model. In application, it has the same structure and uses the same logic as the *AIC*, however, selecting the model that produces the smallest value of the statistic.

Our analysis of the monthly ambient CO_2 time series illustrates the *BIC*. The sample *ACF* for this time series identified a 12th-order *IMA* model with no clear preference between the additive and multiplicative forms. The additive Model 1 was estimated as

$$\nabla\nabla^{12} CO2_t = 0.006 + (1 - 0.29B - 0.53B^{12})a_t$$

---

7. There are actually two Bayesian information criteria. To distinguish it from the other, this one is sometimes called the Schwarz Information Criterion (*SIC*).

and the multiplicative Model 2 was estimated as

$$\nabla\nabla^{12}CO2_t = 0.006 + (1 - 0.32B)(1 - 0.63B^{12})a_t$$

By virtue of its lower *BIC*, the multiplicative model is "better."

$$BIC(\text{Model 2}) = 101.12 < BIC(\text{Model 1}) = 108.74$$

But this is not always the case in our experience. For seasonal *IMA* processes such as this one, we recommend estimating both the additive and multiplicative forms and comparing the two models with *AICs* or *BICs*.

The *AIC* and *BIC* have unique advantages and adherents (Burnham and Anderson, 2002, 2004). The *AIC* and *BIC* do not always select the same model. Due to its more demanding penalty function, the *BIC* selects more parsimonious models. Simulation studies also show that, if a "true" model does exist, and if it is a candidate under consideration, the *BIC* will select it as *N* grows larger. The *AIC* in this situation selects a model with too many components. Otherwise, both the *AIC* and the *BIC* assume identical data for the model. This limits the use of the *AIC* and *BIC* in obvious and non-obvious ways. We have already alluded to the problem of differencing. Obviously, neither the *AIC* nor the *BIC* can tell us *whether* or *how* to difference a time series.

Sample *ACFs* for the quarterly Australian traffic fatality time series identified two very different models. Model 1 was estimated as

$$\nabla AuFtl_t^{1/2} = 0.06 + (1 - 0.83B - 0.29B^3 + 0.32B^4)a_t$$

and Model 2 was estimated as

$$\nabla^4 AuFtl_t^{1/2} = 0.23 + (1 + 0.63B^4 + 0.29B^5)a_t$$

But whereas the *AICs* reported in Table 3.21 select Model 1,

$$AIC(\text{Model 1}) = 254.77 < AIC(\text{Model 2}) = 255.17$$

the *BICs* select Model 2,

$$BIC(\text{Model 2}) = 265.75 < BIC(\text{Model 1}) = 268.13$$

Which selection is correct? Neither is correct, strictly speaking. Because Model 1 and Model 2 are based on different time series— $\nabla AuFtl_t^{1/2}$ vs. $\nabla^4 AuFtl_t^{1/2}$ —and different *Ns*—107 vs. 104—their *AICs* and *BICs* are not comparable. Neither the *AIC* nor the *BIC* can objectively choose between these two models This is not to say that there is *no* way to choose between these two models; but information-theoretic choices are not possible.

The *AIC* and *BIC* do not point to the unique "true" model for a time series or even to the "best" model. Instead, the *AIC* and *BIC* search for "better" models from a set of candidates. One strategy for using the *AIC* and/or the *BIC* is to estimate all of the models in a class of models with the same differencing operators and *N*s and, then, select the model with the smallest *AIC* or *BIC*. For example, one might estimate every possible combination of zero-, first-, and second-order *AR* and *MA* models and use the *AIC* or *BIC* to select the final model from among the nine possible models. Practical considerations should also be weighed, of course, and we will return to this issue.

The last set of statistics reported in Table 3.21 were computed for the Beveridge wheat price time series and are used here to demonstrate a point. Sample *ACF*s for this time series identified an *AR2* model, which was estimated as Model 1:

$$Wheat_t^{-1/2} - 0.10 = \frac{a_t}{1 - 0.82B + 0.35B^2}$$

The residual *ACF* identified an eight-year cycle, which was accommodated with an *MA8* parameter. The resulting Model 2 was estimated as:

$$Wheat_t^{-1/2} - 0.10 = \frac{(1 - 0.16B^8)a_t}{1 - 0.80B + 0.35B^2}$$

Since Model 1 is nested inside Model 2, of course, model equivalence can be tested with the deviance statistic,

$$D = [-2LL(\text{Model } 2)] - [-2LL(\text{Model } 1)$$
$$= 2590.58 + 2601.72 = 11.14$$

Since values of $\chi_1^2 > 11.14$ occur with probability $p < 0.001$, H_0 is rejected. The incremental fit realized by adding a parameter to Model 1 is statistically significant. Model 2 is the "better" model.

The novelty in this example is that $-2LL(\text{Model } 1)$ and $-2LL(\text{Model } 2)$ are *negative*. In our experience, this is a rare occurence but, obviously, *not* an impossible occurence. Although the sign of $-2LL$ has no effect on D, the *AIC* and the *BIC* now have negative values. This does not change their conventional interpretations, however. We still select the model with the smaller *AIC* or *BIC* value. Specifically,

$$AIC(\text{Model } 2) = -2591.72 < AIC(\text{Model } 1) = -2582.58$$
$$BIC(\text{Model } 2) = -2572.16 < BIC(\text{Model } 1) = -2566.92$$

Although the sign reversal may be confusing, Model 2 has smaller *AIC* and *BIC* values and, hence, is the "better" model of the two.

Likelihood ratio tests and information criteria are useful in selecting a model from a set of candidates. Likelihood ratio tests require that the candidate models form a nested sequence. The information criteria are most clearly valuable in selecting between unnested candidates but they also have applications in selecting between nested ones. The tests and criteria have uses as adjuncts in any model selection process. They are perhaps most helpful, however, in borderline situations where two or more models are otherwise satisfactory and fit the time series equally well. In these cases, where the analyst is truly undecided about which model to select, the selection statistics may provide an objective way to make the decision. The methods that we have considered in this section amount to specialized definitions of a desirable model, however, and all closely attend to only one of the model's characteristics. Yet, as we have already suggested, developing a good model requires a balance of many considerations. Likelihood ratios and information criteria play a relatively small role in this process.

3.7.2 Unit Root Tests

In our experience, the simplest, most reliable way to identify a nonstationary model combines a visual inspection of the plotted time series and a reading of the sample ACF. If the plotted time series drifts or trends, and if its sample ACF decays slowly, a nonstationary model is identified. The identification is ordinarily unambiguous. Kroeber's skirt-width time series and the U.S. tuberculosis time series are typical. Nevertheless, formal tests of nonstationarity can be helpful in those rare cases where the simpler methods fail.

In Section 2.4, we derived the bounds of stationarity for AR processes by setting the AR operator to zero and solving it as a polynomial in the backshift operator. If the roots of the polynomial are greater than unity in absolute value, the AR parameters lie within the bounds of stationarity. The model is stationary, in other words, and presumably so is the time series. If the roots are smaller than unity, on the other hand, the model is nonstationary, as is the time series. Formal tests of stationarity rely on this logic. There are many formal tests and the literature grows year by year. We provide only an introduction to these issues, and readers interested in more details can find them in sources such as Hamilton (1994), Maddala and Kim (1998), and Patterson (2011).

We begin with the simplest case, an AR1 model with the single parameter ϕ_1.

$$Y_t = \phi_1 Y_{t-1} + a_t \quad -1 < \phi_1 < +1$$

If $\phi_1 = 1$, the stationary AR1 model is a nonstationary random walk model. This suggests the null hypothesis

$$H_0 : \phi_1 = 1$$

If we cannot reject this H_0, we conclude that the time series is a nonstationary random walk. To simplify the test of this H_0—the unit root test—we rewrite the AR1 model as a difference equation:

$$\nabla Y_t = (\phi_1 - 1)Y_{t-1} + a_t$$

The parameter of this model can be estimated by regressing ∇Y_t on Y_{t-1}. In principle, the t-statistic derived from the ordinary least-squares regression

$$t = \frac{\phi_1 - 1}{\hat{\sigma}_{\phi_1 - 1}}$$

tests the unit root null hypothesis

$$H_0: (\phi_1 - 1) = 0$$

Under this particular H_0, however, the t-statistic is not distributed as Student's t. Dickey and Fuller (1979) derived the form of the distribution and calculated its percentiles by simulation.

Tables of the Dickey-Fuller distribution for finite sample series lengths and a range of significance levels appear in Fuller (1996) and other sources. MacKinnon (1994) developed a computational algorithm for generating Dickey-Fuller critical values for time series of any length and most software packages provide p-values for the test statistic. The limiting critical values for three Dickey-Fuller distributions reported in Table 3.23 will be sufficient for our purposes. Corresponding values of Student's t are reported to illustrate the extreme left-hand skew of the Dickey-Fuller test statistic distributions.

To perform a Dickey-Fuller test, we use the equation with lagged levels and differences, and compare the t-statistic (here called the τ-statistic to avoid confusion) to a Dickey-Fuller critical value. Autocorrelation in the a_t term biases the test, but adding a sufficient number of lagged differences to the equation will remove the problem. The Dickey-Fuller test with lagged differences to control for autocorrelation is called the Augmented Dickey-Fuller, or ADF, test. To use the ADF test, we then estimate the equation

$$\nabla Y_t = (\phi_1 - 1)Y_{t-1} + \beta_1(\nabla Y_{t-1}) + \beta_2(\nabla Y_{t-2}) + \cdots + a_t$$

Table 3.22. CRITICAL VALUES FOR THE UNIT ROOT TEST STATISTICS

α	Student's t	τ	$\tau\mu$	τt
0.10	−1.29	−1.62	−2.57	−3.13
0.05	−1.65	−1.95	−2.86	−3.41
0.01	−2.33	−2.58	−3.42	−3.96

A standard procedure for selecting the number of lagged differences, supported by the work of Ng and Perron (1995), is to begin by overfitting the model with multiple lags. The analysis then sequentially trims the test equation using the t-statistics for the lagged coefficients (which here have Normal limiting distributions) to remove insignificant lags. Said and Dickey (1984) showed that a sufficiently long set of lagged differences also allows use of the Dickey-Fuller distribution when moving average components exist in the error term.

An alternative to the Dickey-Fuller test developed by Phillips and Perron (1988) uses the same distribution but avoids the necessity of choosing a lag order for the regression models. This can be an advantage, since it does not require a possibly incorrect decision about how many lagged differences to include. The Phillips-Perron test nevertheless uses the sample ACF for the differenced time series to adjust the data, and the method for accomplishing this itself introduces an element of judgment.

An extension of unit root testing adds deterministic components and expands the alternative hypothesis beyond a simple AR model. Two variations on the simple model are to allow for a deterministic intercept, and to allow for both a deterministic intercept and a deterministic trend:

$$Y_t - \beta_0 = \phi_1(Y_{t-1} - \beta_0) + a_t$$
$$Y_t - \beta_0 - \beta_t t = \phi_1[Y_{t-1} - \beta_0 - \beta_t(t-1)] + a_t$$

Except for the intercept, the first model is identical in structure to the AR model. An ADF test takes the same form as before except that the test equation includes an intercept term:

$$\nabla Y_t = \beta_0 + (\phi_1 - 1)Y_{t-1} + \beta_1 \nabla Y_{t-1} + \beta_2 \nabla Y_{t-2} + \cdots + a_t$$

The Dickey-Fuller distribution for the test statistic (now called the $\tau\mu$-statistic) is different from that in the previous case and different critical values apply. In particular, more extreme results are necessary to reject the null than in the situation with no intercept, and the 1 percent, 5 percent, and 10 percent limiting critical values are -3.42, -2.86, and -2.57.

The second model differs somewhat from the other two, since it follows a deterministic trend under the alternative hypothesis. The other models are often called "difference stationary," because they require a differencing operation to remove the unit root from a series. The deterministic trend model, in contrast, is "trend stationary" because the levels of the series will be stationary after controlling for the trend. Beyond the addition of the trend variable (a linear counter coded in one-unit increments, such as 1, 2, 3, . . .), the Dickey-Fuller test proceeds in the same manner as with the other two cases:

$$\nabla Y_t = \beta_0 + \beta_t(t) + (\phi_1 - 1)Y_{t-1} + \beta_1 \nabla Y_{t-1} + \beta_2 \nabla Y_{t-2} + \cdots + a_t$$

Again the test statistic (here called τt-statistic) differs from the other cases, and has its own set of critical values. These are the most extreme of the three models, with limit-critical values of -3.96 at the 1 percent level, -3.41 at the 5 percent level, and -3.13 at the 10 percent level.

As with the other two tests, failing to reject

$$H_0: (\phi_1 - 1) = 0$$

supports the existence of a unit root. Rejecting H_0 is consistent with stationarity around a linear trend (trend stationarity), but it does not consider the statistical significance of the intercept term. The overall conclusion in this case is that the series follows a linear trend, with or without an intercept. A separate t-test for the intercept (with Normal limit-critical values) addresses its statistical significance.

In Section 3.3.1, we analyzed an annual time series of Canadian inflation rates between 1956 and 2008. Based on the sample ACF, we concluded that this series was stationary and we fit an AR1 model that passed all standard diagnostic tests. We noted that visual inspection of the plotted time series suggested possible nonstationarity, however, and the series is short enough to make any identification ambiguous. This is a situation in which a formal unit root test can be helpful in deciding whether to conduct the analysis in levels or in differences. The results of a unit root test are not more definitive than are the inferences gained from other methods, but they provide an additional independent source of evidence.

The results of an ADF test for the inflation series, with an intercept and as many as four lagged differences, is reported in Table 3.23. Following the procedure we described earlier, the analysis begins with all four lags, and then successively reduces the model until the last lag is statistically significant. The last lag was not significant at lags 4, 3, 2, or 1, and the preferred test equation is therefore the model with no lagged differences.

The $\tau \mu$-statistic for the test, -1.83, is not enough to reject a unit root at even the 10 percent level.[8] This disagrees with our conclusion about the inflation data in Section 3.3.1 and confirms our initial impression that this is a difficult time series to model. Choosing between a unit root and a stationary model depends on whether we view the inflation rates of the 1970s as a one-time event

---

8. A time series this short does not justify use of limiting critical values, and we would usually consult more detailed tables that report critical values for the exact number of observations. The finite-sample critical values would be larger than the limiting ones, however, and would lead to the same inferences as here.

Table 3.23. UNIT ROOT TEST FOR $Infltn_t$

	$\hat{\beta}_0$	$\hat{\phi} - 1$	$\hat{\beta}_1$	$\hat{\beta}_2$	$\hat{\beta}_3$	$\hat{\beta}_4$
$k=4$	.50	−.12	.20	.01	−.22	.05
	1.28	−1.49	1.30	0.08	−1.49	0.34
$k=3$	.50	−.11	.18	.00	−.21	
	1.36	−1.55	1.28	0.02	−1.47	
$k=2$	.56	−.13	.23	−.04		
	1.57	−1.89	1.62	−0.28		
$k=1$	.53	−.13	.20			
	1.55	−1.98	1.44			
$k=0$	.51	−.12				
	1.52	−1.83				

$$\nabla Infltn_t = \beta_0 + (\phi_1 - 1) + Infltn_t + \sum \beta_k(\nabla Infltn_{t-k}) + a_t$$

or as a characteristic feature. The unit root test implicitly assumes that the large fluctuations in inflations will recur, and that they were not due to a unique set of circumstances.

More generally, very strong evidence against nonstationarity must exist before the Dickey-Fuller test will reject the unit root null hypothesis. Even for the simplest model, the Dickey-Fuller critical values are much larger than are those for the Normal or t distributions and the null will be correspondingly more difficult to reject. The differences between the Dickey-Fuller and Normal or t distributions further increase with the addition of deterministic mean and trend components.

In part due to this situation, the Dickey-Fuller test will often point toward a unit root even when other evidence indicates that a time series follows a stationary process. The test has low statistical power against nonstationarity and this is often a concern when analyzing short series. Several alternatives to the original Dickey-Fuller test, especially a variation developed by Elliott, Rothenberg, and Stock (1996), attempt to mitigate this problem. Low power is nevertheless a generic issue in unit root testing, emphasizing again that the tests are only one source of evidence about stationarity. Unit root tests avoid some of the subjectivity inherent in other approaches to identifying nonstationary time series, but they also have limitations of their own.

To take another example of the Dickey-Fuller test, Section 3.5.2 analyzed the annual incidence of tuberculosis cases in the U.S. Based on the sample ACF, we concluded that the log-transformed incidence series was nonstationary, and we fit a model to the series differences. Another possibility is that the series is trend

Table 3.24. Unit Root Test, $Ln(Tubrc_t)$

	$\hat{\beta}_0$	$\hat{\phi}-1$	$\hat{\beta}_t$	$\hat{\beta}_1$	$\hat{\beta}_2$	$\hat{\beta}_3$	$\hat{\beta}_4$
$k=4$	.51	−.10	−.01	.34	.04	.23	.08
	2.57	−2.66	−2.68	2.70	0.29	1.77	0.59
$k=3$	.47	−.10	−.00	.35	.03	0.25	
	2.57	−2.66	−2.71	2.91	0.24	2.01	

$$\nabla Ln(Tubrc_t) = \beta_0 + (\phi_1 - 1)Ln(Tubrc_t) + \beta_t(t) + \sum \beta_k \nabla Ln(Tubrc_t) + a_t$$

Table 3.25. Unit Root Test for $Infltn_t$

	$\hat{\beta}_0$	$\hat{\phi}-1$	$\hat{\beta}_1$	$\hat{\beta}_2$	$\hat{\beta}_3$	$\hat{\beta}_4$
$k=4$	−.02	−.44	−.20	−.24	−.06	−.12
	−1.83	−2.29	−1.06	−1.32	−.36	−.94
$k=3$	−.02	−.51	−.14	−.16	0.02	
	−2.13	−2.84	−.78	−1.01	0.19	
$k=2$	−.02	−.50	−.16	−.18		
	−2.15	−3.03	−1.07	−1.40		
$k=1$	−.02	−.61	−.04			
	−2.81	−4.27	−.32			
$k=0$	−.03	−.64				
	−3.19	−5.50				

$$\nabla^2 Ln(Tubrc_t) = \beta_0 + (\phi_1 - 1)\nabla Ln(Tubrc_t) + \sum \beta_k \nabla^2 Ln(Tubrc_t) + a_t$$

stationary, in which case we could have modeled it in levels after controlling for a linear trend. The plot of the log-transformed series in Figure 3.23 seems consistent with this possibility.

Table 3.24 presents a sequence of *ADF* equations, beginning as before with four lagged differences and successively reducing the model until the last lag is statistically significant. The coefficient for the final lagged difference was significant in the three-lag model, making this the preferred choice. The τt-statistic of -2.66, although easily large enough to reject H_0 with a t or Normal distribution, falls short of the Dickey-Fuller limit-critical value of -3.41. This is inconsistent with trend stationarity, and supports our decision to analyze the differenced series.

To obtain additional confirmation that the tuberculosis series is difference stationary, Table 3.25 shows the results of *ADF* tests for $\nabla Ln(Tubrc_t)$. If the test did not reject the null of a unit root for the differences, it would suggest the need for second-differencing. If we include an intercept in the test equations, none of the lagged differences (actually, here, differences of differences) are large enough to be statistically significant. The $\tau \mu$-statistic for the final model ($\tau \mu = -5.5$)

easily rejects a unit root at the 1 percent level, and so supports the conclusion that the differenced tuberculosis cases are stationary.

3.7.3 Co-integrated Processes

The time series plotted in Figure 3.35 are the monthly numbers of foreign visitors to Japan broken down by "tourists" and "all others." On March 11, 2011, a violent earthquake in eastern Japan triggered a tsunami that destroyed the Fukushima Daiichi nuclear power plant on the coast. The levels of both time series dropped immediately. Then, over the next year, both time series recovered gradually to their pre-intervention levels (Wu and Hayashi, 2013). The fact that the disaster had a nearly identical impact on the two time series might seem curious at first. Because the two time series follow roughly the same track before and after the disaster, however, their nearly identical responses to the disaster might be expected.

The nearly identical nonstationary tracks of the two time series suggest they share a common set of motivating forces or that they are *co-integrated*. To introduce this concept, suppose that the two time series can be adequately represented by first-order *IMA* models. For $Tourist_t$ and $Other_t$, that is,

$$Tourist_t - Tourist_{t-1} = a_{1,t} = \nabla Tourist_t$$
$$Other_t - Other_{t-1} = a_{2,t} = \nabla Other_t$$

Here $a_{1,t}$ and $a_{2,t}$ are the observations of two distinct white noise processes. Since the two time series are driven by their own white noise processes, they are

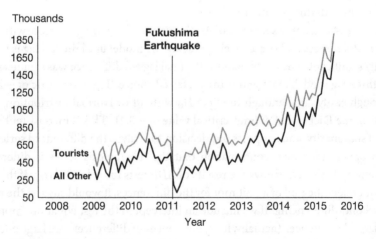

Figure 3.35 Foreign Visitors to Japan

independent—and that is the problem. Independent IMA time series will follow strikingly divergent random walk paths. Their paths would certainly cross from time to time. But for most of their joint history, the two independent *IMA* time series will be separated by a gap that occasionally grows very wide.

Murray (1994) uses the analogy of "a drunk and her dog" to illustrate the random walking behavior of two co-integrated time series. The drunk's dog waits patiently outside a bar until its owner emerges. The two then set off on random walks. Their short-run decisions to stop, go, cross the street, turn the corner, and so on are more or less unpredictable—or random—and uncoordinated. The dog might stop to sniff a weed growing up through the concrete, for example, or the drunk might stop to explore a shop window. These individual decisions—or independent random shocks—tend to separate the drunk and her dog in the short run. In the long run, however, the gap between their two paths remains small. When the gap grows too wide, the dog and/or the drunk adjust their moves to keep the gap small and manageable. The pair eventually arrives at the same place—home, presumably—but their joint arrival is a long-run phenomenon that can be imagined and inferred but *not* observed.

The theory of co-integrated processes was proposed originally by Granger (1981). To coordinate two otherwise independent *IMA* processes, Engle and Granger (1987) incorporate an *error correction mechanism* into the joint random walk model. As the gap between the drunk and her dog grows large, the error correction mechanism pulls the two back together, functioning as an elastic leash that connects the drunk's wrist and her dog's collar.

The literature on co-integrated process models is extensive and technical. Interested readers are directed to Enders (2010) or to Box-Steffensmeier et al. (2015) for accessible introductions to error correction mechanisms for co-integration models. Although there is a growing literature on modeling interventions in co-integrated time series (Johansen, Mosconi, and Nielsen, 2000; Gregory and Hansen, 1996; Gregory, Nason, and Watt, 1996), these models are relatively unimportant for our purposes. The impact of the Fukushima Daiichi disaster on the pair of tourism time series plotted in Figure 3.35 can be estimated without accounting for their co-integration.

While there is no pressing need to develop co-integrated time series models and modeling at this point, however, the causal interpretation of a time series experiment rests heavily on the *idea* of co-integration. When we discuss control time series in Chapter 7, we will argue that the *ideal* control time series is co-integrated with the treated time series. Prior to the intervention, the treated time series and its ideal control share a set of causal forces that keep the pair moving on a common path. After the intervention, the ideal control series stays on the joint pre-intervention path while the treated time series diverges. As two time series diverge, the post-intervention difference between the two can be interpreted as the causal effect of the intervention.

Before leaving this topic, it may be instructive to re-examine the visual evidence. If the intervention of interest is the Fukushima Daiichi disaster, neither of the time series plotted in Figure 3.35 could serve as a control for its mate. Although we will not report the results, this pair of tourism time series is co-integrated *before*, *after*, and *at the precise point* of the disaster. The *ideal* treated-control time series pair must be co-integrated prior to the intervention but then, due to the unique impact of the intervention on the treated time series, will follow parallel paths throughout the post-intervention period.

3.8 CONCLUSION

Box and Jenkins (1970) are widely credited with creating a general *ARIMA* model from existing specialized component models. Though less widely noted, their modeling algorithm was an equally important contribution. Following Box and Jenkins (1970, Figure 1.7), we depict their algorithm as a logical loop that iterates until it locates a "best" *ARIMA* model (Figure 3.1). Within each loop, the algorithm pauses at three decision points— *identification, estimation,* and *diagnosis*—where it waits for the analyst's input. In early iterations, the analyst's input eliminates whole subclasses of *ARIMA* models. In subsequent iterations, the algorithm compares statistically adequate *ARIMA* models on relative criteria such as parsimony and fit. Informed by the analyst's input, the algorithm eliminates statistically adequate models one by one until only the "best" *ARIMA* model remains.

Box and Jenkins (1970, p. 18) describe the *ARIMA* modeling algorithm as a "process of evolution, adaptation or trial and error." Only the fittest model survives. The evolutionary analogy is imperfect, however. Whereas Darwinian evolution works without direction from above, the *ARIMA* modeling algorithm *cannot* work without input from the analyst. Box and Jenkins (1970, p. 495) are explicit on that point:

> The computer has great speed and precision, compared with which the human mind is slow and inaccurate. However, the mind has powers of critical and inductive reasoning, relative to which, those of the present-day computer are minuscule. This makes possible a happy division of labor in which mind and machine each contributes what it does better. Models built entirely automatically by the computer without the intervention of intellectual imagination and restraint are unlikely to be very good, and could be very bad.

Although computing machines have grown exponentially more powerful and versatile, we see no need to retract this early dictum. Most time series software packages include automated modeling algorithms, and since much of the analyst's input to the algorithm consists of statistics printed out by the algorithm, bypassing the analyst may seem economical. This economy comes at the expense of the analyst's wisdom, experience, and sensitivity to subtle cues, however, and that is too steep a price to pay.

If *ARIMA* modeling could be reduced to a rigid application of a simple algorithm, neither we nor Box and Jenkins would object to automated modeling. Rigidly applied algorithms often lead to embarrassing results and missed opportunities. We intend the algorithm in Figure 3.1 to be a loose template that can and should be overridden whenever circumstances warrant. We cannot produce a list of those circumstances; indeed, compiling such a list would amount to replacing one mindless algorithm with another. We used example analyses to illustrate the range of circumstances, and that is the best that we can do.

Each of our example analyses began with a visual inspection of the time series, and that should always be the first step. Visual impressions can be deceiving, even seductive. Hypothetical impacts are not always apparent and visually apparent impacts can arise through an interaction of poorly chosen axis scales and wishful thinking. Nevertheless, visual evidence can suggest the structure of an underlying process. Does the process trend? Is it heteroskedastic? Is it seasonal? Does it generate sporadic "outliers"? If the visual evidence is ambiguous on any of these questions, it can be ignored. Visual evidence should be suggestive and confirmatory but never conclusive. On the other hand, a visual inspection of the time series prior to identification can save hours of frustrating work.

The second step is an investigation of the Normality assumption. If the time series satisfies a high-power goodness-of-fit test, such as a *KS* test, the Normality assumption is plausible. Otherwise, the investigation requires a Box-Cox function defined as

$$Y_t^{(\lambda)} = \frac{Y^\lambda - 1}{\lambda}$$

Most—but *not* all—time series can be made Normal with one of the transformations included in the Box-Cox function. Time series that are made non-Normal by "outliers," for example, are not good candidates for transformation. This reinforces the value of a visual inspection of the time series.

Following a visual inspection of the time series, the variance of $Y_t^{(\lambda)}$ can be plotted against a range of λ-values to see where the Box-Cox function turns. Since the turning point—the "best" value of λ— is usually unknown, finding a proper range of λ-values and locating the minimum value requires several approximations.

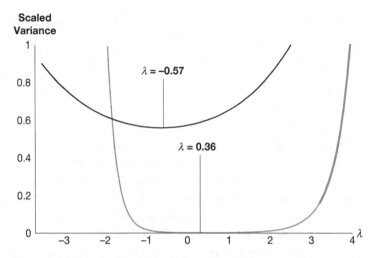

Figure 3.36 Box-Cox Functions for Two Time Series

The visual appearance of the Box-Cox function varies widely across time series for several reasons. To illustrate, Figure 3.36 plots $Y_t^{(\lambda)}$ for the European wheat price time series (Chapter 3.4.1) and the Zurich sunspot time series (Chapter 3.4.2) on a common axis. In addition to their different ranges of λ-values and horizontal incepts, the two Box-Cox functions have very different shapes. The function for the European wheat price time series turns at $\lambda \approx -0.57$ and the inflection point is pronounced. The function for the Zurich sunspot time series turns at $\lambda \approx 0.36$ but the inflection point is imperceptible. There is no simple explanation for the distinctively different shapes of these two Box-Cox functions. Nor is any explanation needed. Regardless of how regular or irregular the function's appearance, if the function has a unique inflection point, it has located the "best" transformation.

The slope of the Box-Cox function on either side of the "best" transformation conveys another useful piece of information. For the European wheat price time series, the Box-Cox function is more or less flat in the segment

$$-0.8 < \lambda < -0.4$$

None of the λ-values in this segment is statistically different than the "best" value of $\lambda \approx -0.57$. On practical and aesthetic grounds, we prefer $\lambda = -0.5$ for the transformation. Likewise, for the Zurich sunspot time series, the Box-Cox function is flat in the segment

$$0.25 < \lambda < 0.5$$

So again, on practical and aesthetic grounds, $\lambda = 0.5$ is the preferred transformation. We revisit this issue in Chapter 5. For now, as a general rule, the simplest transformation that produces a Normal time series is preferred.

Transformations are *always* the first step of any analysis. Following a full Box-Cox analysis, the time series Y_t is either stationary in variance or has been tranformed into the time series Z_t.

$$Z_t = Y_t^\lambda$$

If Y_t is already stationary in variance, of course, then $\lambda = 1$ and $Z_t = Y_t$. But in either case, Z_t is stationary in variance, ready to be modeled.

In its first iteration, the *ARIMA* modeling algorithm (Figure 3.1) determines whether Z_t should be differenced. Visual evidence can inform this decision. A "flat" time series suggests a stationary process, for example, while trend or drift suggests the opposite. Statistical evidence from the *ACF* and the *PACF* should be consulted and weighed. The visual and statistical evidence will identify one specific difference equation in many but not all cases. The Canadian inflation time series (Figure 3.3.1a) illustrates the rare case where the identification is ambiguous. The visual and statistical evidence for that time series was consistent with both a difference equation model and an *AR1* model. Although the *AR1* model was selected on several grounds, there was little difference between the two models. Another analyst might have selected the difference equation model with no substantive consequences.

Seasonal processes are relatively common in the social sciences and many are nonstationary. A comparison of the example time series that we used to demonstrate seasonal models illustrates subtle differences in seasonality. The "best" *ARIMA* model for the Anchorage monthly precipitation time series (Chapter 3.6.1) used 12th-order differencing after a transformation:

$$\nabla^{12} Prcp_t^{1/4} = (1 - 0.86B^{12})a_t$$

The "best" *ARIMA* model for the monthly atmospheric CO_2 time series (Chapter 3.6.2) used first- and 12th-order differencing but no transformation:

$$\nabla\nabla^{12} CO2_t = 0.01 + (1 - 0.32B - 0.63B^{12})a_t$$

And the "best" *ARIMA* model for the quarterly Australian traffic fatality time series (Chapter 3.6.3) used first-order differencing after a transformation:

$$\nabla AuFtl_t^{1/2} = 0.06 + (1 - 0.83B - 0.29B^3 + 0.32B^4)a_t$$

Although we will introduce other seasonal time series in Chapter 5, a careful study of these three examples will demonstrate the variety of modeling decisions presented by seasonal time series.

If it is not apparent, our approach to seasonal *ARIMA* modeling emphasizes parsimony at the expense of effort and uniformity. To illustrate our approach, experience demonstrates that the so-called airline model (Box and Jenkins, 1970, p. 305)

$$\nabla \nabla^{12} Z_t = \theta_0 + (1 - \theta_1 B)(1 - \theta_{12} B^{12}) a_t$$

is statistically adequate for most monthly time series. We considered the airline model for the monthly atmospheric CO_2 time series but rejected it in favor of a simpler linear model that fit the time series better—though not by much. The incrementally better fit of this model outweighed the advantages of using a better-known model.

Our approach does not sacrifice theoretical concerns, however. We dropped the statistically insignificant constant parameter from our model of the Anchorage monthly precipitation time series, for example, because in theory precipitation has no long-range secular trend. For want of a better term, this time series drifts seasonally. We did not drop the statistically insignificant constant from our model of atmospheric CO_2, on the other hand, because in theory this time series has an upward secular trend. Theory trumps parsimony in this case.

Finally, as it applies to the use of auxiliary modeling statistics, our approach is pragmatic and sensible. In our experience, Dickey-Fuller tests provide little information beyond the information that can be gleaned from a visual inspection of the time series and a reading of its *ACF*. Modeling decisions should not be based exclusively on any single piece of information. This is particularly true for short time series. With that said, in our experience, Dickey-Fuller tests, visual evidence, and readings of the *ACF* generally lead to identical modeling decisions. Our opinions of the use of the *AIC* and the *BIC* are similar. In a sense, these information criteria balance model fit and parsimony, which is what the *ARIMA* modeling algorithm aims to do. Of these two information criteria, the *BIC* is preferred. We will make use of the *BIC* in later chapters.

APPENDIX 3A MAXIMUM LIKELIHOOD ESTIMATION

The most popular methods for estimating *ARIMA* model parameters involve maximum likelihood principles. In its simplest, purest form, maximum likelihood estimation of an *ARIMA* model parameter assumes that each of the white noise shocks $a_1, \ldots, a_N$ is drawn from the same Normal population with the probability density function,

$$f(a_t) = \frac{1}{\sqrt{2\pi \sigma_a^2}} e^{-\frac{1}{2\sigma_a^2} a_t^2}$$

Using the multiplication rule for independent events, the joint density of $a_1, \ldots, a_N$ is the product of the individual densities. Thus,

$$f(a_1, \ldots, a_N) = \frac{1}{\sqrt{2\pi\sigma_a^2}} e^{-\frac{1}{2\sigma_a^2} a_1^2} \times \cdots \times \frac{1}{\sqrt{2\pi\sigma_a^2}} e^{-\frac{1}{2\sigma_a^2} a_N^2}$$

Rearranging the terms on the right-hand side of this expression,

$$f(a_1, \ldots, a_N) = \left[\frac{1}{\sqrt{2\pi\sigma_a^2}} \times \cdots \times \frac{1}{\sqrt{2\pi\sigma_a^2}} \right] \left[e^{-\frac{1}{2\sigma_a^2} a_1^2} \times \cdots \times e^{-\frac{1}{2\sigma_a^2} a_N^2} \right]$$

and applying the law of exponents,

$$f(a_1, \ldots, a_N) = \left(\frac{1}{\sqrt{2\pi\sigma_a^2}} \right)^N e^{\left(-\frac{1}{2\sigma_a^2} a_1^2 - \cdots - \frac{1}{2\sigma_a^2} a_N^2 \right)}$$

$$= \left(\frac{1}{\sqrt{2\pi\sigma_a^2}} \right)^N e^{\left(-\frac{1}{2\sigma_a^2} \sum_{t=1}^{N} a_t^2 \right)}$$

The right-hand side of this expression is a version of the *likelihood function* from which *maximum likelihood estimates* of *ARIMA* model parameters are derived.[9] To simplify this function, we take the natural logarithm of both sides.

$$Ln[f(a_1, \ldots, a_N)] = NLn\left(\frac{1}{\sqrt{2\pi\sigma_a^2}} \right) - \frac{1}{2\sigma_a^2} \sum_{t=1}^{N} a_t^2$$

The resulting *log-likelihood function* is the sum of two components. The first is a constant (or intercept) that shifts the function up or down without changing its shape. Dropping this constant and renaming the left-hand side yields a more useful form of the log-likelihood function,

$$LL(\text{parameters}) = -\frac{1}{2\sigma_a^2} \sum_{t=1}^{N} a_t^2$$

The function's new name, *LL*(parameters), acknowledges the explicit relationship between a set of unknown *ARIMA* parameters and the log-likelihood function. Each set of parameter values yields a value of the function. The values

9. The factors on the right-hand side are *densities*, not *probabilities*. Pawitan (2013, p. v.): "Fisher coined the term 'likelihood' in 1921 to distinguish the method of maximum likelihood from the Bayesian or inverse probability argument."

that *maximize* the log-likelihood function are the *maximum likelihood estimates* of the parameters.

For a long time series, maximum likelihood parameter estimates have most of the statistical properties that we like to see in an estimate. Note that with its sign reversed, the log-likelihood function is identical to the sum-of-squares function. That is,

$$SSQ(\text{parameters}) \equiv -LL(\text{parameters}) = \frac{1}{2\sigma^2} \sum_{t=1}^{N} a_t^2$$

The maximum likelihood estimates obtained by maximizing $LL(\text{parameters})$ then are identical to the least-squares estimates obtained by *minimizing* $SSQ(\text{parameters})$. This identity implies that maximum likelihood estimates have least-squares properties and vice versa.

The maximum likelihood estimation algorithm begins by substituting model parameters for a_t in the log-likelihood function. To illustrate this substitution for AR models, consider the $AR1$ model of pediatric trauma admissions reported as Model 1 in Table 3.6. For Model 1, the relationship between a_t and parameters μ and ϕ_1 is

$$a_t = (Admit_t - \mu) - \phi_1(Admit_{t-1} - \mu)$$

Then, by substitution,

$$LL(\mu, \phi_1, \sigma_a^2) = -\frac{1}{2\sigma_a^2} \sum_{t=2}^{130} [(Admit_t - \mu) - \phi_1(Admit_{t-1} - \mu)]^2$$

Note that the index of the summation operator begins with $t = 2$. Due to the lagged observation in the $AR1$ model, the first observation of the time series is lost.

After substituting the $AR1$ model parameters for a_t in $LL(\mu, \phi_1, \sigma_a^2)$, we evaluate the function over a range of parameter values. To simplify our evaluation, we use the value of $RSE = 7.47$, reported in Table 3.6, as an estimate of σ_a. Since $\hat{\sigma}_a = 7.47$,

$$-\frac{1}{2\hat{\sigma}_a^2} = -\frac{1}{2(7.46)^2} = -0.009$$

Substituting this result into the log-likelihood function,

$$LL(\hat{\phi}_1, \hat{\mu} | \hat{\sigma}_a = 7.46) = -0.009 \sum_{t=2}^{130} [(Admit_t - \mu) - \phi_1(Admit_{t-1} - \mu)]^2$$

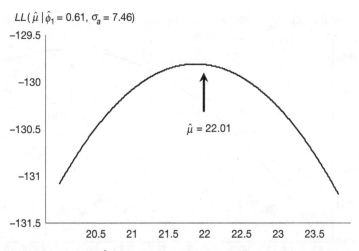

Figure 3.37 $LL(\hat{\mu}|\hat{\phi}_1 = 0.61, \hat{\sigma}_a^2 = 7.47)$ for an AR1 Model of $Admit_t$

Figure 3.37 plots a two-dimensional slice of the three-dimensional log-likelihood function made perpendicular to the $\hat{\mu}$-axis at $\hat{\phi}_1 = 0.61.^{[10]}$ In two dimensions, $LL(\hat{\mu}|\hat{\phi}_1 = 0.61, \hat{\sigma}_a = 7.46)$ is a parabola whose axis of symmetry lies at the maximum likelihood estimate, $\hat{\mu} = 22.01$. Figure 3.38 plots a "slice" made perpendicular to the $\hat{\phi}_1$-axis at $\hat{\mu} = 22.01$. Although $LL(\hat{\phi}_1|\hat{\mu} = 22.01, \hat{\sigma}_a = 7.46)$ is plotted only over the $-1 < \hat{\phi}_1 < +1$ segment—we have no interest in non-invertible values of $\hat{\phi}_1$—this function too is a parabola whose axis of symmetry runs perpendicular to and crosses the $\hat{\phi}_1$-axis at the maximum likelihood estimate $\hat{\phi}_1 = 0.61$. In both cases, the maximum likelihood parameter estimates maximize the log-likelihood function.

Executing the maximum likelihood estimation algorithm for *MA* parameters requires some ingenuity. To illustrate, consider the *MA*1 model of the British GDP time series reported as Model 1 in Table 3.5.

$$UKGDP_t = \theta_0 + a_t - \theta_1 a_{t-1} = \theta_0 + (1 - \theta_1 B) a_t$$

Solving for a_t

$$a_t = \frac{UKGDP_t - \theta_0}{1 - \theta_1 B}$$

10. This two-dimensional slice, or "profile likelihood function," treats σ_a^2 as a nuisance parameter—which, in this instance, it certainly is. See Pawitan (2013, pp. 62-63) for a more complete discussion of nuisance parameters and the methods used to eliminate them

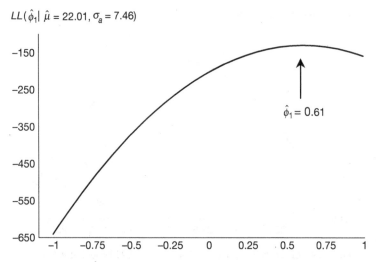

Figure 3.38 $LL(\hat{\phi}_1|\hat{\mu} = 22.01, \hat{\sigma}_a^2 = 7.47)$ for an AR1 Model of $Admit_t$

The MA1 operator in the denominator of the right-hand side term has the series identity

$$(1 - \theta_1 B)^{-1} = \sum_{k=0}^{\infty} \theta_1^k B^k$$

So by substitution

$$a_t = \sum_{k=0}^{\infty} \theta_1^k B^k (UKGDP_t - \theta_0) = \sum_{k=0}^{\infty} \theta_1^k B^k UKGDP_t - \sum_{k=0}^{\infty} \theta_1^k B^k \theta_0$$

Since θ_0 is a constant, the second term on the right-hand side is

$$\sum_{k=0}^{\infty} \theta_1^k B^k \theta_0 = \frac{\theta_0}{1 - \theta_1} \equiv \mu$$

So

$$a_t = \sum_{k=0}^{\infty} \theta_1^k B^k UKGDP_t - \frac{\theta_0}{1 - \theta_1}$$

Substituting the right-hand side into the log-likelihood function,

$$LL(\hat{\theta}_0, \hat{\theta}_1, \hat{\sigma}_a^2) = -\frac{1}{2\sigma_a^2} \left(\sum_{k=0}^{\infty} \theta_1^k B^k UKGDP_t - \frac{\theta_0}{1 - \theta_1} \right)^2$$

To simplify our evaluation, we use the value of $RSE = 2.74$, reported in Table 3.5, to estimate σ_a:

$$-\frac{1}{2\hat{\sigma}_a^2} = -\frac{1}{2(2.74)^2} = -0.066$$

So

$$LL(\theta_0, \theta_1) = -0.066 \left(\sum_{k=0}^{\infty} \theta_1^k B^k UKGDP_t - \frac{\theta_0}{1-\theta_1} \right)^2$$

Figure 3.39 plots a two-dimensional "slice" of the log-likelihood function perpendicular to the $\hat{\theta}_0$-axis at $\hat{\theta}_1 = -0.22$. $LL(\hat{\theta}_0 | \hat{\theta}_1 = -0.22, \hat{\sigma}_a = 2.74)$ is a parabola whose axis of symmetry lies at the maximum likelihood estimate, $\hat{\theta}_0 = 1.46$. Figure 3.40 plots a "slice" of the log-likelihood function made perpendicular to the $\hat{\theta}_1$-axis at $\hat{\theta}_0 = 1.46$. This log-likelihood function has a different appearance than any that we have seen so far. Although it has a peak or mode at $\hat{\theta}_1 = -0.22$, this log-likelihood function is relatively flat at its peak. The shape of this log-likelihood function is due in part to the structure of the model—MA log-likelihood functions have this typical flattened shape—and in part to the nature of this particular time series.

Although visual inspection of a log-likelihood function can be helpful, finding the maximum likelihood estimates of $ARIMA$ parameters requires calculus methods. The $AR1$ log-likelihood function for the pediatric trauma admissions

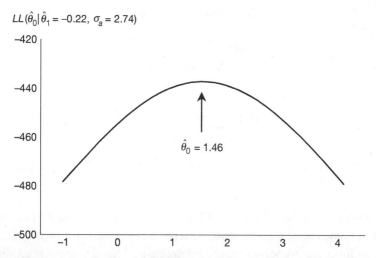

Figure 3.39 $LL(\hat{\theta}_0 | \hat{\theta}_1 = -0.22, \hat{\sigma}_a^2 = 2.74)$ for an $MA1$ Model of $UKGDP_t$

$LL(\hat{\theta}_1 | \hat{\theta}_0 = 1.46, \sigma_a = 2.74)$

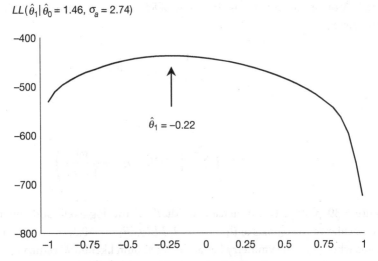

Figure 3.40 $LL(\hat{\theta}_1 | \hat{\theta}_0 = 1.46, \hat{\sigma}_a^2 = 2.74)$ for an MA1 Model of $UKGDP_t$

time series is

$$LL(\hat{\mu}, \hat{\phi}_1) = \sum_{t=2}^{130} [(Admit_t - \mu) - \phi_1(Admit_{t-1} - \mu)]^2$$

Differentiating the log-likelihood with respect to μ and ϕ_1 yields the "score" function, $S(\mu)$.

$$\frac{\partial LL(\hat{\mu}, \hat{\phi})}{\partial \hat{\mu}} = 2(\phi_1 - 1) \sum_{t=2}^{130} [(Admit_t - \mu) - \phi_1(Admit_{t-1} - \mu)]$$

$$\frac{\partial LL(\hat{\mu}, \hat{\phi})}{\partial \hat{\mu}} = 2(\phi_1 - 1) \left[\sum_{t=2}^{130} Admit_t - N\mu \right]$$

$$-2(\phi_1^2 - \phi_1) \left[\sum_{t=2}^{130} Admit_{t-1} - N\mu \right]$$

$$\frac{\partial LL(\hat{\mu}, \hat{\phi})}{\partial \hat{\phi}} = -2(Admit_{t-1} - \mu) \sum_{t=2}^{130} [(Admit_t - \mu) - \phi_1(Admit_{t-1} - \mu)]$$

First derivatives of the log-likelihood functions for the white noise, AR1 and MA1 models, known as "score" functions, are reported in Table 3.26.

Score functions are solved for the maximum likelihood parameter estimates. The simplest, non-trivial model illustrates the nuts and bolts of this procedure.

Table 3.26. ARMA MODEL SCORE FUNCTIONS

White Noise $\quad S(\mu) = -\dfrac{1}{\sigma_a^2} \left(\sum_{t=1}^{N} a_t - N\mu \right)$

AR1 $\quad S(\phi_1, \mu) = -\dfrac{1}{\sigma_a^2} \left(\sum_{t=1}^{N} Y_t + N\mu + \phi_1 \sum_{t=1}^{N} Y_{t-1} - \phi_1 N\mu \right)$

MA1 $\quad S(\theta_1, \mu) = -\dfrac{1}{\sigma_a^2} \left(\sum_{t=1}^{N} Y_t - N\mu - 2\theta_1 \sum_{t=1}^{N} a_{t-1} \right)$

For the white noise model,

$$S(\mu) = -\frac{1}{\sigma_a^2} \sum_{t=1}^{N} a_t - N\mu = 0$$

so

$$\hat{\mu} = \frac{\sum_{t=1}^{N} a_t}{N}$$

The shape of $S(\mu)$ provides a measure of dispersion about the maximum likelihood estimate. Taking the second derivative of the white noise log-likelihood function with respect to $\hat{\mu}$,

$$\frac{\partial^2 LL(\hat{\mu})}{\partial LL(\hat{\mu})^2} = -\frac{N}{\sigma_a^2}$$

This quantity is the "Fisher information" for $\hat{\mu}$. Using $I(\hat{\mu})$ to represent the Fisher information,

$$-I(\hat{\mu})^{-\frac{1}{2}} = \frac{\sigma_a}{\sqrt{N}}$$

which is the standard error of the maximum likelihood estimate.

Some authors divide $LL(\mu)$ by its maximum value to facilitate interpretation of the plotted function. Although this same "trick" might be used to create likelihoods that sum to unity, the resulting "probabilities" would lack some of the most important properties of likelihoods. Ultimately, likelihoods are *not* probabilities and readers should remember that.

It is also important to understand that maximum likelihood estimates offer no obvious degree of control for the common threats to statistical conclusion validity. In particular, when maximum likelihood parameter estimates are used to test null hypotheses, the common threats to statistical conclusion validity associated with p-values are still plausible. We revisit this point in Chapter 6. Readers who are interested in learning more about likelihood are directed to Edwards (1972) for an original development of the underlying theory and to Pawitan (2013) for a large and well-organized collection of illustrative applications.

APPENDIX 3B THE BOX-COX TRANSFORMATION FUNCTION

The *ARIMA* modeling strategy assumes that Y_t is a function of a Gaussian (or Normal) a_t. When this assumption is unwarranted, transformations of Y_t almost always yield a Z_t that satisfies Normality. Useful transformations for that purpose include the powers, roots, reciprocals, and logarithms of Y_t. Choosing the "best" transformation for a particular Y_t may involve aesthetic and/or pragmatic considerations. See Kmenta (1986, pp. 517-521) for an accessible, excellent development of this topic.

Lacking theoretical guidance, two analysts can reasonably disagree on whether a particular Y_t needs transformation and, if so, what the most appropriate transformation might be. Box and Cox (1964) proposed a theory of transformations that answers many of the questions that might be posed and that directs the search for an appropriate transformation. Every Box-Cox transformation is generated by the function

$$Y_t^{(\lambda)} = \frac{Y_t^{\lambda} - 1}{\lambda} \text{ for } \lambda \neq 0; \ Y_t^{(\lambda)} = Ln(Y_t) \quad \text{for} \quad \lambda = 0$$

where λ is a rational number. If it is not obvious, $Y_t^{(\lambda)}$ generates all of the better-known transformations. Ignoring the constant terms, for example, $Y_t^{(\lambda=1)}$ leaves Y_t untransformed; $Y_t^{(\lambda=-1)}$ returns the reciprocal, $1/Y_t$; $Y_t^{(\lambda=2)}$ and $Y_t^{(\lambda=1/2)}$ return the square and square root of Y_t respectively.

The utility of the Box-Cox transformation function lies in the fact that its single parameter, λ, generates all of the common, useful transformations. Finding the "best" transformation then reduces to finding the "best" λ-value, which amounts, ordinarily, to plotting Box-Cox functions as we did throughout this chapter. Before demonstrating the method used to generate these plots, however, we explain two structural features of the Box-Cox function that may seem odd, curious, unnecessary, or problematic.

First, dividing $Y_t^{\lambda} - 1$ by λ seems unnecessary and, worse, would seem to cause problems when $\lambda = 0$. Division by λ is required to ensure that Y_t^{λ} is a *monotonic* function of Y_t. To demonstrate this crucial property, consider a time series of three numbers: $Y_1 = 1$, $Y_2 = 2$, and $Y_3 = 3$. The three observations of Y_t have a definite order:

$$Y_1 < Y_2 < Y_3$$

A monotonic transformation *preserves* this order. When $\lambda > 0$, $(Y_t)^\lambda$ is a monotonic transformation. Let $\lambda = 2$, for example:

$$(1^2 = 1) < (2^2 = 4) < (3^2 = 9)$$

The simple power function maintains the original order of the observations. When $\lambda < 0$, however, $(Y_t)^\lambda$ is no longer a monotonic transformation. When $\lambda = -2$, for example, $(Y_t)^\lambda$ reverses the original order of the observations:

$$\left(1^{-2} = \frac{1}{1^2} = 1\right) > \left(2^{-2} = \frac{1}{2^2} = \frac{1}{4}\right) > \left(3^{-2} = \frac{1}{3^2} = \frac{1}{9}\right)$$

If we divide $(Y_t)^\lambda$ by λ, however, the original order of the observations is preserved:

$$\left(\frac{1^{-2}}{-2} = -\frac{1}{2}\right) < \left(\frac{2^{-2}}{-2} = -\frac{1}{8}\right) < \left(\frac{3^{-2}}{-2} = -\frac{1}{18}\right)$$

Division by λ ensures that $Y_t^{(\lambda)}$ is a *monotonic* transformation. Lacking this property, the Box-Cox functions used in this chapter would be more difficult to generate and interpret. Once the "best" value of λ is found, of course, simpler power, root, reciprocal, and log transformations should be used. We use $Y_t^{(\lambda)}$ only to find a "best" transformation.

The second feature of $Y_t^{(\lambda)}$ that may seem unnecessary is the numerator term, $Y_t^\lambda - 1$. Why not just Y_t^λ? Though not obvious, $Y_t^\lambda - 1$ is required if $Y_t^{(\lambda=0)}$ is to return the natural logarithm, $Ln(Y_t)$. Although on the face of it, $Y_t^{(\lambda=0)}$ involves division by zero, a little manipulation proves the limiting identity of $Y_t^{(\lambda=0)}$ and $Ln(Y_t)$. Begin by rewriting Y_t^λ as the identity

$$Y_t^\lambda = e^{Ln(Y_t^\lambda)}$$

The right-hand side of this expression can be expanded as the MacLaurin series

$$e^{Ln(Y_t^\lambda)} = \sum_{j=0}^{\infty} \frac{[Ln(Y_t^\lambda)]^j}{j} = 1 + Ln(Y_t^\lambda) + \frac{[Ln(Y_t^\lambda)]^2}{2} + \frac{[Ln(Y_t^\lambda)]^3}{6} + \cdots$$

Equating Y_t^λ and this series,

$$Y_t^\lambda = 1 + Ln(Y_t^\lambda) + \frac{[Ln(Y_t^\lambda)]^2}{2} + \frac{[Ln(Y_t^\lambda)]^3}{6} + \cdots$$

Subtract one from each side of the expression:

$$Y_t^\lambda - 1 = Ln(Y_t^\lambda) + \frac{[Ln(Y_t^\lambda)]^2}{2} + \frac{[Ln(Y_t^\lambda)]^3}{6} + \cdots$$

Rewrite $Ln(Y_t^\lambda)$ as $\lambda Ln(Y_t)$ and simplify:

$$Y_t^\lambda - 1 = \lambda Ln(Y_t) + \frac{[\lambda Ln(Y_t)]^2}{2} + \frac{[\lambda Ln(Y_t)]^3}{6} + \cdots$$

$$= \lambda Ln(Y_t) + \frac{\lambda^2 Ln(Y_t)}{2} + \frac{\lambda^3 Ln(Y_t)}{6} + \cdots$$

Then divide by λ.

$$\frac{Y_t^\lambda - 1}{\lambda} = Ln(Y_t) + \lambda \frac{Ln(Y_t)}{2} + \lambda^2 \frac{Ln(Y_t)}{6} + \cdots$$

As λ grows smaller, only the first right-hand-side term remains constant. All of the other right-hand-side terms approach zero, so we substitute that value for these terms:

$$\lim_{\lambda \to 0} \frac{Y_t^\lambda - 1}{\lambda} = Ln(Y_t)$$

In practice, of course, when $Y_t^{(\lambda=0)}$ is the "best" transformation—the meaning of "best" will be made clear shortly—we simply take the natural logarithm of Y_t. Again, $Y_t^{(\lambda)}$ is used only to find a "best" transformation.

Because the transformation is motivated by the Normality assumption, the "best" transformation corresponds to the maximum likelihood estimate of λ derived from the Normal likelihood function:

$$L(\lambda) = (\lambda - 1) \sum_{t=1}^{N} Ln(Y_t) - \frac{1}{2\sigma_Y^2} \sum_{t=1}^{N} \left(\frac{Y^\lambda - 1}{\lambda} \right)^2$$

We developed maximum likelihood estimation methods in Appendix 3A for *ARMA* parameters. We do not recommend formal maximum likelihood methods for estimating λ, however. Spitzer (1982) gives an algorithm for deriving $\hat{\lambda}$ from $L(\lambda)$. But unless the standard errors of $\hat{\lambda}$ are needed—to test $\hat{\lambda}$ for statistical significance, for example—that is overkill. This simpler method is preferred in practice.

First, compute the geometric mean of Y_t:

$$\mu_{g(Y)} = \sqrt[N]{\prod_{t=1}^{N} Y_t}, \qquad Y_t \neq 0$$

Second, scale Y_t by its geometric mean:

$$Z_t = \frac{Y_t}{\mu_{g(Y)}}$$

This "trick" simplifies $L(\lambda)$ considerably. Ignoring constant terms, $L(\lambda)$ for Z_t is

$$L(\lambda \text{ for } Z_t) = -\sum_{t=1}^{N} \left(\frac{Z^\lambda - 1}{\lambda} \right)^2$$

which is minus the sum of squares function. The "best" value of λ coincides with the maximum value of $L(\lambda \text{ for } Z_t)$ or, alternatively, with the minimum value of the variance of Z_t. All of the Box-Cox transformation functions plotted in this chapter used this simple method.

Pawitan (2013, p. 102) derives the Box-Cox likelihood functions and discusses their use and interpretation. "Flat" Box-Cox likelihood functions can be difficult to interpret. In general, a "flat" likelihood function suggests uncertainty—that the time series holds little or no information about the value of its mean. The high degree of uncertainty can be particularly troublesome when the likelihood function is centered about $\lambda = 1$. The likelihood functions plotted in Figure 3.36 illustrate the general problem. One of the likelihood functions is nearly ideal. The other is less than ideal and more difficult to interpret. Since its center is a reasonable distance from $\lambda = 1$, we interpret the function to support the value of $\lambda \approx 0.5$.

It would be a mistake to assume that *all* time series can be made Normal by a Box-Cox transformation. Time series that cannot be made Normal with a Box-Cox transformation are exceedingly rare in our experience, however.

4

Forecasting

In view of the record of forecasters, it hardly needs to be argued that it would be better to shun forecasting and rely instead on as prompt an evaluation of the current situation as possible.

—Friedman (1948)

Business is not that interested in forecasts. They use them a bit like wallpaper, you know, to feel respectable.

—Evans (1999)

Forecasting may be the most widely used (and abused) application of *ARIMA* modeling. *ARIMA* models perform only to their limits and, depending on model structure, forecasts tend to be reliable only in the short-run. Long-range forecasts are often unreliable and, worse, trivial. In forecasting and most other applications, knowledge of models and modeling is no substitute for substantive knowledge. It takes a canny arbitrageur less time to learn the mechanics of *ARIMA* modeling than it takes a bright student to learn the intricacies of markets and trading. This is a word to the wise.

In this chapter, we introduce the principles of forecasting to expand on concepts developed in the preceding chapters and, to a lesser extent, to set the stage for concepts yet to be introduced. To motivate our development of forecasting, write out the realization string explicitly as:

$$\ldots Y_{-m}, \ldots, Y_0, [Y_1, \ldots Y_N], Y_{N+1}, \ldots, Y_m \ldots$$

The string is fully determined by mean and covariance, μ_Y and γ_k—which we now call the process *information*. Modeling aims at estimating μ_Y and γ_k from the observed string, $Y_1, \ldots Y_N$—which we now call the process *history*. Since $\ldots Y_{-m}, \ldots, Y_0$ is unobserved and because $Y_{N+1}, \ldots, Y_m \ldots$ lie in the future, this is not entirely accurate. For accuracy's sake, $\ldots Y_{-m}, \ldots, Y_0$ and $Y_1, \ldots, Y_N$ might be called, respectively, the *unobserved* and *observed* parts of the process history. In any event, the history–information relationship is analogous to the process–realization relationship. Process information is estimated from process history.

A forecast uses the process information to find the expected values of future realizations, $Y_{N+1}, Y_{N+2} \ldots$. Process information is estimated from process history, and the information is then extrapolated into the future. Implicit in forecasting are the assumptions that the process information has been correctly estimated, and that the process will continue to operate in the future as it has in the past. Both assumptions are obviously more reasonable in some situations than in others, but they are assumptions that the forecaster must always be willing to make.

There are two ways in which process information may be used to generate a forecast of the ℓth future observation, denoted $Y_{N+\ell}$. One may base the forecast on the unconditional expected value of the process, $E(Y_{N+\ell})$, or one may use the expected value conditional on process history, $E(Y_{N+\ell} \mid Y_N)$. The unconditional expected value ignores information that might be gleaned from γ_k; forecasts are based on the information provided by μ. Since unconditional forecasts do not use the process information optimally, they are generally of limited value. The information of an *MA*1 process, for example, includes μ and θ_1. Taking unconditional expected values of the *MA*1 process for Y_{N+1}, however,

$$E(Y_{N+1}) = \mu + E(a_{N+1}) + \theta_1 E(a_N) = \mu$$

The information contained in θ_1 is lost, and the unconditional forecast of Y_{N+1} will be the process mean, μ. This result holds in general. Solving the most general *ARIMA* model for $Y_{N+\ell}$,

$$Y_{N+\ell} = \mu + \phi(B)^{-1} \nabla^{-d} \theta(B)^{-1} a_{N+\ell} \qquad \text{so}$$
$$E(Y_{N+\ell}) = \mu + \phi(B)^{-1} \nabla^{-d} \theta(B)^{-1} E(a_{N+\ell}) = \mu$$

The unconditional forecast for each and every future value of an *ARIMA* process will always be the process mean (or trend parameter, if the process is nonstationary in level). This outcome is due to the fact that unconditional forecasts ignore the information supplied by past shocks. Each shock in the history of the series is expected to be zero, and unconditional forecasts are based on these expected shocks. Most actual shocks will not be zero, of course, and therein lies the major limitation of unconditional forecasting.

In contrast, forecasts based on the conditional expected value use the information of both μ and γ_k. For the $MA1$ process, Y_N is known and

$$a_N = Y_N + \theta_1 a_{N-1} - \mu$$

so by substitution,

$$Y_{N+1} = \mu + a_{N+1} - \theta_1(Y_N + \theta_1 a_{N-1} - \mu)$$
$$= (1 + \theta_1)\mu + a_{N+1} - \theta_1 Y_N + \theta_1^2 a_{N-1}$$

Then by backward substitution,

$$Y_{N+1} = \sum_0^N \theta_1^k \mu + a_{N+1} - \sum_0^N \theta_1^k Y_{N-k+1} + \theta_1^{N+1} a_0 \text{ and}$$

$$E(Y_{N+1} \mid Y_N) = \sum_0^N \theta_1^k \mu + Ea_{N+1} - \sum_0^N \theta^k Y_{N-k+1} + \theta^{N+1} a_0$$

$$Y_{N+1} = \sum_0^N \theta_1^k \mu - \sum_0^N \theta_1^k Y_{N-k+1} + \theta_1^{N+1} a_0$$

Since this conditional expected value of Y_{N+1} uses the process information contained in θ_1, it seems intuitively plausible that it provides a "better" forecast than the unconditional expected value. In fact, we show in the next section that the conditional expected value is the "best" univariate forecast possible.

The conditional forecast will generally be a power series of the history of Y, estimated from $Y_1, \ldots, Y_N$, plus the expected value of future shocks, $a_{N+1}, \ldots, a_{N+\ell}$. As the forecast horizon, ℓ, grows larger, then, the known values of $Y_1, \ldots, Y_N$ weigh smaller and smaller in the conditional forecast. The forecast will eventually be dominated by the future shocks, $a_{N+1}, \ldots, a_{N+\ell}$, which are unknown, and the conditional and unconditional forecasts will become identical. It is for this reason that even the "best" univariate forecasts become trivial in the long run.

4.1 "BEST" UNIVARIATE FORECASTS

In the preceding section we claimed that the "best" forecast of an $ARIMA$ process is given by the conditional expected value, $E(Y_{N+\ell} \mid Y_N)$. Obviously, there are many possible ways to define "best" (see Granger and Newbold, 1977, Chapter 4). For most purposes, however, a reasonable definition is that the "best" forecast will be the one that minimizes mean square forecast error (*MSFE*), defined as

$$MSFE = E[Y_{N+\ell} - Y_{N(\ell)}]^2$$

where $Y_{N+\ell}$ is the actual value of the series at time $N + \ell$, and $Y_{N(\ell)}$ is the value that has been forecasted. By this definition, then, the "best" forecast will be the one that produces squared forecast errors with the smallest possible expected values.

In this and the following sections, the exposition will be considerably simplified by assuming that $\mu = 0$, or, alternatively, that μ has been subtracted from each realization. No loss of generality is involved in this assumption, since $Y_t + \mu$ can be substituted in all expressions involving Y_t.

It is easy to demonstrate that the conditional expected value satisfies the requirement of minimum mean square forecast error. To do this, we first solve the general *ARIMA* model for its shocks; this involves writing the model as an *MA* process of infinite order:

$$Y_N = \theta(B)\phi(B)^{-1}\nabla^{-d}a_N$$

Evaluating the inverse operators as infinite series, this is

$$Y_N = a_N + \psi_1 a_{N-1} + \psi_2 a_{N-2} + \cdots + \psi_\infty a_{N-\infty} = \sum_{j=1}^{\infty} \psi_j a_{N-j}$$

where the ψ-weights express the dependence of Y_N on $a_{N-1}, \ldots, a_{N-\infty}$. Then

$$Y_{N+\ell} = \psi_0 a_{N+\ell} + \psi_1 a_{N+\ell-1} + \cdots + \psi_{\ell-1} a_{N+1} + \sum_{j=0}^{\infty} \psi_{\ell+j} a_{N-j}$$

The values $a_{N+\ell}, \ldots, a_{N+1}$ will be unknown when the forecasts are made, of course, and must be set to their expected values (zero). The forecasts will then be based on the weighted sum of current and past shocks,

$$Y_N(\ell) = \sum_{j=0}^{\infty} \psi_{\ell+j} a_{N-j}$$

Now suppose that the "best" forecast of $Y_{N+\ell}$ is

$$Y_{N(\ell)} = \sum_{j=0}^{\infty} \tilde{\psi}_{\ell+j} a_{N-j}$$

where the values of $\widetilde{\psi}_{\ell+j}$ will be chosen to minimize *MSFE*. The *MSFE* of this forecast will be

$$
\begin{aligned}
MSFE &= E[Y_{N+\ell} - Y_N(\ell)]^2 \\
&= E[(\psi_0 a_{N+\ell} + \psi_1 a_{N+\ell} + \cdots + \psi_{\ell-1} a_{N+1})^2 \\
&\quad + \sum_{j=0}^{\infty} (\psi_{\ell+j} a_{N-j} - \widetilde{\psi}_{\ell+j} a_{N-j})^2]
\end{aligned}
$$

Since the shocks are independent, all cross-product terms drop out, leaving the simplified expression

$$
MSFE = (\psi_0^2 + \psi_1^2 + \cdots + \psi_{\ell-1}^2)\sigma_a^2 + \sum_{j=0}^{\infty}(\psi_{\ell+j} - \widetilde{\psi}_{\ell+j})\sigma_a^2
$$

So the *MSFE* will be smallest when $\widetilde{\psi}_{\ell+j} = \psi_{\ell+j}$. The "best" forecast of $Y_{N+\ell}$ is then just the expected value of $Y_{N+\ell}$ conditioned on $Y_1, \ldots, Y_N$:

$$
\begin{aligned}
Y_N(\ell) &= E[Y_{N+\ell} \mid Y_N] \\
&= \psi_0 E a_{N+\ell} + \psi_1 E a_{N+\ell-1} + \cdots + \psi_{\ell-1} E a_{N+1} + \sum_{j=0}^{\infty} \psi_{\ell+j} a_{N-j} \\
&= \sum_{j=0}^{\infty} \psi_{\ell+j} a_{N-j}
\end{aligned}
$$

The mean square error of a forecast may be divided into two components: the variance of the forecast and the square of the forecast bias. The expected forecast error is zero.

$$
E(\psi_0 E a_{N+\ell} + \psi_1 E a_{N+\ell-1} + \cdots + \psi_{\ell-1} E a_{N+1}) = 0
$$

Forecasts based on the conditional expected value are, thus, unbiased. From this it follows that the variance of the conditional forecasts will be smaller than that of any other unbiased univariate forecasts possible.

4.2 COMPUTING A FORECAST

In practice, the conditional expected values of future realizations can be computed from the *ARIMA* model in several ways. Although the analyst will ordinarily use a computer program to obtain the forecasts, developing the details of the two possible methods illuminates the logic of forecasting. The simplest computational method for obtaining forecasts is the so-called difference equation or π-weight identity of the *ARIMA* model. The difference equation identity expresses the current realization in terms of a current shock and a weighted sum of past realizations and shocks. In general,

$$Y_t = \pi_1 Y_{t-1} + \cdots + \pi_{p+d} Y_{t-p-d} + a_t - \psi_1 a_{t-1} - \cdots - \psi_q a_{t-q}$$

There will be one π-weight in this expression for each of the p *AR* parameters and d differences. For example, the π-weight identity of an *AR2* model is simply

$$Y_t = \pi_1 Y_{t-1} - \pi_2 Y_{t-2} + a_t$$

where $\pi_1 = \phi_1$ and $\pi_2 = \phi_2$. In contrast, an integrated *AR1* model

$$(1 - \phi_1)(1 - B)Y_t = a_t$$
$$Y_t = (\phi_1 + 1)Y_{t-1} - \phi_1 Y_{t-2} + a_t$$

also has a second-order π-weight identity but with $\pi_1 = (\phi_1 + 1)$ and $\pi_2 = -\phi_1$.

In general, the π-weight identity of a model is derived by solving the model for Y_t and collecting the common powers of B on the right-hand side. Table 4.1 lists the π-weight identities of several *ARIMA* models. Conditional forecasts of future realizations can be computed recursively from the π-weight identity of an *ARIMA* model. $Y_{N(1)}$ is computed conditional on $Y_N, \ldots, Y_{N-p-d+1}$ and $a_N, \ldots, a_{N-q+1}$. Setting a_{N+1} to its expected value of zero, the forecast for Y_{N+1} is

$$Y_{N(1)} = \sum_{j=0}^{p+d} \pi_{j+1} Y_{N-j} - \sum_{j=0}^{q} \theta_{j+1} a_{N-j}$$

Table 4.1. π-Weight Identities of *ARIMA* Models

ARIMA Model		π-Weight Identity
ARp	$\phi(B)Y_N = +a_N$	$Y_N = \sum_{j=1}^{p} \phi_j Y_{N-j} + a_N$
MA1	$Y_N = a_N - \theta_1 a_{N-1}$	$Y_N = a_N - \sum_{j=1}^{\infty} \theta_1^j Y_{N-j}$
Integrated AR1	$(1 - \phi_1)\nabla Y_N = a_N$	$Y_N = (\phi_1 + 1)Y_{N-1} - \phi_1 Y_{N-2} + a_N$
Integrated MA1	$\nabla Y_N = a_N - \theta_1 a_{N-1}$	$Y_N = a_N + \sum_{j=1}^{\infty} (1 - \theta_1) a_{N-j}$

In the same way, $Y_{N(2)}$ is computed conditional on $Y_{N(1)}, \ldots, Y_{N-p-d+2}$ and $a_N, \ldots, a_{N-q+2}$:

$$Y_{N(2)} = \pi_1 Y_{N(1)} + \sum_{j=0}^{p+d+1} \pi_{j+1} Y_{N-j} - \sum_{j=1}^{q-1} \theta_{j+1} a_{N-j}$$

Continuing this algorithm, the forecast for $Y_{N+\ell}$ will be

$$Y_{N(\ell)} = \sum_{j=0}^{\ell-1} \pi_{j+1} Y_{N(j+\ell-1)} + \sum_{j=1}^{p+d+\ell-1} \pi_{j+1} Y_{N-j} - \sum_{j=1}^{q-\ell-1} \theta_{j+1} a_{N-j}$$

Using the π-weight identity in Table 4.1, for example, the first three forecasts of an integrated $AR1$ model are

$$Y_{N(1)} = \pi_1 Y_N - \pi_2 Y_{N-1} = (1+\phi_1)Y_N - \phi_1 Y_{N-1}$$
$$Y_{N(2)} = \pi_1 Y_{N(1)} - \pi_2 Y_N = (1+\phi_1)Y_{N(1)} - \phi_1 Y_N$$
$$Y_{N(3)} = \pi_1 Y_{N(2)} - \pi_2 Y_{N(1)} = (1+\phi_1)Y_{N(2)} - \phi_1 Y_{N(1)}$$

In practice, the forecasts from the difference equation form of the *ARIMA* model can be computed by substituting the known and forecasted values of $Y_{N+\ell-1}, \ldots, Y_{N+\ell-p-d}$ and the known values of $a_N, \ldots, a_{N-1+\ell}$ into the model. The shocks, $a_N, \ldots, a_{N-1+\ell}$, are unobserved, but estimates of their values are provided by the residuals from the fitted model.

The difference equation form of the *ARIMA* model expresses each realization in terms of previous realizations and current and previous shocks. An alternative method of generating conditional forecasts is to express the model in terms of current and previous shocks only. This form of the model is called the random shock or ψ-weight identity. The random shock form solves the model for its shocks:

$$Y_N = a_N + \psi_1 a_{N-1} + \psi_2 a_{N-2} + \cdots + \psi_\infty a_{N-\infty} = \sum_{j=0}^{\infty} \psi_j a_{N-j}$$

Table 4.2 lists the ψ-weight identities of several *ARIMA* models. The ψ-weights are found by writing the model for its shocks and then collecting the common powers of B. Once the ψ-weights are found, it is easy (though tedious) to compute the forecasts. For example, using the ψ-weight identity of the integrated $AR1$ model in Table 4.2,

$$Y_{N(1)} = E(a_{N+1}) + (1+\phi_1)a_N + (1+\phi_1+\phi_1^2)a_{N-1} + \cdots$$

Table 4.2. ψ-WEIGHT IDENTITIES OF ARIMA MODELS

	ARIMA Model	ψ-Weight Identity
AR1	$(1 - \phi_1 B)Y_N = a_N$	$Y_N = \displaystyle\sum_{j=0}^{\infty} \phi_1^j a_{N-j}$
MAq	$Y_N = \theta(B)a_N$	$Y_N = a_N - \displaystyle\sum_{j=1}^{\infty} \theta_j a_{N-j}$
Integrated AR1	$(1 - \phi_1)\nabla Y_N = a_N$	$Y_N = \displaystyle\sum_{j=0}^{\infty} [\sum_{k=0}^{j} \phi_1^k] a_{N-j}$
Integrated MA1	$\nabla Y_N = a_N - \theta_1 a_{N-1}$	$Y_N = a_N + \displaystyle\sum_{j=1}^{\infty} (1 - \theta_1) a_{N-j}$

The first term of this forecast is zero. The second forecast is

$$Y_{N(2)} = E(a_{N+2}) + (1 + \phi_1)E(a_{N+1}) + (1 + \phi_1 + \phi_1^2)a_N + \cdots$$

The first two terms of this forecast are zero. The third forecast is

$$Y_{N(3)} = E(a_{N+3}) + (1 + \phi_1)E(a_{N+2}) + (1 + \phi_1 + \phi_1^2)E(a_{N+1}) + \cdots$$

and so forth.

The π- and ψ-weight identities generate the same forecasts. Since the ψ-weight identity usually requires more computational effort, the π-weight identity would be preferred if one were forced to calculate a set of forecasts with paper and pencil. The ψ-weight identity is quite useful, nevertheless. We will use it to demonstrate two additional points.

First, the random shock form of the model makes it clear that each forecast depends on the values of shocks that occurred before observation of the process began. For example, the conditional one-step forecast of an MA1 process is

$$Y_{N(1)} = E(a_{N+1}) - \theta_1 a_N$$

By backward substitution, this is

$$Y_{N(1)} = E(a_{N+1}) + \sum_{j=1}^{N-1} \theta_1^j Y_{N-j} - \theta_1^N a_0$$

The forecast for Y_{N+1} thus depends partly on a_0, which is unobserved. Similarly, for an $AR1$ process

$$Y_{N(1)} = E(a_{N+1}) + \sum_{j=1}^{N-1} \phi_1^j a_{N-j} + \sum_{j=N}^{\infty} \phi_1^j a_{N-j}$$

Only a finite string of realizations is available from the process history, however, and all shocks before a_1 are unknown. A decision must therefore be made about how to allow for shocks that occurred before observation of the process began.

One possibility is to set the unobserved shocks to their unconditional expected values of zero. If the ϕ- and θ-parameters of the $ARIMA$ model satisfy the bounds of stationarity-invertability, the sequence of ψ-weights, $\psi_1, \psi_2, \ldots, \psi_k$ will eventually converge to zero, and shocks from the distant past will have essentially no influence on the forecasts. Therefore, if the series is long compared to the order of the process ($N > 50$ is usually sufficient), we can be sure that

$$E(a_0) \approx E(a_1) \approx \ldots \approx 0$$

So realizations that occurred before the series began to be observed may be safely ignored.

Alternatively, shocks prior to a_1 may be back forecasted—or backcasted—from the model. In this case, the methods of forecasting are reversed, and the model is used to estimate the conditional expected values of past realizations rather than those of future ones. After forecasts have been developed for the past observations, the model is re-estimated using both the observed realizations and the back forecasts. This procedure of generating back forecasts and then re-estimating the model may be continued iteratively until the model estimates converge (see Box and Jenkins, 1976, pp. 215-220). In practice, unless the realization string is short or the values of ϕ- and θ-parameters are close to the stationarity-invertability bounds, the unconditional expected value and the back forecasting approaches should produce very similar results.

The ψ-weight identity of an $ARIMA$ model also provides a way to compute the forecast variance and, thus, to construct confidence intervals for the forecasts. The conditional expected value, $E(Y_{N+\ell} \mid Y_N)$, provides the single "best" point forecast of $Y_{N+\ell}$. Point forecasts are seldom if ever "on the button," however, and for this reason interval forecasts are often more useful. Constructing an interval forecast requires, first, estimating the variance of the conditional expected value, and then using this estimate to form a confidence interval.

For a long time series and nominal 95 percent confidence, the "best" interval forecast of $Y_{N+\ell}$ is

$$E(Y_{N+\ell} \mid Y_N) \pm 1.96\sigma_{N(\ell)}$$

The value 1.96 is taken from a Normal distribution table, since the process shocks are assumed to be Normally distributed. If the parameters of the process were known exactly, such an interval would include $Y_{N+\ell}$ 95 percent of the time. Since the parameters are estimated, $\sigma_{N(\ell)}$ is not known exactly, and the interval is only approximate. The approximation becomes more accurate as the length of the series increases and, thus, as in other applications of *ARIMA* modeling, long realization strings are preferred to short ones.

The variance of $E(Y_{N+\ell} \mid Y_N)$ required for the interval forecast is defined as

$$\sigma_{N(\ell)}^2 = E[Y_{N+\ell} - E(Y_{N+\ell} \mid Y_N)]^2$$

The value of $Y_{N+\ell}$ is unknown, of course, and as a practical matter, the forecaster cannot wait until $Y_{N+\ell}$ is realized to draw forecast intervals. The forecast variance is easy to derive, however, by writing the model in random shock form. The error made in using $E(Y_{N+\ell} \mid Y_N)$ to forecast Y_{N+1} is

$$Y_{N+1} - Y_{N(1)} = a_{N+1}$$

That is, the error of the first forecast is equal to the actual value of Y_{N+1} minus its forecasted value. Similarly, the error made in forecasting Y_{N+2} is

$$Y_{N+2} - Y_{N(2)} = a_{N+2} + \psi_1 a_{N+1}$$

And in general, the forecast error of $Y_{N+\ell}$ is

$$Y_{N+\ell} - Y_{N(\ell)} = a_{N+\ell} + \psi_1 a_{N+\ell-1} + \cdots + \psi_{\ell-1} a_{N+1}$$

The variance of the forecast error is thus

$$\sigma_{N(\ell)}^2 = E(a_{N+\ell} + \psi_1 a_{N+\ell-1} + \cdots + \psi_{\ell-1} a_{N+1})^2$$
$$= E a_{N+\ell}^2 + \psi_1^2 E a_{N+\ell-1}^2 + \cdots + \psi_{\ell-1}^2 E a_{N+1}^2$$
$$= (1 + \psi_1^2 + \cdots + \psi_{\ell-1}^2) \sigma_a^2$$

The variance of the first forecast will always equal the variance of the shocks driving the process. Depending on model structure, the variance (and confidence intervals) will remain constant or grow larger with successive forecasts, reflecting the degree of uncertainty associated with extrapolating process history further and further into the future.

4.3 FORECAST PROFILES

The general principles of forecasting an *ARIMA* process using the conditional expectation of $Y_{N+\ell}$ apply to any type of *ARIMA* model structure. Each *ARIMA* model class will generate conditional forecasts that follow a unique pattern, however. Consideration of these characteristic patterns, or forecast profiles, provides additional insight into forecasting and into the model structures themselves. Accordingly, we next derive the forecast profiles of each major class of *ARIMA* models.

The best forecast of a white noise process is the unconditional expected value of $Y_{N+\ell}$

$$Y_{N(\ell)} = E(a_{N+\ell}) = 0 \quad \text{for} \quad \ell = 1, 2, \ldots$$

This follows from the white noise definition. No matter how long the forecast horizon (ℓ) might be, furthermore, the variance of this forecast is the white noise variance

$$\sigma^2_{N(\ell)} = \sigma^2_a \quad \text{for} \quad \ell = 1, 2, \ldots$$

This is consistent with our understanding of white noise.

Figure 4.1 plots the last 30 observations of the β-particle time series that was analyzed and modeled as a white noise process (see Section 3.1). Forecasts of this model begin with the 250th observation. The time series mean ($\mu = 75.506$) is the best forecast for any value of ℓ. The variance of the forecast is the white noise variance. The 95 percent confidence intervals plotted in Figure 4.3a are set at $\pm 1.96\sigma^2_a$. In the future, we expect 95 percent of the time series' observations to lie within these bounds. Since the forecast and process variances are equal, of course, 95 percent of the past observations will also lie within these bounds.

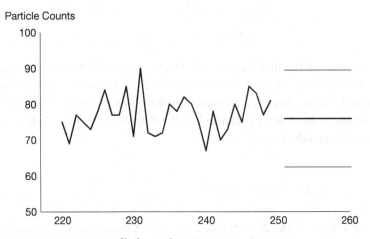

Figure 4.1 Forecast Profile for a White Noise Time Series

For an $AR1$ process, the value of $Y_{N+\ell}$ is given by the ψ-weight identity

$$Y_{N(\ell)} = \sum_{j=0}^{\infty} \phi_1^j a_{N+\ell-j} \text{ for } \ell = 1, 2, \dots$$

Separating this forecast into future and past components

$$Y_{N(\ell)} = \sum_{j=N+1}^{N+\ell} \phi_1^{N+\ell-j} a_j + \sum_{j=N}^{\infty} \phi_1^{N+\ell-j} a_{N-j}$$

The first series in this expression consists of future and, hence, unobserved shocks; we can substitute the expected value of zero for these shocks. And although the second series goes back to the infinite past, it is recognized as an $AR1$ identity of Y_N. That is,

$$Y_N = (1 - \phi_1 B)^{-1} a_N = \sum_{j=N}^{\infty} \phi_1^{N-j} a_{N-j}$$

So by substitution,

$$Y_{N(\ell)} = \sum_{j=N+1}^{N+\ell} \phi_1^{N+\ell-j} E a_j + \phi_1^\ell Y_N = \phi_1^\ell Y_N \quad \text{for} \quad \ell = 1, 2, \dots$$

The "best" forecast of an $AR1$ process for any ℓ is the last observation of the series, Y_N, weighted by the ℓth power of ϕ_1. The variance of the $AR1$ forecast is a simple function of ℓ and σ_a^2. Specifically

$$\sigma_{N(\ell)}^2 = E\left(\sum_{j=N+\ell}^{N+1} \phi_1^{N+\ell+j} a_j \right)^2 = E\left(a_{N+\ell} + \phi_1 a_{N+\ell-1} + \cdots + \phi_1^{\ell-1} a_{N+1} \right)^2$$

Since the expected value of the cross-product terms are zero, this simplifies to

$$\sigma_{N(\ell)}^2 = E a_{N+\ell}^2 + \phi_1^2 E a_{N+\ell-1}^2 + \cdots + \phi_1^{2\ell-2} E a_{N+1}^2$$

For $\ell = 1, 2$, and 3, then,

$$\sigma_{N(\ell=1)}^2 = \sigma_a^2$$
$$\sigma_{N(\ell=2)}^2 = \sigma_a^2 (1 + \phi_1^2)$$
$$\sigma_{N(\ell=2)}^2 = \sigma_a^2 (1 + \phi_1^2 + \phi_1^4)$$

The forecast variance increases, but by smaller and smaller increments. As ℓ grows larger and larger, the $AR1$ forecast variance approaches the limit of

$$\sigma^2_{N(\ell \to \infty)} = \frac{\sigma^2_a}{1 + \phi_1}$$

This is the variance of the $AR1$ process, of course.

Figure 4.2 plots the weekly pediatric trauma admissions time series that was analyzed and modeled as an $AR1$ process in Chapter 3.3.3. Rates for 20 weeks beginning with the 131st week were forecasted from the $AR1$ model. The forecasts approach the series mean ($\hat{\mu} = 27.87$) as ℓ grows longer. The 95 percent confidence interval around the forecasts grows wider as ℓ grows longer, approaching the limit determined by the values of ϕ_1 and σ^2_a. The distinctive geometric decay of $AR1$ forecasts is visually apparent in Figure 4.2. For values of ℓ greater than, say, 10 weeks, the $AR1$ forecasts and the unconditional forecast are the same.

As an aside, Figure 4.2 reveals a salient weakness of "classical" forecast confidence intervals: The 95 percent confidence interval includes negative values, which make no substantive sense at all. Truncating the lower-bound confidence interval at zero provides a crude but effective solution to the problem. Transforming the time series prior to modeling provides another solution. Bayesian forecasting models lack this salient weakness and might be preferred for that reason alone. Although we discuss Bayesian approaches to hypothesis testing in Chapter 6, we will not discuss Bayesian forecasting models. Zellner (1971) is the original source for Bayesian forecasting; see Geweke and Whiteman (2006) for a review and an interesting history.

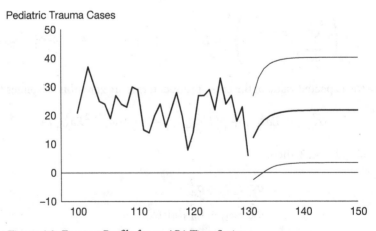

Figure 4.2 Forecast Profile for an $AR1$ Time Series

The conditional expected value of a random walk follows from the $AR1$ result. Since the random walk is a special $AR1$ case where $\phi_1 = 1$, its ψ-weight identity is

$$Y_{N(\ell)} = \sum_{j=0}^{\infty} a_{N+\ell-j} \quad \text{for} \quad \ell = 1, 2, \ldots$$

Separating this forecast into past and future parts

$$Y_{N(\ell)} = \sum_{j=0}^{\ell+1} a_{N+\ell-j} + \sum_{j=0}^{\infty} a_{N-j}$$

The first series in this expression consists of unknown future shocks whose expected value is zero. The second series of this expression is an identity of Y_N. By substitution, then,

$$Y_{N(\ell)\} } = \sum_{j=0}^{\ell+1} E(a_{N+\ell-j}) + Y_N = Y_N \quad \text{for} \quad \ell = 1, 2, \ldots$$

The "best" forecast of a random walk is the last observation, Y_N. From our $AR1$ result, the variance of this forecast is

$$\sigma^2_{N(\ell \to \infty)} = E(a^2_{N+\ell} + a^2_{N+\ell-1} + \cdots + a^2_{N+1}) = \ell \sigma^2_a$$

In contrast to the $AR1$ process, the random walk forecast interval grows larger with each unit increment in ℓ.

The forecast profile of a random walk process is plotted in Figure 4.3. The series consists of 50 observations of the coin-flip gambling experiment described

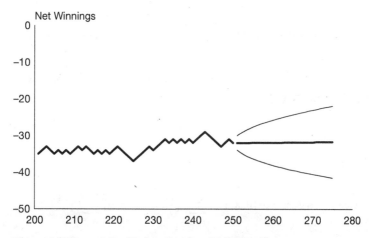

Figure 4.3 Forecast Profile for a Random Walk Time Series

in Section 2.6. At this point, "tails" has lost \$32 but, assuming that "tails" has enough capital to stay in the game, the tables will be turned. Since the random walk's history has no useful information, the best forecast for any horizon is the last observation, Y_N. The 95 percent confidence interval about this point forecast grow larger with N. This reflects the fact that, although we know that a random walk always returns to its starting point—zero in this case—the timing of its return is unpredictable by definition.

The conditional expected value of an $MA1$ process has a more complicated derivation. By definition,

$$Y_{N(\ell)} = a_{N+\ell} - \theta_1 a_{N+\ell-1} \quad \text{for} \quad \ell = 1, 2, \ldots$$

But by backward substitution, we can show that

$$Y_{N+\ell} = a_{N+\ell} - \theta_1 Y_{N+\ell-1} - \theta_1^2 Y_{N+\ell-2} - \cdots$$

To illuminate this expression, consider $\ell = 1$ and backward substitution to the first observation, Y_1.

$$Y_{N+1} = a_{N+1} - \theta_1 Y_N - \theta_1^2 Y_{N-1} - \cdots - \theta_1^N Y_1 - \theta_1^{N+1} a_0$$

The value of a_0 is unknown but as N grows larger, the weight of this shock approaches zero. So for a reasonably long time series, say, $N > 50$, we know that

$$Y_{N+1} \approx a_{N+1} - \sum_{j=1}^{N} \theta_1^j Y_{N-j+1}$$

and taking expected values,

$$Y_{N(1)} = E(a_{N+1}) - \sum_{j=1}^{N} \theta_1^j Y_{N-j+1} = - \sum_{j=1}^{N} \theta_1^j Y_{N-j+1}$$

The "best" forecast of Y_{N+1} for an $MA1$ process is a series of all observations weighted by powers of θ_1. For $\ell = 2$, however,

$$Y_{N+2} = a_{N+2} - \theta_1 Y_{N+1} - \theta_1^2 a_N$$

Substituting for Y_{N+1} and a_N in this expression,

$$Y_{N+2} = a_{N+2} - \theta_1 [a_{N+1} - \sum_{j=1}^{\infty} \theta_1^j Y_{N-j+1}] - \theta_1^2 \sum_{j=1}^{\infty} \theta_1^{j-1} Y_{N-j+1}$$

$$= a_{N+2} - \theta_1 a_{N+1}$$

Taking expected values

$$Y_{N(2)} = E(a_{N+2}) - \theta_1 E(a_{N+1}) = 0$$

Following the same logic, we can show that, for $\ell > 1$, the best forecast is zero. That is

$$Y_{N(\ell)} = 0 \quad \text{for} \quad \ell = 2, 3, \ldots$$

This reflects the fact that an $MA1$ process "forgets" all shocks prior to a_{t-1}. Two periods into the future, the entire past of the process has been "forgotten," and the conditional and unconditional forecasts are identical. The variance of this best $MA1$ forecast is

$$\sigma^2_{N(1)} = \sigma^2_a \quad \text{and} \quad \sigma^2_{N(\ell>1)} = \sigma^2_a(1+\theta_1)$$

Comparing the "best" $MA1$ and $AR1$ forecasts reinforces our understanding of MA and AR processes. Otherwise, as ℓ grows larger, $MA1$ and $AR1$ forecasts both decay to the process mean, $EY_{N+\ell}$. As the forecast horizon increases, in other words, the quality of even these "best" $MA1$ and $AR1$ forecasts declines rapidly.

Figure 4.4 plots the U.K. GDP growth rate series that was modeled as an $MA1$ process in Chapter 3.3.2. Rates for 2011–2020 were forecasted from the $MA1$ model. The forecast for $\ell = 1$ takes advantage of the information in the last shock, a_N. But for $\ell > 1$, the best forecast is the series mean ($\hat{\mu} = 1.46$). The 95 percent confidence interval makes a discrete jump from $\ell = 1$ to $\ell = 2$ but then does not increase for horizons $\ell > 2$. This profile generalizes to the MAq case. The best forecast of an MAq model uses the information in the last q shocks, $a_{N-q}, \ldots, a_N$. But for $\ell > q$, the series mean is the best forecast. Confidence intervals around

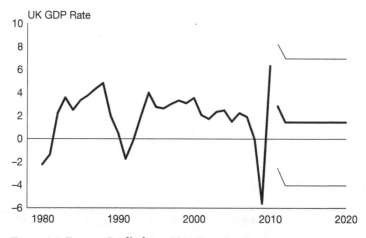

Figure 4.4 Forecast Profile for an $MA1$ Time Series

the best MAq forecasts increase in discrete jumps at $\ell = 1, \ldots, q$ but then remain constant for horizons of $\ell > q$.

Judging from these forecast profiles, univariate $ARIMA$ forecasts may not be useful for many purposes. The best point forecasts are often the process mean and confidence intervals are often large for even relatively short time series. Moreover, many practitioners seem to have a "feel" for their fields, rivaling the predictive ability of a univariate model. This is particularly true when the process can be modeled as a random walk. In that case, an experienced "insider" might be able to predict the turning points of the random walk, a feat that no $ARIMA$ model can match.

Higher-order models or models with strong seasonal or trend components are an exception to the general rule. The best forecast of these models are often nontrivial for relatively long values of ℓ. Seasonal models in particular carry information forward, extending the useful forecasting horizon at least one (and sometimes two) seasonal periods. Figure 4.5 plots the forecasts of the CO_2 series modeled as

$$\nabla \nabla^{12} Y_t = \theta_0 + (1 - \theta_1 B)(1 - \theta_{12} B^{12}) a_t$$

As shown, the forecasts of this model track the pattern of seasonal variation quite well for the $\ell = 36$ months plotted in Figure 4.5. Furthermore, although this model has a nonstationary mean, 95 percent confidence intervals around the forecasts stay within reasonable (i.e., helpful) bounds for this horizon. Because the model is nonstationary, of course, confidence intervals will grow steadily wider.

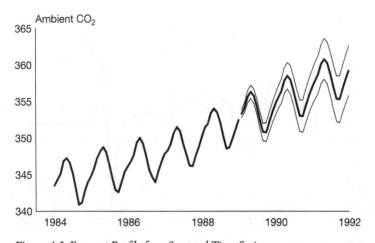

Figure 4.5 Forecast Profile for a Seasonal Time Series

Table 4.3. FORECAST PROFILES

	Best Forecast	Forecast Variance
$Y_t = a_t$	$Y_{N(\ell)} = 0 \; \ell = 1, 2, \ldots$	$\sigma^2_{N(\ell)} = \sigma^2_a \; \ell = 1, 2, \ldots$
$(1 - \phi_1 B) Y_t = a_t$	$Y_{N(\ell)} = \phi_1^\ell Y_N \; \ell = 1, 2, \ldots$	$\sigma^2_{N(\ell)} = \sigma^2_a \sum_{j=0}^{\ell} \phi_1^j \; \ell = 1, 2, \ldots$
$\nabla Y_t = a_t$	$Y_{N(\ell)} = Y_N \; \ell = 1, 2, \ldots$	$\sigma^2_{N(\ell)} = \ell \sigma^2_a \; \ell = 1, 2, \ldots$
$Y_t = (1 - \theta_1 B) a_t$	$Y_{N(1)} = -\sum_{j=1}^{N} \theta_1^j Y_{N-j+1}$	$\sigma^2_{N(1)} = \sigma^2_a$
	$Y_{N(\ell > 1)} = 0$	$\sigma^2_{N(\ell > 1)} = (1 + \theta_1) \sigma^2_a$

4.4 FORECASTING APPLICATIONS

Our view of univariate *ARIMA* forecasting is gloomy. Although the principles of forecasting help provide deeper insight into the nature of *ARIMA* models and modeling, the forecasts themselves are ordinarily of limited practical value. By contrast, in this last section, we discuss one situation in which univariate forecasting can in fact be extremely useful: as a tool in model diagnosis.

Often the analyst will find it difficult to choose between two competing univariate models. Support for either model may be found in the series *ACF* and *PACF*, and both models may provide a satisfactory fit to the data. For example, an *AR*1 process with a large ϕ_1 coefficient can produce realizations that are nearly identical to those of a random walk over a relatively short series. In cases like these, forecasting accuracy can help guide the decision about which of the competing models to select.

An analysis of U.S. birth rates by Dickey *et al.* (1986) illustrates this use. For an annual series of births per thousand 20- to 24-year-old women during 1948–80, Dickey *et al.* considered two models:

$$\nabla Y_t = .622 \nabla Y_{t-1} + a_t$$
$$\nabla^2 Y_t = a_t - .459 a_{t-1}$$

One of these models is based on the first differences of the birth rate time series, while the other is based on second differences. The purpose of the Dickey *et al.* analysis was to illustrate a test designed to select the appropriate degree of differencing. With only 33 observations the test did not provide clear-cut results in this example, however, and Dickey *et al.* conclude that "analysts with very different opinions about the future behavior of fertility rates could pick a model corresponding to their opinion." First-order models are preferred to second-order models on ground of parsimony except, of course, when the true model is second-order. Although the analyst can never know the true process generating a time series, there are many procedures that can be helpful in ruling out competing alternatives. One of these is forecasting. Using 1980 as the origin, forecasts of the two birth rate models are:

	∇	∇^2	Actual
1981	114.7	115.3	111.8
1982	114.5	115.5	111.3
1983	114.4	115.7	108.3
1984	114.3	115.9	107.3
1985	114.2	116.2	108.9

The forecasts of both models are quite close and both are consistently above the observed birth rate. The first-order model predicts declining birth rates, however, while the second-order model predicts increasing birth rates. In fact, except for 1985, birth rates decreased every year over the forecast period. The forecast errors of the first-order model are also smaller for each of the five years and the *MSFE* of the first-order model is only 63 percent as large as that of the second-order model for the period (26.59 vs. 42.38). Based on forecasting performance, then, the first-order model appears to be the "best" one for this series.

Forecasting accuracy should never be used as the sole criterion for choosing between competing models. Model selection is based on many statistical and substantive concerns. Forecasting is only one of many criteria that might be considered. Nevertheless, forecasts can provide useful guidance in ambiguous situations. Other things being equal, it is fair to say that a statistically adequate model of a process should provide reasonable forecasts of the future. Forecast accuracy depends on other factors, however, including many that lie outside the grasp of model adequacy. More important, unlike information criteria and other statistical measures of model adequacy, forecast accuracy has no universally accepted metric.

4.5 CONCLUSION

Our introduction to forecasting downplayed its role in the design and analysis of time series experiments and emphasized its potential abuses. Readers who are interested in forecasting for its own sake are directed to sources that focus on forecasting. Now for short-run horizons, the "best" *ARIMA* model will generally outperform non-*ARIMA* forecasting models. Even for medium-run horizons, the "best" *ARIMA* forecast may be as good as or better than the forecasts of more sophisticated, cumbersome models (Lin et al. 1986). This is particularly true when the underlying causal processes are stable.

As horizons grow longer, however, some non-*ARIMA* forecasting models will often outperform the "best" *ARIMA* model. The confidence intervals around *ARIMA* point-forecasts emphasize this long-run property. Long-horizon *ARIMA* forecasts grow increasingly inaccurate with diminishing utility for the forecaster. Readers who are interested in forecasting per se are advised then "to break away from simple linear univariate *ARIMA* or multivariate transfer functions" (Granger, 1992, p. 11) as well as the iterative, conservative *ARIMA* modeling strategy (Figure 3.1). We cannot recommend an alternative modeling strategy, unfortunately, but direct the reader instead to one of the many sources written for forecasters.

A fair reading of our views on forecasting begs the question of why we would cover forecasting at all. Glass *et al.* (1975), McCain and McCleary (1979), and McDowall et al. (1980) develop the design and analysis of time series experiments with no attention paid to *ARIMA* forecasting; McCleary et al. (1980) do so with only a cursory, superficial development of *ARIMA* forecasting. The answer to this question, put simply, is that the π- and ψ-weight identities used to calculate forecast variance and confidence intervals further illuminate *ARIMA* algebra (Chapter 2) and modeling (Chapter 3). Readers who have taken the time and effort to understand π- and ψ-weight identities will have a more complete understanding of *ARIMA* models:

The calculation of *ARIMA* forecasts and backcasts is straightforward. Calculation begins with a statistically adequate *ARIMA* model built from the modeling strategy described in Chapter 3. The information about the underlying process is coded in the *ARIMA* model, though with some error. The *ARIMA* model structures dictate a set of ℓ forecasts. Within this structure, the variance of the white noise driving process, σ_a^2, dictates the corresponding confidence intervals. While there is some didactic value in calculating forecasts and confidence intervals by hand, in practice, time series software packages routinely calculate and print out these statistics.

We will have little to say about forecasting in subsequent chapters. In Chapter 6, we discuss models and methods that have been proposed to *detect* interventions. Although these models and methods are often confused with forecasting, they are distinct from *ARIMA* forecasting, at least in terms of their motivation.

Intervention Modeling

Data of potential value in the formulation of public and private policy frequently occur in the form of time series. Questions of the following kind often arise: "Given a known intervention, is there evidence that change in the series of the kind expected actually occurred, and, if so, what can be said of the nature and magnitude of the change?"

—Box and Tiao (1975)

Allowing for commonsense modifications, the strategy for building an intervention model parallels the strategy for building an *ARIMA* noise model diagrammed in Figure 3.1. To motivate the modification, recall that the general *ARIMA* model can be written as the sum of the noise and exogenous components

$$Y_t = N(a_t) + X(I_t)$$

If the impact of $X(I_t)$ is trivially small, $N(a_t)$ can be identified with the conventional modeling strategy. If the impact is *not* small, however, or if its magnitude is *unknown*, the sample ACF will be distorted in unknown ways. Jump-started with a rough approximation of $N(a_t)$, the iterative modeling strategy will converge sooner or later on the "best" *ARIMA* model. But even a rough approximation of $N(a_t)$ may not be possible when the impact of $X(I_t)$ is large.

There are two solutions to this problem. When Y_t is long and well behaved, $N(a_t)$ can be identified from an unaffected pre- or post-intervention segment. Long, well-behaved time series are not common, unfortunately. Alternatively, when the structure of $X(I_t)$ is known, $N(a_t)$ can be identified from the residualized time series,

$$\hat{N}(a_t) = Y_t - X(I_t)$$

This second solution is more practical. Thus, although we will demonstrate both methods, the second is preferred—even in those rare instances where Y_t is a long, well-behaved time series. The requirement that the structure of $X(I_t)$ be known seems to pose an obstacle to the second method. Indeed, few substantive theories specify the "true" model of $X(I_t)$. But most substantive theories specify the dichotomous *onset* and *duration* of an impact, and these two impact properties are sufficient for our purposes.

It will be important to keep the terms "intervention" and "impact" distinct. The four impacts diagammed in Figure 5.1 are the most widely used in our experience. In each of the four, the *intervention* is represented by a step function or dummy variable, I_t, defined as

$$I_t = 0 \text{ when } t \leq N_{pre}$$
$$= 1 \text{ when } t > N_{pre}$$

I_t breaks Y_t into segments of N_{pre} and N_{post} observations. The *impact* of I_t on Y_t is estimated by comparing the N_{pre} and N_{post} observations. In the general model, I_t and Y_t are connected by a *transfer function* of I_t. The simplest transfer function of I_t is a *zero-order* transfer function:

$$X(I_t) = \omega_0 I_t \quad \text{for} \quad -1 \leq \delta \leq 1 \quad \text{and} \quad j = 1, 0$$

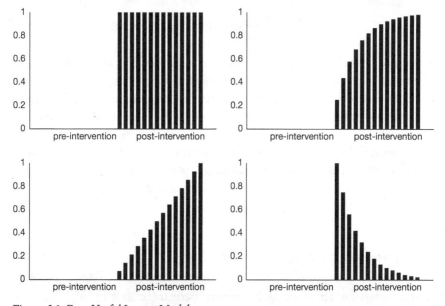

Figure 5.1 Four Useful Impact Models

The zero-order transfer function of I_t passes on a one-time change of ω units in the level of Y_t. The impact of the change in I_t is the *abrupt, permanent* shift in level of Y_t shown in the upper left-hand panel of Figure 5.1.

The impact of I_t need not be abrupt in onset. The *first-order* transfer function of I_t,

$$X(I_t) = \frac{\omega_0}{1 - \delta_1 B} I_t \quad \text{for} \quad -1 \le \delta_1 < 1$$

accrues gradually at a rate determined by the parameter δ_1. In j successive post-intervention observations, the level of Y_t responds to the unit change in I_t with increments of $\omega_0, \delta_1 \omega_0, \delta_1^2 \omega_0, \ldots, \delta_1^{k-1} \omega_0$. When $|\delta_1| < 1$, δ_1^{k-1} approaches zero, the series converges on the limit of $\omega/(1 - \delta)$. An impact of this type is shown in the upper right-hand panel of Figure 5.1. When $\delta^{k-1} = 1$, the series does not converge and the impact takes the form of a post-intervention secular trend. An impact of this type is shown in the lower left-hand panel of Figure 5.1.

Finally, the duration of an impact need not be permanent. Differencing I_t transforms the step function into a pulse function:

$$\nabla I_t = 0 \text{ when } t \le N_{pre}$$
$$= 1 \text{ when } t = N_{pre} + 1$$
$$= 0 \text{ when } t > N_{pre} + 1$$

When ∇I_t changes from zero to one, the first-order transfer function of ∇I_t,

$$X(I_t) = \frac{\omega_0}{1 - \delta_1 B} \nabla I_t \quad \text{for} \quad -1 \le \delta_1 < 1$$

transmits an abrupt change of ω_0 units to Y_t. When ∇I_t returns to zero, Y_t returns to its pre-intervention level at an exponential rate. After k observations, the difference between the pre- and post-intervention levels of Y_t is $\delta_1^{k-1} \omega_0$ units. An example of this type of impact is shown in the lower right-hand panel of Figure 5.1.

The modified modeling strategy and the dynamics of the four common impact models are better understood in the context of practical examples. We begin with one of the better-known time series experiments and the simplest impact model, the zero-order transfer function of I_t.

5.1 ABRUPT, PERMANENT IMPACTS

The simplest impact model is the abrupt, permanent shift in level shown in the upper left-hand panel of Figure 5.1. The impact is realized *abruptly*, or instantaneously, and persists *permanently*. Representing the intervention as a step function that changes from zero to one at $t = N_{pre}+1$, the impact of I_t on Y_t is realized through the zero-order transfer function,

$$X(I_t) = \omega_0 I_t$$

If it is not clear, the *order* of a transfer function is determined by the highest power of B, which is zero in this instance. Although this simple impact model may not fit some of the more interesting social phenomena, the model is eminently interpretable. We return to the issue of interpretability shortly.

5.1.1 Directory Assistance Calls

The Cincinnati Directory Assistance time series, plotted in Figure 5.2, has the most dramatic and apparently interpretable impact that most readers have ever seen. For that reason, the time series has been widely used to illustrate the logic of time series experiments. The abrupt collapse of the time series level in March 1974 coincides with the onset of a change in the cost of local calls to Directory Assistance. McSweeney (1978, p. 50) interprets the impact of this change in policy as evidence of "the power of response cost procedures." McSweeney's interpretation is not entirely convincing, however. Although the sheer magnitude of the March 1974 impact may render the common threats to internal validity implausible, other impacts in this time series are more difficult to explain.

The time series level also drops abruptly seven months earlier, in August 1973, when the Ohio Utilities Commission approved the policy change. This earlier

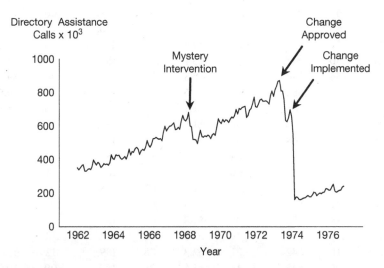

Figure 5.2 Directory Assistance Calls (McSweeney, 1978)

impact raises an alternative explanation. Perhaps the March 1974 impact was a continuation of a downward trend that began seven months earlier. Perhaps the *real* causal agent was the August 1973 public announcement of the policy, not the implementation itself. Some readers might see this alternative explanation as hair-splitting, of course, arguing that an unannounced, invisible policy change could not possibly affect behavior. But even granting this argument, there is no explanation for an earlier impact. In May 1968, due to some "mystery intervention," the level of the Directory Assistance time series drops by approximately 25 percent. We assume that the May 1968 impact is not a chance fluctuation. That would question McSweeney's causal interpretations of the August 1973 and March 1974 impacts. Causal interpretation aside, the interruptions in this time series will pose an obstacle to identification.

The seasonal sample *ACFs* reported in Table 5.1 were estimated from the first 76 observations of the Directory Assistance time series, $Calls_t$. Based on the

Table 5.1. DIRECTORY ASSISTANCE CALLS, IDENTIFICATION

	$Calls_t$		$\nabla Calls_t$		$\nabla^{12} Calls_t$		$\nabla \nabla^{12} Calls_t$	
k	r_k	Q_k	r_k	Q_k	r_k	Q_k	r_k	Q_k
1	.93	69.1	−.11	0.9	.71	33.8	−.25	4.1
2	.88	131.	−.39	13.0	.58	57.0	−.28	9.2
3	.85	190.	.10	13.9	.61	82.8	.13	10.4
4	.81	245.	.04	14.0	.54	103.	.00	10.4
5	.77	293.	−.11	15.0	.44	117.	−.19	12.9
6	.72	338.	.04	15.2	.48	134.	.08	13.4
7	.69	379.	−.02	15.2	.47	150.	.11	14.3
8	.66	417.	.03	15.3	.40	162.	.06	14.5
9	.63	452.	.04	15.4	.30	170.	−.12	15.6
10	.59	484.	−.33	24.9	.28	175.	−.06	15.9
11	.56	513.	.04	25.1	.25	180.	.28	22.3
12	.54	540.	.51	48.8	.07	181.	−.46	39.5
13	.49	562.	−.09	49.6	.15	183.	.01	39.5
14	.44	580.	−.14	51.4	.20	186.	.30	46.8
15	.40	595.	.01	51.5	.08	187.	−.11	47.9
16	.36	608.	.02	51.5	.06	187.	−.14	49.5
17	.31	618.	.04	51.6	.11	188.	.24	54.5
18	.26	625.	−.06	51.9	.02	188.	−.14	56.2
19	.24	631.	−.05	52.2	.02	188.	.02	56.2
20	.21	635.	.06	52.6	.01	188.	−.01	56.2
21	.18	638.	.05	52.8	.01	188.	−.05	56.4
22	.14	641.	−.29	62.3	−.00	188.	.17	59.2
23	.11	642.	−.01	62.3	−.08	189.	−.12	60.8
24	.09	643.	.45	85.1	−.08	189.	−.00	60.8

$N_{pre} = 76$ pre-intervention observations, we model the first- and twelfth-order differences of $Calls_t$. Spikes at r_1 and r_{12} of the sample ACF of $\nabla\nabla_t^{12}Calls_t$ identify the multiplicative seasonal model

$$\nabla\nabla^{12}Calls_t = \theta_0 + (1 - \theta_1 B)(1 - \theta_{12}B_{12})a_t$$

For reasons to be explained shortly, we solve this model for $Calls_t$ as

$$Calls_t = \frac{\theta_0 + (1 - \theta_1 B)(1 - \theta_{12}B_{12})a_t}{\nabla\nabla^{12}}$$

Other $ARIMA$ models are possible, of course, but this multiplicative seasonal IMA model is a reasonable first approximation to $N(a_t)$.

To model the intervention, we use step functions $I_{77,t}$, $I_{141,t}$, and $I_{148,t}$ that change from zero to one respectively in the 77th, 141st, and 148th months of the time series. Based on the appearance of the impacts and on the substantive theory, we use zero-order transfer functions to link $I_{77,t}$, $I_{141,t}$, and $I_{148,t}$ to $Calls_t$. The full model is thus

$$Calls_t = \left(\frac{\theta_0 + (1 - \theta_1 B)(1 - \theta_{12}B^{12})a_t}{\nabla\nabla^{12}}\right) + \left(\omega_{0,1}I_{77,t} + \omega_{0,2}I_{141,t} + \omega_{0,3}I_{148,t}\right)$$

Parameter estimates for this model are reported in Table 5.2. Our first approximation of $N(a_t)$ turns out to be the "best" $ARIMA$ noise model. The value of $Q_{24} = 18.3$ for the residuals is too small to reject a white noise hypothesis, so the model is adequate. The MA parameter estimates are statistically significant and lie inside the invertibility bounds. Prudent analysts might want to estimate the additive seasonal IMA model before judging the multiplicative model "best." But we leave that as an exercise for the reader. If the multiplicative seasonal IMA model reported in Table 5.2 is not "best" for this time series, it is certainly "good enough" for our purposes, which, in this instance, are focused narrowly on interpreting the impacts.

The zero-transfer function has a straightforward interpretation. In May 1968, the level of $Calls_t$ drops by $\hat{\omega}_{0,1} = -78,929$ calls. Although the causal agent is

Table 5.2. ESTIMATION AND DIAGNOSIS, $Calls_t$

	Estimate	SE	t	Diagnosis
$\hat{\theta}_0$	−.1478	.2228	−0.66	$RSE = 21.0771$
$\hat{\omega}_{0,1}$	−78.9292	20.2849	−3.89	$Q_{24} = 18.3$
$\hat{\omega}_{0,2}$	−85.5987	20.4239	−4.19	$Z_{KS} = 0.72$
$\hat{\omega}_{0,3}$	−425.0217	22.6645	−18.75	
θ_1	.2425	.0842	2.88	
$\hat{\theta}_{12}$	.9047	.0328	27.57	

a mystery, the impact persists throughout the post-intervention period. So far as we can tell, it is permanent. Five years later, in August 1973, when the Ohio Utilities Commission approves a charge for local Directory Assistance calls, the level of $Calls_t$ drops again by $\hat{\omega}_{0,2} = -85,599$ calls. The impact persists for seven months. In March 1974, the charge goes into effect and the level of $Calls_t$ drops by a staggering $\hat{\omega}_{0,3} = -425,022$ calls. Like the two preceding impacts, this one persists throughout the post-intervention segment.

5.1.2 Rest Breaks and Productivity

Another simple impact is plotted in Figure 5.3. These are 80 weekly productivity measures from the Hawthorn Bank Wiring Room experiment. During the 32-week pre-intervention segment, the five Bank Wiring Room workers received 25-minute rest breaks each day. Rest breaks were eliminated in the 33rd week and then reinstated in the 45th week. Franke and Kaul (1978) argue that productivity fell when the rest breaks were eliminated because the unrested workers were fatigued. Although the visual evidence seems to support their claim, they arrived at this conclusion without benefit of an analysis.

Unlike the Cincinnati Directory Assistance time series, this impact seems too small to cause the same identification problem. Sample $ACFs$ for the time series and its first difference, estimated from all 80 observations, are plotted in Figure 5.4. The sample $ACFs$ identify an IMA model as a first approximation:

$$PRD_t = \frac{\theta_0 + (1 - \theta_1)B}{\nabla} a_t$$

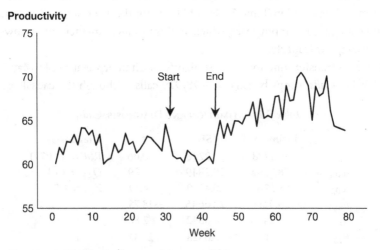

Figure 5.3 Weekly Productivity Measures, PRD_t

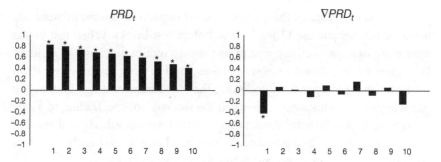

Figure 5.4 Sample *ACFs, PRD*$_t$, and ∇PRD_t

Table 5.3. ESTIMATION AND DIAGNOSIS, ∇PRD_t

	Estimate	SE	t	Diagnosis
$\hat{\theta}_0$	.0454	.0750	0.60	$RSE = 1.3611$
$\hat{\theta}_1$	.5082	.0982	5.18	$Q_{10} = 12.3$
$\hat{\omega}_0$	-2.8287	.8263	-3.42	$Z_{KS} = 0.805$

To represent the intervention, we define the step function

$$I_t = 0 \text{ for } 0 < t \le 32$$
$$= 1 \text{ for } 33 \le t > 45$$
$$= 0 \text{ for } t \ge 45$$

Using a zero-order transfer function to link I_t to Y_t specifies the full model as:

$$PRD_t = \frac{\theta_0 + (1 - \theta_1)B}{\nabla} a_t + \omega_0 I_t$$

Parameter estimates for this model are reported in Table 5.3. The model's *MA* parameter is statistically significant and invertible and its residuals are not different than white noise. The value of $\hat{\theta}_0 = 0.0454$ is not statistically significant and should be dropped from the model. We leave that exercise to the reader, however. The model reported in Table 5.3 is "good enough" for our purposes. When rest breaks were eliminated, the five Bank Wiring Room workers' productivity dropped by $\hat{\omega} = -2.8287$ units. Compared to the 32 pre-intervention weeks, this amounts to a 5 percent drop in productivity. Since *PRD*$_t$ is nonstationary, of course, a comparative interpretation is a rough approximation.

Though perhaps substantively small, the drop in productivity is statistically significant. A formal null hypothesis test rules out chance explanations without favoring any of the alternative explanations. The reduction may have been due to worker fatigue, as Franke and Kaul (1978) suggest, or to a planned slowdown by the workers. Whatever the explanation, the impact was abrupt in onset and persisted throughout the 12-week period of no rest breaks. When rest breaks were reinstated, productivity rose to its pre-intervention level just as abruptly. Inspection of the plotted time series raises another question, however. PRD_t seems to have a steeper trend following the reinstatement of rest breaks. Is it possible that the reinstatement boosted the workers' morale, leading to a new rising trend in productivity? Readers may want to investigate this hypothesis. For now, what appears to be a post-intervention trend proves, after analysis, to be a continuation of the pre-intervention trend in this series.

5.1.3 Prophylactic Vancomycin and Surgical Infection

The time series plotted in Figure 5.5 consists of monthly surgical site infection rates for coronary artery bypass graft patients at a large hospital (Garey et al., 2008). For $N_{pre} = 20$ months, patients are treated with prophylactic cefuroxime and for the next $N_{post} = 35$ months, with prophylactic vancomycin. Modeling this time series will be especially difficult. The inherent difficulty of identifying $N(a_t)$ from a short time series is aggravated in this instance by the unruly appearance of this time series and the possibility of a large impact. We start the iterative $ARIMA$ modeling strategy with the simplest possible model:

$$SSI_t = \theta_0 + a_t + \omega_0 I_t$$

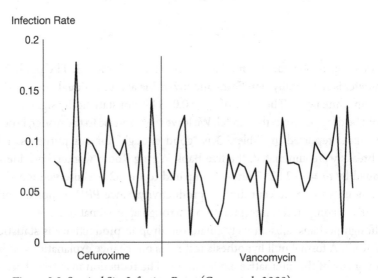

Figure 5.5 Surgical Site Infection Rates (Garey et al., 2008)

where

$$I_t = 0 \text{ for } 0 < t \le 20$$
$$= 1 \text{ for } 21 \le t \le 55$$

Parameter estimates for this simplest model are reported as Model 1 in Table 5.4. Although the Model 1 residuals could pass for white noise ($Q_{10} = 7.4$), given the relatively small N for SSI_t, we withhold judgment.

The sample ACF and $PACF$ for the Model 1 residuals are plotted in Figure 5.6. The values $r_1 = -.27$ and $r_2 = .15$ identify an $AR1$ model for $N(a_t)$ and the $PACF$ confirms the identification. Parameter estimates are reported as Model 2 in Table 5.4. All of the estimates are statistically significant; the $AR1$ parameter estimate is invertible; and the value of $Q_{10} = 3.9$ for the model's residuals is too small to reject a white noise hypothesis. We accept Model 2.

To interpret the estimated Model 2, we use the infinite series identity of the inverse $AR1$ operator. That is,

$$SSI_t = 0.084 - 0.014I_t + \frac{a_t}{1 + .27B}$$

$$= 0.084 - 0.014I_t + \sum_{k=0}^{\infty} 0.27^k a_t$$

$$= 0.084 - 0.014I_t + a_t + 0.27a_{t-1} + 0.07a_{t-2} + 0.02a_{t-3} + \cdots$$

Table 5.4. Surgical Site Infection Rates, Estimation and Diagnosis

	Estimate	SE	t	Diagnosis
Model 1	$\hat{\theta}_0$	.0833	.0075	11.04	$RSE = 0.03373$
	$\hat{\omega}_0$	−.0141	.0095	−1.49	$Q_{10} = 7.4$
					$Z_{KS} = 0.805$
Model 2	$\hat{\theta}_0$	.0836	.0059	14.11	$RSE = 0.03277$
	$\hat{\phi}_1$	−.2710	.1312	−2.07	$Q_{10} = 3.9$
	$\hat{\omega}_0$	−.0144	.0074	−1.95	$Z_{KS} = 0.805$

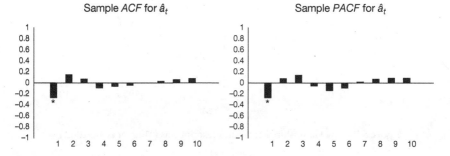

Figure 5.6 Surgical Site Infection Rates, Residual ACFs

Taking the expected value of the infinite series, only the first two terms are nonzero. Prior to the intervention, the infection rate is $\hat{\theta}_0 = 0.084$. After the intervention, the infection rate drops by $\hat{\omega}_0 = -0.014$. This impact is approximately 16 percent of the pre-intervention level. Given this relatively small impact, we were able to identify a first approximation to $N(a_t)$ directly from the time series.

5.1.4 New Hampshire Medicaid Prescriptions

Figure 5.7 plots a time series of the monthly mean number of prescriptions for a sample of New Hampshire Medicaid enrollees (Wagner et al., 2002). In an attempt to reduce Medicaid expenditures, beginning in September 1981, the 21st month of the time series, the number of monthly prescriptions was capped at three per enrollee. Judging from the visual evidence, this intervention was effective. The level of the time series dropped abruptly beginning that month and did not return to the pre-intervention level. Eleven months later, the three-prescription cap was replaced by a co-payment provision. Compared to rigid caps, co-payments are more easily enforced but theoretically less effective. The visual evidence seems to corroborate the theory. The level of the time series rose abruptly in response to this intervention but the increment was not large enough to return the time series to its pre-intervention level.

There are two potential obstacles to the identification of an *ARIMA* model for this time series. First, this time series may be too short to support a confident identification. $N = 48$ observations is sufficient for some purposes, especially if the underlying process is *non*seasonal and *un*complicated. This is a monthly

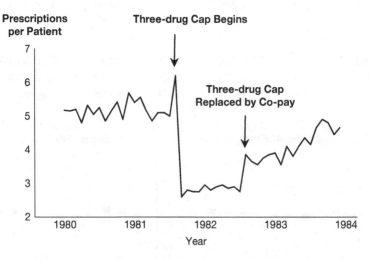

Figure 5.7 New Hampshire Medicaid Prescriptions (Wagner et al., 2002)

time series from a region with long winters, however, so we should not be surprised if the time series has a strong seasonal component. Second, the two visually apparent impacts in this time series are large enough to complicate the identification. The impacts seem to be abrupt and permanent, on the other hand, and easily modeled.

To represent the two interventions, we define a step function that changes from zero to one in the 32nd month, coinciding with the onset of the second intervention:

$$I_t = 0 \text{ for } 0 < t \leq 31$$
$$= 1 \text{ for } 32 \leq t \leq 48$$

Since the first intervention occurred 11 months earlier, we represent it with the 11th lag of I_t. Using zero-order transfer functions to link I_t and Y_t and assuming a white noise disturbance, our initial model is

$$Prscrp_t = \theta_0 + a_t + \omega_{0,1}B^{11}I_t + \omega_{0,2}I_t$$
$$= \theta_0 + a_t + (\omega_{0,1}B^{11} + \omega_{0,2})I_t$$

Parameter estimates for the initial model are reported as Model 1 in Table 5.5. The parameter estimates are all statistically significant and consistent with the visual evidence. The value of $Q_{12} = 37.2$ for the model's residuals rejects the white noise hypothesis, however, so Model 1 is not statistically adequate. That is no surprise, of course, because Model 1 was specified for the sole purpose of jump-starting the modeling algorithm.

The first 12 lags of the sample ACF and $PACF$ for the Model 1 residuals are plotted in Figure 5.8. We report 12 lags because $Prescrip_t$ is a monthly time series. The seasonal process is relatively weak, however, and the time series too short. Although the seasonal component cannot be identified, the sample ACF and

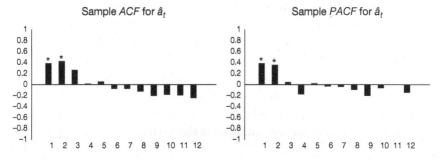

Figure 5.8 Sample ACF and $PACF$ for $\hat{a}_t = Prescrip_t - 5.21 + 2.4I_{t-11} - 1.3I_t$

Table 5.5. MEDICAID PRESCRIPTIONS, ESTIMATION AND DIAGNOSIS

		Estimate	SE	t	Diagnosis
Model 1	$\hat{\theta}_0$	5.2145	.0740	70.50	$RSE = 0.3308$
	$\hat{\omega}_{0,1}$	−2.3963	.1242	−19.30	$Q_{12} = 37.2$
	$\hat{\omega}_{0,2}$	1.3024	.1280	10.18	$Z_{KS} = 0.86$
Model 2	$\hat{\theta}_0$	6.3088	.8528	7.40	$RSE = 0.2846$
	$\hat{\omega}_{0,1}$	−3.0267	.2815	−10.75	$Q_{12} = 7.1$
	$\hat{\omega}_{0,2}$	.9799	.2600	3.77	$Z_{KS} = 0.97$
	$\hat{\phi}_1$	.4249	.1405	3.02	
	$\hat{\phi}_2$	.5012	.1367	3.67	
Model 3	$\hat{\theta}_0$	4.7714	.2943	16.21	$RSE = 0.3617$
	$\hat{\omega}_0$	−2.0223	.1395	−14.50	$Q_{12} = 10.0$
	$\hat{\phi}_1$	.4536	.1189	3.81	$Z_{KS} = 0.88$
	$\hat{\phi}_2$	.3726	.1326	2.81	

PACF identify an *AR2* model:

$$Prscrp_t = \frac{\theta_0 + a_t}{(1 - \phi_1 B - \phi_2 B^2)} + (\omega_{0,1} B^{11} + \omega_{0,2}) I_t$$

Parameter estimates for this model are reported as Model 2 in Table 5.5. All of the parameter estimates are statistically significant and invertible. The values of $Q_{12} = 7.1$ and $Z_{KS} = 0.97$ are too small to reject a white noise hypothesis for the model's residuals. Nor do we see evidence of seasonality in the model residuals. Model 2 is statistically adequate, so we accept it.

Model 2 has a simple interpretation. Prior to the 21st month, the time series fluctuated more or less randomly about the pre-intervention mean of $\hat{\theta}_0 = 6.31$ prescriptions per Medicaid enrollee. In the 21st month, the number of prescriptions was capped at three per enrollee. The level of the series changed by $\hat{\omega}_{0,1} = -3.03$ in response to this intervention. Eleven months later, when the three-prescription cap was replaced by a co-pay provision, the level of the time series changed by $\hat{\omega}_{0,2} = 0.98$. In sum, although the co-pay intervention was effective, it was not as effective—apparently—as the three-prescription cap.

We say "apparently" because we have not tested a model equivalence hypothesis. Is the difference between $\hat{\omega}_{0,1}$ and $\hat{\omega}_{0,2}$ small enough to be attributed to chance? To investigate this possibility, we test the null hypothesis that the two impacts have equal magnitudes but opposite signs. Thus,

$$H_0: \omega_{0,1} - \omega_{0,2} = 0$$

To test this H_0, we re-estimate Model 2 with one parameter:

$$Prescrip_t = \frac{\theta_0 + a_t}{(1 - \phi_1 B - \phi_2 B^2)} + \omega_0 (B^0 - B^{11}) I_t$$

$$= \frac{\theta_0 + a_t}{(1 - \phi_1 B - \phi_2 B^2)} - \omega_0 I_{t-11} + \omega_0 I_t$$

Parameter estimates for the constrained model are reported as Model 3 in Table 5.5. The parameter estimates are significant and invertible and the residuals are not different than white noise. Since Model 3 is statistically adequate, we can use it to test H_0. Note here that H_0 is identical to the model equivalence hypothesis

$$H_0: \text{Model 2} \approx \text{Model 3}$$

Since Model 3 is nested within Model 2, H_0 can be tested with the deviance statistic,

$$D = -2LL(\text{Model 3}) - 2LL(\text{Model 2}) \text{ where}$$
$$-2LL(\text{Model 3}) = 39.6401 \text{ and}$$
$$-2LL(\text{Model 2}) = 16.5939$$

Under H_0, D is distributed as χ^2 with one degree of freedom. That is,

$$D = -2LL(\text{Model 3}) - 2LL(\text{Model 2}) = 23.05$$

Since $Pr(\chi^2_{df=1} \geq 23.05) < 0.00001$, the hypothesis that Model 2 and Model 3 are equivalent is rejected with a high degree of confidence. By logical implication, the hypothesis that the two impacts have the same magnitude but opposite signs is also rejected.

5.1.5 Methadone Maintenance Treatments

The time series data plotted in Figure 5.9 are the proportions of cocaine-free ("clean") urine samples collected from 10 methadone maintenance patients (Kirby et al., 2008). The first 25 samples are used to estimate a baseline control level for the time series. Beginning with the 26th sample and continuing through the 54th sample, the patients are rewarded for multiple behaviors, including cocaine abstinence (Treatment A). Beginning with 55th sample and continuing through the 73rd sample, the patients are rewarded for cocaine abstinence only (Treatment B). Treatment A begins again with the 74th sample and continues through the 91st. Finally, Treatment B begins again with the 92nd sample and continues through the 105th sample.

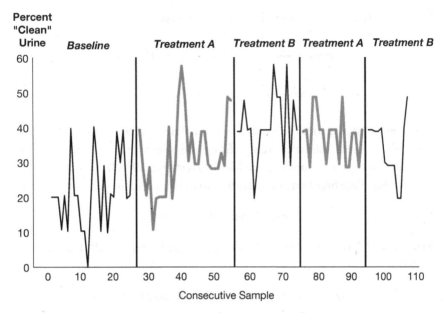

Figure 5.9 Percent "Clean" Urine Samples (Kirby et al., 2008)

The design of this time series experiment is so common that it has a name: ABAB. Our analysis aims to determine whether either treatment has any effect whatsoever and, if so, whether the effects of Treatments A and B are different. Toward that end, we define step functions $IA_t = IB_t = 0$ except that

$$IA_t = 1 \text{ when } 26 \leq t \leq 54 \text{ and } 74 \leq t \leq 91$$
$$IB_t = 1 \text{ when } 55 \leq t \leq 73 \text{ and } 92 \leq t \leq 105$$

Assuming that $N(a_t)$ is white noise and using zero-order transfer functions to link the step functions to the time series, our initial model is

$$Clean_t = (\theta_0 + a_t) + (\omega_{0,A} IA_t + \omega_{0,B} IB_t)$$

Parameter estimates for this model are reported as Model 1 in Table 5.6. The value of $Q_{10} = 22.5$ rejects the white noise hypothesis, so Model 1 is not statistically adequate. This is not too big a disappointment, of course: Model 1 was specified only for the purpose of jump-starting the iterative modeling strategy.

Ten lags of the sample *ACF* and *PACF* for the Model 1 residuals, plotted in Figure 5.10, identify an *MA2* model:

$$Clean_t = \left[\theta_0 + (1 - \theta_1 B - \theta_2 B^2)a_t\right] + (\omega_{0,A} IA_t + \omega_{0,B} IB_t)$$

Parameter estimates for this model are reported as Model 2 in Table 5.6. All of the parameter estimates are statistically significant and the *MA* parameter estimates

Table 5.6. ESTIMATION AND DIAGNOSIS, *Clean$_t$*

		Estimate	SE	t	Diagnosis
Model 1	$\hat{\theta}_0$	21.2189	1.9697	10.77	$RSE = 9.8487$
	$\hat{\omega}_{0,1}$	12.8139	2.4379	5.26	$Q_{10} = 22.5$
	$\hat{\omega}_{0,2}$	16.6468	2.6113	6.37	$Z_{KS} = 0.84$
Model 2	$\hat{\theta}_0$	20.9138	2.6303	7.95	$RSE = 9.3256$
	$\hat{\omega}_{0,1}$	13.4337	3.2296	4.16	$Q_{10} = 7.5$
	$\hat{\omega}_{0,2}$	16.9206	3.4736	4.87	$Z_{KS} = 0.56$
	$\hat{\theta}_1$	−.2713	.0972	−2.79	
	$\hat{\theta}_2$	−.1959	.0982	−2.00	
Model 3	$\hat{\theta}_0$	20.9244	2.6862	7.79	$RSE = 9.3861$
	$\hat{\omega}_0$	14.8753	3.0747	4.84	$Q_{10} = 6.9$
	$\hat{\theta}_1$	−.2840	.0971	−2.92	$Z_{KS} = 0.68$
	$\hat{\theta}_2$	−.2086	.0983	−2.12	

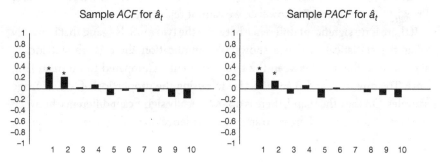

Figure 5.10 Sample *ACF* and *PACF*, $\hat{a}_t = Clean_t - 21.2 - 12.8IA_t - 16.6IB_t$

are invertible. The values of $Q_{10} = 7.5$ and $Z_{KS} = 0.56$ do not reject the white noise hypothesis, so Model 2 is statistically adequate.

Rounding to two decimal places and ignoring the error terms, Model 2 is

$$Clean_t = 20.91 + 13.43IA_t + 16.92IB_t$$

Approximately 21 percent of the urine samples collected during the baseline period are "clean." During Treatments A and B, the proportion rises to approximately 34 percent and 38 percent respectively. Both treatments are effective, but is one *more* effective? To address this question, we re-estimate Model 2 with the constraint that $\omega_{0,1} = \omega_{0,2}$. Parameter estimates for the constrained model are reported as Model 3 in Table 5.6. Since Model 3 is "nested" within Model 2, the null hypothesis

$$H_0: \omega_{0,1} = \omega_{0,2}$$

is identical to the model equivalence hypothesis

$$H_0: \text{Model } 2 \approx \text{Model } 3$$

Since Model 3 is nested within Model 2, H_0 can be tested with the same deviance statistic used in our analysis of New Hampshire Medicaid prescriptions. Where

$$-2LL(\text{Model } 3) = 768.3518 \text{ and}$$
$$-2LL(\text{Model } 2) = 766.9796$$

the deviance statistic for these two models is

$$D = -2LL(\text{Model } 3) - 2LL(\text{Model } 2) = 1.36$$

Under H_0, D is distributed as χ^2 with one degree of freedom Since $\Pr(\chi^2_{df=1} \geq 1.36) = 0.76$, however, we cannot reject H_0.

If there is no significant difference between the two models—and that is exactly what the statistical evidence shows—by implication there is no statistically significant difference between the two treatments. Compared to no treatment, both Treatments A and B are effective in raising the proportion of "clean" urine samples. On the other hand, there is no statistically significant difference between the two treatments—there is no statistical evidence that either treatment is more effective than the other.

5.2 GRADUALLY ACCRUING IMPACTS

Not all interventions have immediate impacts. Some accrue *gradually* over the post-intervention segment. This property of the impact can be modeled with a lagged rate parameter that weights the scalar impact. Representing the intervention as a step function, the impact of I_t on Y_t is realized through the first-order transfer function,

$$X(I_t) = \frac{\omega_0}{1 - \delta_1 B} I_t$$

The post-intervention rate of accrual is determined by the value of δ_1, which ordinarily lies in the interval $0 \leq \delta_1 \leq 1$. The first-order stability bounds for δ_1 are identical to the $AR1$ stationarity bounds and they play the same role. When δ_1 falls outside these bounds, the post-intervention time series is nonstationary.

When $\delta_1 = 0$, the first-order transfer function reduces to a zero-order transfer function. The impact accrues instantaneously. When $\delta_1 = 1$, on the other hand, the first-order transfer function reduces to ∇^{-1}. The impact accrues at a constant rate, interpreted as a post-intervention linear trend. Values of δ_1 between zero and one accrue at a diminishing rate.

Figure 5.11 shows several first-order transfer functions with a range of useful δ_1-values. The value of δ_1 is constrained to the open interval $-1 \le \delta_1 \le 1$. The so-called bounds of system stability for δ-parameters are identical to the AR stationarity bounds again and with the same rationale. Values of δ_1 outside the stability bounds imply that the intervention has made a stationary process nonstationary. Although an impact of this type is not unimaginable, it may require an idiosyncratic interpretation if $|\delta_1|$ is too large. Values of $\delta_1 = 1$ are tolerable, of course, but require a cautious interpretation. Finally, negative values of δ_1,

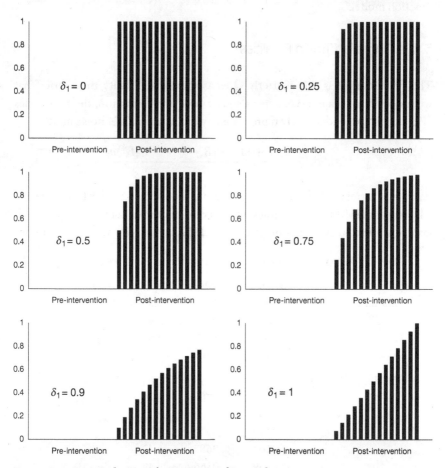

Figure 5.11 First-Order Transfer Functions of I_t, $0 \le \delta_1 \le 1$

which imply an *oscillating* impact, pose the same problem. Because these types of impacts are rare in our experience, we postpone their discussion, focusing instead on the range shown in Figure 5.11.

The parameter δ_1 is often called the "rate of gain" and this is a neatly descriptive term. As δ_1 grows larger, approaching $\delta_1 = 1$, the impact accrues more slowly. As δ_1 grows smaller, approaching $\delta_1 = 0$, the impact accrues more rapidly. Excluding the boundary endpoints, when $0 < \delta_1 < 1$, the model impact approaches the limit of

$$\frac{\omega_0}{1 - \delta_1}$$

We call this limit the "steady gain state" or the "asymptotic impact." The model impacts shown in Figure 5.11 have identical one-unit steady gain states. A few examples will illustrate the interpretation of the dynamic first-order transfer function model.

5.2.1 Australian Traffic Fatalities

The first example is the quarterly Queensland Road Fatality time series that we modeled in Chapter 3.6. After a square-root transformation, the time series (Figure 3.31) was adequately represented by the seasonal *IMA* noise model,

$$AuFtl_t^{1/2} = \frac{\theta_0 + (1 - \theta_1 B - \theta_3 B^3 - \theta_4 B^4) a_t}{\nabla}$$

Parameter estimates for this "best" model are reported as Model 1 in Table 5.7. The seasonal *IMA* model assumes no intervention. In fact, a mandatory seatbelt law took effect in Australia on January 1, 1972. Although the U.S. experience

Table 5.7. Australian Traffic Fatalities, Estimation and Diagnosis

		Estimate	SE	t	Diagnosis
Model 1	$\hat{\theta}_0$	.0553	.0154	3.58	$RSE = 0.7603$
	$\hat{\theta}_1$	.8233	.0690	11.94	$Q_8 = 4.2$
	$\hat{\theta}_3$	.2932	.1023	2.87	$Z_{KS} = 0.72$
	$\hat{\theta}_4$	−.3118	.0915	−3.41	
Model 2	$\hat{\theta}_0$	.0701	.0055	12.84	$RSE = 0.7087$
	$\hat{\theta}_1$	.9629	.0714	13.49	$Q_8 = 5.3$
	$\hat{\theta}_3$	.3399	.1090	3.12	$Z_{KS} = 0.72$
	$\hat{\theta}_4$	−.3270	.0972	−3.36	
	$\hat{\omega}_0$	−.1662	.0687	−2.42	
	$\hat{\delta}_1$	.9339	.0566	−16.49	

leads us to expect a reduction in traffic fatalities (Ross and McCleary, 1983), Bhattacharyya and Layton (1979) found no impact. A visual inspection of the time series is at least ambiguous. Some readers may see a modest impact—we do—but other readers may see no impact. A formal analysis will resolve this disagreement.

To capture the hypothetical impact of the mandatory seatbelt law, we define a step function I_t that changes from zero to one in the first quarter of 1972, the 89th quarterly observation. Because the hypothetical impact of I_t is expected to accrue gradually, we link I_t to $AUFtl_t^{1/2}$ with a first-order transfer function. Adding this impact model to the seasonal IMA component yields the full model:

$$AuFtl_t^{1/2} = \frac{\theta_0 + (1 - \theta_1 B - \theta_3 B^3 - \theta_4 B^4)}{\nabla} a_t + \frac{\omega_0}{1 - \delta_1 B} I_t$$

Because the seatbelt law is expected to reduce the level of the time series, we hypothesize $\omega_0 < 0$. Because the impact of the law is expected to accrue gradually over the post-intervention period, we further hypothesize $0 < \delta_1 < 1$. Parameter estimates for the full model, reported as Model 2 in Table 5.7, confirm our expectations. All six estimates are statistically significant; estimates of the MA parameters are invertible; and the Q-statistic is too small to reject a white noise hypothesis for the model residuals. Because Model 2 has a lower RSE than Model 1, it is the "better" model.

Estimates of the intervention parameters are statistically significant and in the expected direction—i.e., $\hat{\omega}_0 = -.1662$ corresponds to a *reduction* in the level of time series and $\hat{\delta}_1 = .9339$ corresponds to the expected *gradual* accrual of the impact. Strictly speaking, any estimate of the rate parameter that lies in the stable interval $-1 < \delta_1 < 1$ is acceptable. Negative values of δ_1 are less interpretable, however. To facilitate interpretation of Model 2, we subtract $N(a_t)$ from $AuFtl_t^{1/2}$, leaving the residualized time series Z_t:

$$Z_t = \frac{-.1662}{1 - .9339B} I_t$$

Z_t and I_t are linked deterministically by the first-order transfer function. The denominator of the first-order transfer function has an infinite series identity.

$$Z_t = -.1662 \left(\sum_{j=0}^{\infty} .9339B^j \right) I_t$$

$$= (-.1662) \left(.9339^0 B^0 + .9339^1 B^1 + .9339^2 B^2 + \cdots + .9339^{j-1} B^{j-1} + \cdots \right) I_t$$

$$= (-.1662)I_t + (-.1662)(.9339)I_{t-1} + (-.1662)(.9339^2)I_{t-2} + \cdots$$
$$+ (-.1662)(.9339^{j-1})I_{t-j} + \cdots$$

Prior to the first quarter of 1972, $I_t = 0$ and all terms of the infinite series are zero, so

$$Z_t = 0 \qquad \text{for} \qquad 0 \le t \le N_{pre}$$

In the first post-intervention quarter, $I_{N_{pre}+1} = 1$, so the first term of the infinite series is nonzero.

$$\begin{aligned} Z_{N_{pre}+1} &= (-.1662)I_{N_{pre}+1} \\ &= -.1662 \end{aligned}$$

In the second post-intervention quarter, $I_{N_{pre}+2} = I_{N_{pre}+1} = 1$. The first two terms of the infinite series are nonzero.

$$\begin{aligned} Z_{N_{pre}+2} &= (-.1662)I_{N_{pre}+2} + (-.1662)(.9339)I_{N_{pre}+1} \\ &= (-.1662) + (-.1662)(.9339) \\ &= -.1662(1 + .9339) \end{aligned}$$

In the third post-intervention quarter, $I_{N_{pre}+3} = I_{N_{pre}+2} = I_{N_{pre}+1} = 1$, so the first three terms of the infinite series are nonzero.

$$\begin{aligned} Z_{N_{pre}+3} &= (-.1662)I_{N_{pre}+3} + (-.1662)(.9339)I_{N_{pre}+2} \\ &\quad + (-.1662)(.9339^2)I_{N_{pre}+1} \\ &= (-.1662) + (-.1662)(.9339) + (-.1662)(.9339^2) \\ &= -.1662(1 + .9339 + .9339^2) \end{aligned}$$

In general, in the jth post-intervention quarter, the first j terms of the infinite series are nonzero. Thus

$$Z_{N_{pre}+j} = (-.1662)(1 + .9339 + .9339^2 + \cdots + .9339^{j-1})$$

Given the relatively large rate parameter, $\hat{\delta}_1 = .9339$, the impact accrues gradually over the post-intervention segment. Indeed, it is only after years of accrual that the impact becomes visually apparent—to the extent that it is visually apparent at all.

Given the slow rate of accrual, a quarter-to-quarter report of the impact would involve tedious details. Instead, Table 5.8 reports the *incremental* and *cumulative* impacts for the first quarter of 14 post-intervention years, beginning with 1972. In the jth post-intervention quarter, the *incremental* impact of the mandatory seatbelt law is

$$\hat{\delta}_1^{j-1}\hat{\omega}_0 = (.9339^{j-1})(-.1662)$$

Table 5.8. IMPACT OF THE AUSTRALIAN SEATBELT LAW

Year	j	$\hat{\delta}_1^{j-1}\hat{\omega}_0$	$\displaystyle\sum_{i=1}^{j}\hat{\delta}_1^{j-1}\hat{\omega}_0$	$\dfrac{\displaystyle\sum_{i=1}^{j}\hat{\delta}_1^{j-1}\hat{\omega}_0}{\dfrac{\hat{\omega}_0}{1-\hat{\delta}_1}}$
1972	1	−.1662	−0.1662	0.0661
1973	5	−.1264	−0.7282	0.2896
1974	9	−.0962	−1.1556	0.4596
1975	13	−.0732	−1.4808	0.5889
1976	17	−.0556	−1.7282	0.6873
1977	21	−.0423	−1.9163	0.7621
1978	25	−.0322	−2.0594	0.8191
1979	29	−.0245	−2.1683	0.8624
1980	33	−.0186	−2.2511	0.8953
1981	37	−.0142	−2.3141	0.9204
1982	41	−.0108	−2.3734	0.9439
1983	45	−.0082	−2.4098	0.9584
1984	49	−.0063	−2.4376	0.9694
1985	53	−.0047	−2.4587	0.9778

These increments are reported in the third column of Table 5.8. As j grows larger, $\delta_1^{j-1}\omega_0$ approaches zero. Added to the preceding $j-1$ increments, the cumulative impact of the mandatory seatbelt law is

$$\sum_{i=1}^{j}\hat{\delta}_1^{j-1}\hat{\omega}_0 = \sum_{i=1}^{j}(.9339^{j-1})(-.1662)$$

Cumulative increments are reported in the fourth column of Table 5.8. So long as the rate parameter lies in the stable interval, $0 < \delta_1 < 1$, as j grows larger, the cumulative impact approaches the limit

$$\frac{\hat{\omega}_0}{1-\hat{\delta}_1} = \frac{-.1662}{1-.9339} \approx -2.5144$$

This *asymptotic impact* suggests a useful standardization. The fifth column of Table 5.8 reports the *cumulative impact* as a proportion of the *asymptotic impact*. Fifty percent of asymptotic impact is realized in the 10th post-intervention quarter, the second quarter of 1974; 90 percent of the asymptotic impact is realized in the 34th post-intervention quarter, the second quarter of 1980; and 95 percent of the asymptotic impact is realized in the 42nd post-intervention quarter, the second quarter of 1982.

5.2.2 British Traffic Fatalities

Figure 5.12 plots a monthly time series of British traffic fatalities from January 1969 through December 1984 (Harvey, 1989). When a mandatory seatbelt law takes effect in February 1983, fatalities seem to drop abruptly. Nevertheless, to demonstrate a point, we will try to fit the same first-order transfer function to this British time series. Unlike the Queensland time series, which had noticeable trends in mean and variance, this British time series seems to be homogeneous in mean and variance. Judging from the visual evidence, this time series will not require a Normalizing transformation. The pattern of monthly seasonality is stronger, of course, suggesting a need for seasonal differencing.

Sample ACFs estimated from the $N_{pre} = 169$ observations of the U.K. traffic fatality time series and its differences are reported in Table 5.9.

Based on Q-statistics, 12th-order differencing is appropriate. The sample ACF for $\nabla^{12}UKFtl_t$ identifies $N(a_t)$ as a low-order AR and seasonal MA model. The sample PACF for $\nabla^{12}UKFtl_t$, not reported here, identifies the low-order AR model as AR2. We write this model as:

$$UKFtl_t = \frac{\theta_0 + \left(1 - \theta_{12}B^{12}\right)}{\nabla^{12}\left(1 - \phi_1 B - \phi_2 B^2\right)} a_t$$

Parameter estimates for this model, based on the $N_{pre} = 169$ observations, are reported in Table 5.10 as Model 1. Except for the constant, all of the parameter estimates are statistically significant and stationary-invertible and the residuals are not different than white noise. The next step is to add a first-order transfer

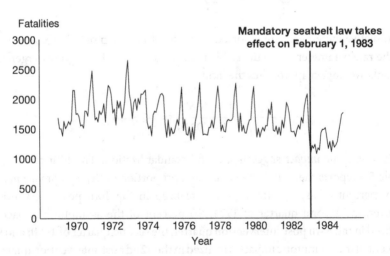

Figure 5.12 Monthly British Traffic Fatalities (Harvey, 1989)

Table 5.9. BRITISH TRAFFIC FATALITIES, IDENTIFICATION

	$UKFtl_t$		$\nabla UKFtl_t$		$\nabla^{12} UKFtl_t$		$\nabla\nabla^{12} UKFtl_t$	
k	r_k	Q_k	r_k	Q_k	r_k	Q_k	r_k	Q_k
1	.63	68.9	−.10	1.6	.36	20.4	−.50	40.5
2	.35	89.8	−.10	3.2	.36	40.9	.13	43.1
3	.13	92.8	−.12	5.6	.19	46.9	−.07	43.9
4	−.00	92.8	−.17	10.9	.12	49.2	−.13	46.7
5	−.01	92.8	.06	11.7	.22	56.9	.19	52.5
6	−.07	93.7	−.12	14.2	.07	57.7	−.14	56.0
7	−.04	94.0	.04	14.5	.11	59.7	.04	56.2
8	−.04	94.3	−.18	20.2	.10	61.3	−.05	56.6
9	.09	95.7	−.07	21.0	.15	64.9	.06	57.3
10	.26	108.	−.12	23.5	.11	66.9	.02	57.3
11	.53	160.	.11	25.6	.05	67.4	.14	60.6
12	.72	254.	.54	79.1	−.19	73.7	−.41	89.8
13	.51	302.	.12	81.8	.10	75.4	.31	106.
14	.22	311.	−.16	86.3	−.00	75.4	−.14	110.
15	.04	311.	−.11	88.6	.08	76.5	.04	110.
16	−.05	311.	−.09	90.1	.11	78.7	.08	111.
17	−.08	313.	−.04	90.4	.03	78.9	−.21	119.
18	−.09	314.	.01	90.4	.24	88.8	.30	135.
19	−.10	317.	−.02	90.5	.06	89.4	−.16	140.
20	−.11	319.	−.14	94.3	.08	90.6	.09	141.
21	−.00	319.	−.06	95.0	.00	90.6	.04	141.
22	.14	323.	−.16	100.	−.13	93.6	−.24	152.
23	.41	356.	.18	107.	.05	94.2	.28	166.
24	.54	415.	.47	151.	−.12	96.9	−.17	172.

function to Model 1. Where $I_t = 0$ for $1 \le t \le 169$ and $I_t = 1$ for $t > 169$, the full model is:

$$UKFtl_t = \frac{\theta_0 + \left(1 - \theta_{12}B^{12}\right)}{\nabla^{12}\left(1 - \phi_1 B - \phi_2 B^2\right)} a_t + \frac{\omega_0}{1 - \delta_1 B} I_t$$

Parameter estimates for this model, based on all $N = 192$ observations, are reported as Model 2 in Table 5.10 The ARMA parameter estimates of Model 2 are statistically significant and stationary-invertible and the residuals are not different than white noise. The transfer function parameter estimates are a mixed bag. The value of $\hat{\omega}_0 = -312.2608$ is statistically significant and negative, as expected. The value of $\hat{\delta}_1 = -.2847$ is not statistically significant, however, and, worse, lies outside the range of useful values. We will return to this point shortly. Dropping

Table 5.10. BRITISH TRAFFIC FATALITIES, ESTIMATION AND DIAGNOSIS

		Estimate	SE	t	Diagnosis
Model 1	$\hat{\theta}_0$	−16.5153	11.2047	−1.47	$RSE = 142.67$
	$\hat{\phi}_1$	.4013	.0776	5.17	$Q_{24} = 30.3$
	$\hat{\phi}_2$	.2957	.0768	3.85	$Z_{KS} = 0.66$
	θ_{12}	.7732	.0551	14.03	
Model 2	$\hat{\theta}_0$	−14.9446	10.1430	−1.47	$RSE = 137.61$
	$\hat{\phi}_1$	.4032	.0729	5.53	$Q_{24} = 30.5$
	$\hat{\phi}_2$	.2812	.0723	3.89	$Z_{KS} = 0.55$
	$\hat{\theta}_{12}$	.7658	.0496	15.43	
	$\hat{\omega}_0$	−328.6481	118.3753	−2.78	
	$\hat{\delta}_1$	−.2847	.3983	−0.71	
Model 3	$\hat{\phi}_1$	.4151	.0730	5.69	$RSE = 138.59$
	$\hat{\phi}_2$	.2862	.0722	3.96	$Q_{24} = 30.6$
	$\hat{\theta}_{12}$	.7525	.0494	15.24	$Z_{KS} = 0.49$
	$\hat{\omega}_0$	−312.2608	81.6807	−3.82	

the statistically insignificant parameters leaves

$$UKFtl_t = \frac{1 - \theta_{12}B^{12}}{\nabla^{12}\left(1 - \phi_1 B - \phi_2 B^2\right)} a_t + \omega_0 I_t$$

Parameter estimates for this model, based on all $N = 192$ observations, are reported as Model 3 in Table 5.10. Model 3 satisfies the conventional criteria and is accepted. Ignoring the *ARMA* parameters, which have no substantive interpretations, the value of $\hat{\omega}_0 = -312.2608$ is interpreted as an abrupt, permanent drop in traffic fatalities. This effect is consistent with the Queensland effect in that in both instances a mandatory seatbelt law produced a permanent reduction in fatalities. We cannot explain why the impact accrued gradually in one instance and abruptly in another.

The statistically insignificant value of $\hat{\delta}_1 = -.2847$ in Model 2 is instructive. To be useful, a rate parameter must ordinarily be a *positive* fraction. Though admissible, a *negative* fraction like $\hat{\delta}_1 = -.2847$ is not often useful. Ignoring the issue of statistical significance, the estimated first-order transfer function in Model 2 specifies alternating positive and negative changes. In the first six post-intervention months,

$$\hat{\delta}_1^0 \hat{\omega}_0 = (-.2847)^0(-328.6481) = -328.65$$
$$\hat{\delta}_1^1 \hat{\omega}_0 = (-.2847)^1(-328.6481) = 93.57$$
$$\hat{\delta}_1^2 \hat{\omega}_0 = (-.2847)^2(-328.6481) = -26.54$$
$$\hat{\delta}_1^3 \hat{\omega}_0 = (-.2847)^3(-328.6481) = 7.58$$
$$\hat{\delta}_1^4 \hat{\omega}_0 = (-.2847)^4(-328.6481) = -2.16$$
$$\hat{\delta}_1^5 \hat{\omega}_0 = (-.2847)^5(-328.6481) = 0.61$$

At the end of the first six post-intervention months, the net impact amounts to −255.69. This interpretation of Model 2 is consistent with the interpretation of Model 3, at least to the extent that both are interpreted as reductions. There is no theoretical reason to expect alternating positive and negative changes, however, so Model 2 is not useful as a time series experiment. We revisit this point—and this time series—in Chapter 6.

5.2.3 "Talking Out" Incidents

The time series plotted in Figure 5.13 is a daily count of disruptive "talking out" incidents in a second-grade inner-city classroom (Hall et al., 1971). When a behavioral intervention was introduced on the 21st day, the number of incidents dropped on that day and continued to drop steadily over the next 20 days, approaching a new post-intervention level. Without the benefit of a formal statistical analysis, Hall et al. concluded that their intervention was effective. Parsonson and Baer (1986) argue that statistical analyses are unnecessary when

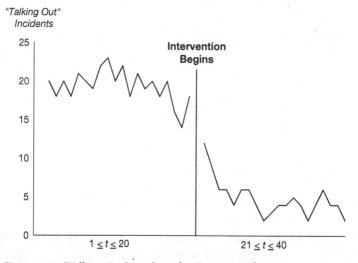

Figure 5.13 "Talking Out" Incidents (Hall et al., 1971)

the visual evidence is unambiguous and, in this instance, we agree. A formal statistical analysis would not enhance the credibility of the visual evidence. Given the difficulty of modeling a short time series, moreover, the formal analysis might produce discrepant statistical results that challenged the credibility of the visual evidence.

The obstacles to *ARIMA* identification in the "talking out" time series are common to experimental behavioral interventions. Put simply, the time series is too short and the interruption too large for direct identification of $N(a_t)$. Accordingly, we propose a white noise disturbance as a first approximation to $N(a_t)$. Using the first-order transfer function to link I_t to the time series, the full model is

$$Talk_t = a_t + \theta_0 + \frac{\omega_0}{1 - \delta_1 B} I_t$$

where $I_t = 0$ for $1 \leq t \leq 20$ and $I_t = 1$ for $21 \leq t \leq 40$. This is an unrealistic model, of course. But if all goes well, we can identify a closer approximation to $N(a_t)$ from the residuals of this model.

Parameter estimates for the initial model are reported in Table 5.11 as Model 1. There are no surprises in these estimates. The values of $\hat{\omega}_0 = -6.7945$ and $\hat{\delta}_1 = .5606$ are consistent with the visual evidence. Under a white noise hypothesis, $Q_{10} = 15.0$ occurs with $p < 0.13$, so the initial model is statistically adequate. It is *barely* adequate, however. Given the weak statistical power inherent to analyses of short time series and arbitrary choice of $k = 10$ lags for the sample *ACF*, we look for a "better" *ARIMA* model.

Sample *ACFs* for the Model 1 residuals are plotted in Figure 5.14. For $\hat{a}_t$, only two of the first 10 lags are statistically significant. Three other lags are large but not statistically significant. Although the sample *ACF* for $\hat{a}_t$ is ambiguous, it is not wholly inconsistent with a nonstationary process. The sample *ACFs* for the differenced residuals, $\nabla \hat{a}_t$, are consistent with the *IMA* model:

$$Talk_t = \frac{a_t + \theta_0}{\nabla} + \frac{\omega_0}{1 - \delta_1 B} I_t$$

Parameter estimates for the *IMA* model are reported in Table 5.11 as Model 2. All of the parameter estimates are statistically significant and the value of $Q_{10} = 8.8$ for the model residuals is an improvement. Model 2 is acceptable, so we move on to the next step, interpretation.

The estimated impact of the behavioral intervention is reported in Table 5.12. On the 21st day, or the first post-intervention day, the level of the "talking out" time series drops by more than 5.6 incidents. On successive post-intervention

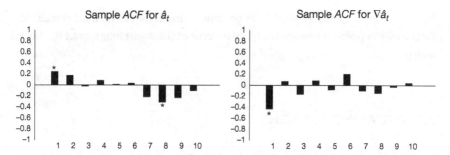

Figure 5.14 Identification, $\hat{a}_t = Talk_t - 19.3 + 6.8(1 + .56)^{-1}I_t$

Table 5.11. "Talking Out," Estimation and Diagnosis

		Estimate	SE	t	Diagnosis
Model 1	$\hat{\theta}_0$	19.3381	.3697	52.31	$RSE = 1.6575$
	$\hat{\omega}_0$	−6.7945	.8915	−7.62	$Q_{10} = 15.0$
	$\hat{\delta}_1$	.5606	.0597	9.40	$Z_{KS} = 0.86$
Model 2	$\hat{\theta}_0$	−.1060	.0844	−1.26	$RSE = 1.6440$
	$\hat{\theta}_1$	.7957	.1190	6.68	$Q_{10} = 8.8$
	$\hat{\omega}_0$	−5.6511	1.1295	−5.00	$Z_{KS} = 0.86$
	$\hat{\delta}_1$	.5497	.0941	5.84	

Table 5.12. Impact of the "Talking Out" Intervention

Day	j	$\hat{\delta}_1^{j-1}\hat{\omega}_0$	$\sum_{i=1}^{j}\hat{\delta}_1^{j-1}\hat{\omega}_0$	$\dfrac{\sum_{i=1}^{j}\hat{\delta}_1^{j-1}\hat{\omega}_0}{\dfrac{\hat{\omega}_0}{1-\hat{\delta}_1}}$
21	1	−5.6511	−5.6511	0.4504
22	2	−3.1064	−8.7575	0.6980
23	3	−1.7076	−10.4651	0.8341
24	4	−.9387	−11.4038	0.9089
25	5	−.5160	−11.9198	0.9500
26	6	−.2836	−12.2034	0.9726
27	7	−.1559	−12.3593	0.9850
28	8	−.0857	−12.4450	0.9919

days, the time series level continues to drop but by smaller and smaller increments, approaching the *asymptotic impact*

$$\frac{\omega_0}{1-\delta_1} = \frac{-5.6511}{1-.5497} \approx -12.5468$$

By the fifth post-intervention day, 95 percent of this *asymptotic impact* is realized. By the eighth post-intervention day, 99 percent of the *asymptotic impact* has been realized.

5.3 DECAYING IMPACTS

Figure 5.15 shows daily cholera deaths in the vicinity of London's Broad Street pump for six weeks in late summer, 1854. About 15 years earlier, cholera appeared suddenly and mysteriously in Britain, probably brought back from India by returning troops. By 1850, annual British cholera deaths numbered in the tens of thousands. Cholera is caused by a water-borne bacterium, *V. cholerae*, but that was unknown in 1854. Indeed, although Victorian medical scientists knew that microbes flourished in air and water, the central role played by microbes in disease was unknown.

In the 1850s, the state-of-the-art *miasma* theory held that cholera was transmitted through air by the odor of decaying organic matter—corpses. The miasma theory explained the spatial clustering of cholera deaths as well as the higher death rates in low-lying slum areas near the Thames. The summer air was stagnant near the river. Wealthier areas uphill from the river were vented by summer breezes and had lower death rates. These facts were also consistent with the water transmission theory proposed by John Snow (1855). At the end of August 1854, Snow observed an epidemic of cholera deaths near the Broad Street water pump.

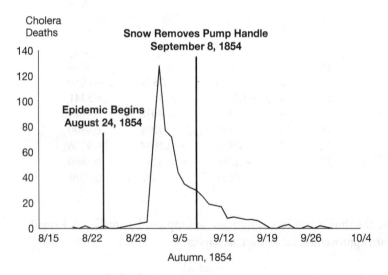

Figure 5.15 Cholera Deaths Near the Broad Street Pump, 1854 (Lai, 2013)

When Snow disabled the pump, the epidemic subsided. A few days later, Snow discovered that raw sewage had leaked into the Thames at the pump inlet.

Three decades after Snow demonstrated the causal link between cholera and contaminated drinking water, Robert Koch isolated water-borne *V. cholerae* (Ewald, 1994). Snow's inquiry involved more than the crude experimental intervention described in our account. The descriptions found in epidemiology textbooks are questionable, moreover, and apocryphal. For our purposes, the important point is that the cholera epidemic peaked on August 31, 1854. When Snow confiscated the handle of the Broad Street pump on September 8, 1854, the epidemic had already begun to subside. This revisionist timeline, due to Lai (2013), weakens the popular causal interpretation of Snow's experimental intervention. Nevertheless, the decaying spike in Figure 5.15 is typical of interventions that effect temporary changes in the equilibrium levels of time series.

One of the clearest examples of this type of intervention is the recovery of a local economy from a natural disaster (Friesema et al., 1978). The immediate economic impact of a tornado or flood occurs when bridges, highways, and power lines are destroyed. As these infrastructure components are replaced or repaired, the local economy returns to its pre-disaster equilibrium. If the damage is not too severe and if the governmental response is immediate and adequate, the local economy returns to its pre-disaster equilibrium level in a few months. If the damage is too severe, of course, or if the governmental response is slow and/or inadequate, the local economy may never return to normal.

Political "honeymoons" present another well-studied example. When a new president takes office, presidential popularity (or "approval") spikes upward and then decays quickly over time (Norpoth, 1984, 1986, 1987a, 1987b; Norpoth and Yantek, 1983). This phenomenon is apparent in Figure 5.16. This time series

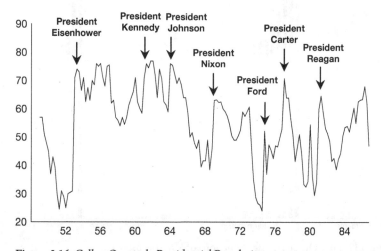

Figure 5.16 Gallup Quarterly Presidential Popularity

consists of quarterly Gallup Poll presidential approval ratings for 1968 through 1983. In the first quarter of 1973, President Nixon fired Attorney General Elliot Richardson and Watergate Special Prosecutor Archibald Cox. President Nixon's popularity declines precipitously. Presidential popularity rebounds in the fourth quarter of 1974, when President Ford takes office, but then drops immediately, due presumably to the pardon of President Nixon. When Presidents Carter and Reagan take office in 1976 and 1980, popularity spikes and decays. Allowing for the unusual circumstances faced by President Ford, the rate of decay in presidential popularity is roughly the same for each new administration.

To model any temporary impact, we represent the intervention as a pulse function that turns "on" at the point of intervention and then turns "off." For reasons that will become clear shortly, we use the differenced step function, ∇I_t,

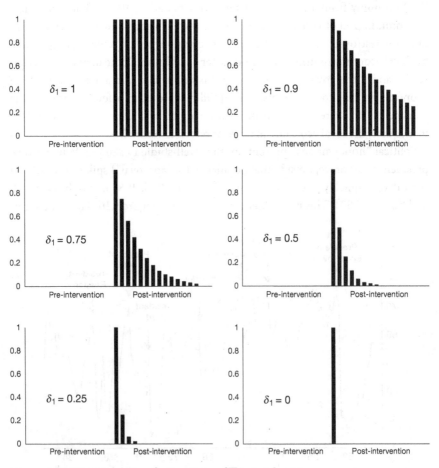

Figure 5.17 First-Order Transfer Functions of ∇I_t, $0 \le \delta_1 \le 1$

as the pulse intervention.

$$\nabla I_t = 0 \text{ for } 1 \leq t \leq N_{pre}$$
$$= 1 \text{ for } t = N_{pre} + 1$$
$$= 0 \text{ for } N_{pre} + 2 \leq t \leq N_{post}$$

The impact of ∇I_t on Y_t is realized through the same first-order transfer function,

$$X(I_t) = \frac{\omega_0}{1 - \delta_1 B} \nabla I_t$$

Although the rate parameter, δ_1, can take any value in the stable interval, the most useful values once again lie in the interval $0 \leq \delta_1 \leq 1$.

Figure 5.17 shows the expected impacts for values of δ_1 in the useful interval. When $\delta_1 = 1$, the first-order transfer function of ∇I_t reduces to the zero-order transfer function:

$$\frac{\omega}{1 - \delta_1 B} \nabla I_t = \omega \frac{1 - B}{1 - B} I_t = \omega I_t$$

This identity allows for a straightforward hypothesis test, which we will demonstrate shortly. When $\delta_1 = 0$, on the other hand, the first-order transfer function shifts the level of Y_t by ω units for one post-intervention observation. Values of δ_1 between these two extremes decay at exponential rates.

5.3.1 Self-Injurious Behavior

The time series plotted in Figure 5.18 are daily self-injurious behavior counts for two institutionalized patients before and after an intervention. These data were introduced in Chapter 1 and were plotted in Figures 1.6 and 1.9 on ordinal scales. The time series are plotted on a common axis in Figure 5.18 to highlight similarities between the patients' immediate reactions to the intervention. In the first few post-intervention days, both patients have similar reactions to the new regime. Thereafter, self-injurious behavior counts for the treated patient drop while the placebo patient returns to the pre-intervention level.

Based on physiological theory, the most reasonable impact model for the patient treated with naltrexone is a zero-order transfer function of I_t:

$$SIB_{Naltrexone,t} = N(a_t) + \omega_0 I_t$$

It may be comforting to note that the visual evidence is consistent with this model. The validity of a null hypothesis test assumes that $\omega_0 I_t$ is specified on the basis of substantive theory, however. As part of the design, a control patient

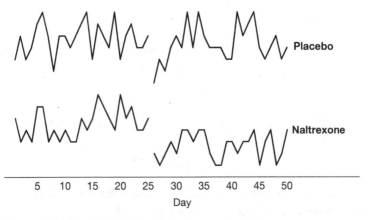

Figure 5.18 Daily Self-Injurious Behavior for Two Patients

receives a placebo on the 26th day. This patient's self-injurious behavior also drops abruptly but returns to the pre-intervention level within a few days. Based on our theory of placebo effects, a reasonable model for this impact is

$$SIB_{Placebo,t} = N(a_t) + \frac{\omega_0}{1 - \delta_1 B} \nabla I_t$$

Compared to the physiological theory of opioid antagonists, the theory of placebo effects is controversial. A meta-analysis of clinical trials (Hróbjartsson and Gotzsche, 2001) finds little evidence that placebo effects exist in most medical fields; but see the review by Price, Finniss, and Benedetti (2008). We take no stand on this controversy. Because the control patient received a physiologically inert placebo, there is no theoretical reason to expect any impact other than a placebo effect—or something very much *like* a placebo effect.

To jump-start the *ARIMA* modeling strategy, we used white noise disturbances as first approximations to $N(a_t)$ for both patients. Q-statistics for the residuals of both models are too small to reject white noise hypotheses. Parameter estimates for the naltrexone patient's *abrupt, permanent* impact model are reported in Table 5.13 as Model 1. Rounded to two decimal places, we write this model as

$$SIB_{Naltrexone,t} = 4.56 + a_t - 1.92 I_t$$

This model has the following straightforward interpretation: When $I_t = 0$, the patient's self-injurious behavior occurs at the daily rate of $\hat{\theta}_0 = 4.56$ incidents. When $I_t = 1$, the daily rate drops abruptly. The difference between the pre- and post-intervention rate is $\hat{\omega}_0 = -1.92$ incidents. Parameter estimates for the control patient's *abrupt, temporary* impact model are reported in Table 5.13 as

Table 5.13. SELF-INJURIOUS BEHAVIOR, ESTIMATION AND DIAGNOSIS

		Estimate	SE	t	Diagnosis
Model 1	$\hat{\theta}_0$	4.5599	.2331	19.56	$RSE = 1.1655$
	$\hat{\omega}_0$	−1.9198	.3297	−5.82	$Q_{10} = 9.2$
					$Z_{KS} = 0.86$
Model 2	$\hat{\theta}_0$	4.7141	.2022	23.32	$RSE = 1.3155$
	$\hat{\omega}_0$	−3.8326	1.2427	−3.08	$Q_{10} = 10.7$
	$\hat{\delta}_1$	.5610	.1925	2.91	$Z_{KS} = 0.86$
Model 3	$\hat{\theta}_0$	4.5600	.2328	19.59	$RSE = 1.1640$
	$\hat{\omega}_0$	−2.0567	.5052	−4.07	$Q_{10} = 8.7$
	$\hat{\delta}_1$	.9944	.0148	67.29	$Z_{KS} = 0.86$

Table 5.14. IMPACT OF A PLACEBO INTERVENTION

j	$\hat{\omega}_0\hat{\delta}_1^{j-1}$	$\hat{\theta}_0 - \hat{\omega}_0\hat{\delta}_1^{j-1}$	$\dfrac{\hat{\theta}_0 - \hat{\omega}_0\hat{\delta}_1^{j-1}}{\hat{\theta}_0}$
1	$-3.83 \times .56^0 = -3.83$	$4.71 - 3.83 = 0.88$	0.186
2	$-3.83 \times .56^1 = -2.14$	$4.71 - 2.14 = 2.57$	0.546
3	$-3.83 \times .56^2 = -1.20$	$4.71 - 1.20 = 3.51$	0.745
4	$-3.83 \times .56^3 = -0.67$	$4.71 - 0.67 = 4.04$	0.858
5	$-3.83 \times .56^4 = -0.38$	$4.71 - 0.38 = 4.33$	0.896
6	$-3.83 \times .56^5 = -0.21$	$4.71 - 0.21 = 4.50$	0.955
7	$-3.83 \times .56^5 = -0.12$	$4.71 - 0.12 = 4.59$	0.974

Model 2. Rounded to two decimal places,

$$SIB_{Placebo,t} = 4.71 + a_t - \frac{3.83}{1 - .56B}\nabla I_t$$

When $\nabla I_t = 0$, the control patient's self-injurious behavior occurs at the daily rate of $\hat{\theta}_0 = 4.71$ incidents. On the first post-intervention day, when $\nabla I_t = 1$, the rate drops abruptly. But on the second post-intervention day, when $\nabla I_t = 0$ again, the impact begins to decay quickly. Six days after the intervention, the time series has returned to 95 percent of the pre-intervention level.

To illustrate the dynamics of the placebo impact, Table 5.14 estimates the impact for the first seven post-intervention days. The first column indexes the post-intervention day, $j = 1, 2, 3, 4, 5, 6, 7$. The second column estimates the *scalar* impact for the jth post-intervention day as $\hat{\omega}_0\hat{\delta}_1^{j-1}$. The third column estimates the *relative* impact as the difference of the *scalar* impact and $\hat{\theta}_0$, the pre-intervention level. Finally, the fourth column standardizes the relative impact as a proportion of the pre-intervention time series level. As reported in Table 5.14, the level of self-injurious behavior has returned to 95 percent of its pre-intervention level by the j =6th post-intervention day.

To complete our demonstration of the first-order transfer function of ∇I_t, ignoring physiological theory, we estimate the abrupt, *temporary* model for the naltrexone patient's time series. Parameter estimates of this model are reported as Model 3 in Table 5.13. Rounded to two decimal places,

$$SIB_{Naltrexone,t} = -4.56 + a_t - \frac{-2.06}{1 - .99B}\nabla I_t$$

The interpretation of Model 3 is virtually identical to the interpretation of Model 1. But since $\hat{\delta}_1 = .9944$ lies in the stable interval—though just barely—Model 3 could be interpreted as an *abrupt, temporary* impact. The impact would persist for years, of course, decaying at a rate so slow that it would escape notice. Alternatively, since the standard error of $\hat{\delta}_1$ is too small to reject the null hypothesis that $\delta_1 = 1$, we invoke the rule of parsimony. Accepting the fact that $\delta_1 = 1$, we can rewrite the model as

$$SIB_{Naltrexone,t} = -4.56 + a_t - 2.06\left(\frac{1-B}{1-B}\right)I_t = -4.56 + a_t - 2.06I_t$$

This suggests a simple null hypothesis test to distinguish between permanent and temporary effects. If the value of $\hat{\delta}_1$ is not significantly different than unity, the first-order transfer function of ∇I_t should be reduced to a zero-order transfer function of I_t.

Placebo-like effects are also found in aggregate-level time series. When a new law is enacted, for example, general deterrence theory holds that people will obey the law if they perceive, correctly or incorrectly, that breaking the law will incur a punishment. The drunk-driving literature gives the best evidence for this proposition. Drunk driving is so common in many Western nations that only a small fraction of lawbreakers are apprehended and punished. Given the trivially small probability of punishment, we are surprised to find any impact from a drunk-driving law. But this is not the case. Evaluating the effects of drunk-driving laws in several nations, Ross (1984), Homel (1988), and others find that most of the laws have some impact on traffic fatality time series. The impacts often decay over time, however, suggesting that drunk-driving laws have placebo-like effects.

5.4 COMPLEX IMPACTS

Under ideal circumstances—strong *theories*, long *series*— simple impact models can be combined in a single complex model. The most useful combinations combine zero-order and first-order transfer functions of I_t. For example,

$$X(I_t) = \omega_{0,1}I_t + \frac{\omega_{0,2}}{1-\delta_1}\nabla I_t$$

$$= \left(\omega_{0,1} + \frac{\omega_{0,2}}{1-\delta_1}\nabla\right)I_t$$

In this complex model, the first component describes an abrupt change of $\omega_{0,1}$ units that persists permanently. The second component describes an abrupt change of $\omega_{0,2}$ units that decays geometrically at the rate of δ_1 units per observation.

5.4.1 Australian Family Law Act of 1975

Figure 5.19 plots annual divorces in Australia from 1901 to 2009. The striking intervention in this time series is the 1975 Family Law Act, which provided, among other things, for no-fault divorce. In an evaluation of the 1975 Act, Ozdowski and Hattie (1981, p. 11) concluded that the Act had no *permanent* impact on divorces, that "one may expect the divorce rate to return to 'normal' in the near future." This conclusion was based on a comparison of post-1975 time series to the least-squares quadratic trend line. Since the numbers of divorces in 1976–80 were smaller than predicted by the least-squares quadratic trend line, the researchers concluded that, after a brief period of instability, divorces had returned to normal.

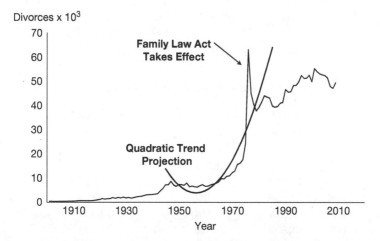

Figure 5.19 Australian Divorce Rates (Ozdowski and Hattie, 1981)

While the 1975 Family Law Act did have a temporary impact on divorces, it also had a permanent impact. Although a least-squares quadratic trend might seem to fit the pre-intervention time series—though not very well—it is not a reasonable model of the underlying process. Extrapolated to the end of the century, for example, the quadratic trend predicts a 10-fold increase in divorce rates. Figure 5.19 illustrates and reinforces the distinction between *fitting* and *modeling* a time series.

Reanalyzing these data, McCleary and Riggs (1982) used a zero-order transfer function of I_t and a first-order transfer function of ∇I_t to create a complex impact composed of an abrupt, permanent impact and an abrupt, temporary impact. To replicate and update their reanalysis, we estimated the same complex intervention model from the 1946–2009 segment of the time series with a white noise disturbance. The residuals of this model identified $N(a_t)$ as an integrated white noise disturbance. Parameter estimates for

$$AuDvrc_t = \frac{\theta_0 + a_t}{\nabla} + \omega_{0,1}I_t + \frac{\omega_{0,2}}{1 - \delta_1 B}\nabla I_t$$

are reported as Model 1 in Table 5.15. All of the parameter estimates are statistically significant and the model residuals are not different than white noise.

The permanent effect $(\hat{\omega}_{0,1}I_t)$, temporary effect $(\hat{\omega}_{0,2}\hat{\delta}_1^{j-1}\nabla I_t)$, and net total effect— the sum of the permanent and temporary effects— are reported in Table 5.16 for eight post-intervention years. By the start of the ninth year, the

Table 5.15. AUSTRALIAN DIVORCES, ESTIMATION AND DIAGNOSIS

		Estimate	SE	t	Diagnosis
Model 1	$\hat{\theta}_0$	.4747	.2289	2.07	$RSE = 1.7483$
	$\hat{\omega}_{0,1}$	12.3090	3.9185	3.14	$Q_{10} = 10.7$
	$\hat{\omega}_{0,2}$	26.1393	3.4442	7.59	$Z_{KS} = 0.97$
	$\hat{\delta}_1$	.2909	.0841	3.46	

Table 5.16. IMPACT OF THE 1975 FAMILY LAW ACT

Year	$\hat{\omega}_{0,1}I_t$	$\hat{\omega}_{0,2}\hat{\delta}_1^{j-1}\nabla I_t$	$\hat{\omega}_{0,1}I_t + \hat{\omega}_{0,2}\hat{\delta}_1^{j-1}\nabla I_t$
1976	12,309	26,139	38,448
1977	12,309	7,604	19,913
1978	12,309	2,212	14,521
1979	12,309	643	12,952
1980	12,309	187	12,496
1981	12,309	54	12,363
1982	12,309	16	12,325
1983	12,309	5	12,314

temporary part of the effect has decayed to zero while the permanent part persists indefinitely.

There are at least two lessons to be learned from this time series experiment. First, quadratic trend lines will almost always provide a good fit to short time series segments. Extrapolating the quadratic trend line beyond the short segment is risky, however, because very few social science processes follow quadratic trends. There is a fundamental difference between *fitting* a time series and modeling the underlying time series process. We list this fundamental difference as a threat to construct validity in Chapter 8. Until then, the reader might draw a lesson from the visual evidence in Figure 5.19.

The second lesson informs the theory of legal interventions. In our experience, legal interventions often have complex impacts. The hybrid model that we used to evaluate the 1975 Australian Family Law Act is widely applicable to legal interventions and reforms. Whenever a new law is introduced to encourage positive behavior or to discourage negative behavior, post-intervention instability should be expected. If the instability dies out quickly—say, in a week or two—it might be lost in temporal aggregation. Otherwise, the pattern of instability can be realized as a spike that decays to a new post-intervention level. Another example illustrates this phenomenon.

5.4.2 Decriminalization of Public Drunkenness

Figure 5.20 shows a monthly time series of public drunkenness arrests for Washington D.C. In January 1969, the 37th month, public drunkenness was

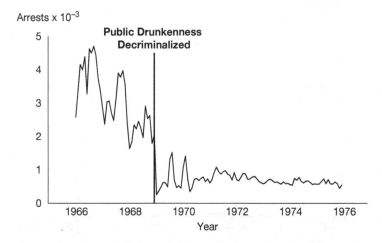

Figure 5.20 Monthly Public Drunkenness Arrests, Washington D.C.

decriminalized with the apparent impact shown. Aaronson *et al.* (1978) argue
that the postintervention reduction in the level of this time series is the crude
impact of a policy change by the Washington D.C. Police Department. After
decriminalization, police officers were instructed to give public drunkenness
cases low priority and, hence, the monthly number of cases dropped. Like any
bureaucratic innovation, however, the impact of the policy change accumulated
gradually and, for this reason, we hypothesize an exponential response to the
intervention.

A visual inspection of the time series is often informative. Monthly fluctuations
in the plotted time series are relatively large in the pre-intervention segment
and relatively small in the post-intervention segment. This suggests variance
nonstationarity and the need for a transformation.

Figure 5.21 plots the variance of the transformed time series, $PubDrnk_t^{(\lambda)}$,
for a range of λ-values. The minimum variance occurs when $\lambda = -0.6$ but
the function is relatively flat in the vicinity of this "best" Box-Cox value. If
the intervention were smaller—or if the time series were longer—variance in
the function would shrink, allowing for a more confident inference. The "best"
λ-value would probably move as well. In any event, this "best" λ-value is not
significantly different than $\lambda = 0$. Since natural logarithms are recommended for
"floor effects" such as this one, we use the natural log transformation but resolve
to revisit this decision at a later point in the analysis.

The log-transformed time series, plotted in Figure 5.22, is smoother and more
nearly homogeneous. Given the magnitude of the intervention, however, model
identification is still problematic. Accordingly, we begin the analysis with the

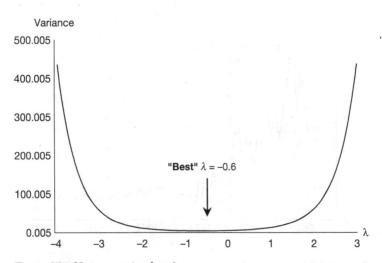

Figure 5.21 Variance, $-4 \leq \lambda \leq 3$

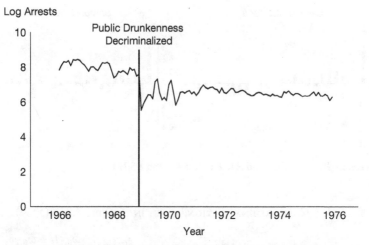

Figure 5.22 Log-Transformed Monthly Public Drunkenness Arrests, Washington D.C.

Table 5.17. LOG PUBLIC DRUNKENNESS ARRESTS, ESTIMATION AND DIAGNOSIS

		Estimate	SE	t	Diagnosis
Model 1	$\hat{\theta}_0$	7.9925	.0429	186.50	$RSE = 0.2571$
	$\hat{\omega}_{0,1}$	-1.4575	.0520	-28.05	$Q_{24} = 86.5$
	$\hat{\omega}_{0,2}$	-1.0651	.2437	-4.37	$Z_{KS} = 0.92$
	$\hat{\delta}_1$	.5029	.1410	3.57	
Model 2	$\hat{\theta}_0$	7.9942	.0749	106.72	$RSE = 0.1956$
	$\hat{\omega}_{0,1}$	-1.4548	.0901	-16.14	$Q_{24} = 22.6$
	$\hat{\omega}_{0,2}$	$-.9150$	.2003	-4.57	$Z_{KS} = 0.54$
	$\hat{\delta}_1$	.6439	.1828	3.52	
	$\hat{\phi}_1$	.7313	.0888	8.23	
	$\hat{\phi}_2$	$-.2620$	.0911	-2.87	
	$\hat{\theta}_6$	$-.2410$	.0918	-2.62	

white noise model

$$Ln(PubDrnk_t) = \theta_0 + a_t + \omega_{0,1}I_t + \frac{\omega_{0,2}}{1-\delta_1}\nabla I_t$$

Parameter estimates are reported in Table 5.17 as Model 1. The value of $Q_{24} = 86.5$ rejects the white noise model, but that was not unexpected. The *ACF* and *PACF* for the Model 1 residuals, plotted in Figure 5.23, identify the *ARMA* model

$$Ln(PubDrnk_t) = \frac{\theta_0 + (1 - \theta_6 B^6)}{1 - \phi_1 B - \phi_2 B^2}a_t + \omega_{0,1}I_t + \frac{\omega_{0,2}}{1-\delta_1}\nabla I_t$$

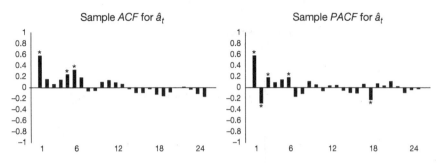

Figure 5.23 Residual *ACF* and *PACF* (Model 1, Table 5.17)

Table 5.18. DECRIMINALIZATION IMPACT IN THE FIRST YEAR (1969)

	$\hat{\omega}_{0,1} I_t$	$\hat{\omega}_{0,2} \hat{\delta}_1^{j-1} \nabla I_t$	$\hat{\omega}_{0,1} I_t + \hat{\omega}_{0,2} \hat{\delta}_1^{j-1} \nabla I_t$	$\dfrac{\hat{\omega}_{0,1} I_t + \hat{\omega}_{0,2} \hat{\delta}_1^{j-1} \nabla I_t}{\hat{\omega}_{0,1} I_t}$
January	−1.4548	−.9150	−2.3698	1.6290
February	−1.4548	−.5892	−2.0440	1.4050
March	−1.4548	−.3794	−1.8342	1.2608
April	−1.4548	−.2443	−1.6991	1.1679
May	−1.4548	−.1573	−1.6121	1.1081
June	−1.4548	−.1013	−1.5561	1.0696
July	−1.4548	−.0652	−1.5200	1.0448
August	−1.4548	−.0420	−1.4968	1.0289
September	−1.4548	−.0270	−1.4818	1.0186
October	−1.4548	−.0174	−1.4722	1.0120
November	−1.4548	−.0112	−1.4660	1.0077
December	−1.4548	−.0072	−1.4620	1.0050

The parameter estimates reported in Table 5.17 as Model 2 are significant and lie within the stationarity-invertibility bounds. The residuals of Model 2 are not different than white noise, so we accept this model.

The estimated impact of decriminalization for the first post-intervention year is reported in Table 5.18. A permanent impact of $\hat{\omega}_{0,1} = -1.4548$ units is realized in the first post-intervention month, January 1969, and continues unchanged throughout the post-intervention segment. A temporary impact of $\hat{\omega}_{0,2} = -0.915$ units is also realized in January 1969 but begins to decay immediately. By August 1969, 95 percent of the temporary effect has decayed. By end of the first post-intervention year, less than 1 percent remains.

What are these impact "units"? To simplify the arithmetic, wait until the temporary effect has vanished. Then exponentiate both sides of the model.

$$e^{PubDrnk_t} = e^{N(a_t) - 1.4548} = e^{N(a_t)} e^{-1.4548}$$

The first exponential factor in this expression is the pre-intervention level of the time series level. We can represent this level as an arbitrary constant, say,

$$e^{N(a_t)} = 1$$

The second exponential factor is the ratio of the post-intervention level to the pre-intervention level. In this instance,

$$\frac{\text{Post-Intervention}}{\text{Pre-intervention}} = e^{-1.4548} = 0.2334$$

The asymptotic impact of decriminalization amounts to a 76.66 percent reduction in public drunkenness arrests.

This analysis illustrates the easy interpretability of the natural logarithm transformation. For that reason alone, we recommend natural logarithms whenever possible. Would the analysis arrive at substantively different results if we had used $\lambda = -0.6$, the "best" Box-Cox transformation, instead of natural logarithms? In fact, though less interpretable, the analysis would have yielded nearly identical results. We leave that demonstration as an exercise for the reader.

5.5 CONCLUSION

The strategy developed in this chapter for building an *ARIMA* intervention model is a modified version of the strategy developed in Chapter 3 for building an *ARIMA* noise model. The modifications reflect the potentially distorting effects of the intervention on the identification statistics. If the intervention has a small impact on the time series, the conventional noise modeling strategy (Figure 3.1) will converge quickly on the "best" intervention model. If the impact is *not* small, on the other hand, the conventional strategy may iterate endlessly without converging on the "best" model.

This problem has two potential solutions. When Y_t is long and well-behaved, $N(a_t)$ can be identified from the pre-intervention segment. Since long, well behaved time series are rare, this solution is not generally feasible. The alternative solution identifies a model from the residualized time series. That is,

$$\hat{N}(a_t) = Y_t - X(I_t)$$

where $X(I_t)$ is a theoretically specified intervention model. Generating the residualized time series requires an a priori specification of $X(I_t)$, of course, but with that done, the time series residuals can be used to identify $N(a_t)$.

Theoretical specification of the intervention model requires at least some sense of the *onset* and *duration* of the impact. Most of the applications that we reviewed for this chapter use one of three intervention models. The simplest model produces an abrupt, permanent shift in the time series level. This impact is shown in the upper left-hand panel of Figure 5.5. For an intervention that changes from zero to one instantly and persistently, this impact is represented by the zero-order transfer function

$$X(I_t) = \omega_0 I_t$$

The Cincinnati Directory Assistance time series plotted in Figure 5.2 illustrates this type of impact. The coefficients of the zero-order transfer function listed in Table 5.2 are interpreted to mean that the three interventions each had abrupt and persistent impacts on Directory Assistance calls.

The time series of weekly productivity measures plotted in Figure 5.3 use the same zero-order transfer function model to model the elimination and reinstatement of rest breaks in the 33rd and 45th weeks. The parameter estimates reported in Table 5.3 must be reasonably interpreted to mean that the effect of eliminating rest breaks was a 5 percent drop in productivity. Following reinstatement of the rest breaks, productivity rose just as abruptly, returning to pre-intervention levels. What appeared to be a post-intervention trend proved, after analysis, to be a continuation of the pre-intervention trend in this time series.

The surgical infection time series analyzed in Chapter 5.1.3 demonstrates the difficulty of identifying $N(a_t)$ from short, noisy time series. Given the relatively small impact, $N(a_t)$ was identifiable directly from the time series. Proper identification of $N(a_t)$ in a short, seasonal time series is another matter. With only $N = 48$ monthly observations, proper identification of the New Hampshire Medicaid prescription time series plotted in Figure 5.7 required ingenuity.

The New Hampshire Medicaid prescription time series also introduced model equivalence tests. Under the equivalence null hypothesis, the deviance statistics reported in Table 5.5 are distributed approximately as χ^2 with degrees of freedom equal to the number of parameters in Model 2 minus the number in Model 1. The methadone maintenance time series plotted in Figure 5.9, known colloquially as an "ABAB" design, provided another illustration of model equivalence hypothesis tests. In this design, two distinct treatments are applied to subjects in a repeated sequence. The parameter estimates reported in Table 5.6 suggest that both treatments were effective but that there was no evidence that either treatment was more or less effective than the other.

Not all impacts are abrupt in onset and permanent in duration, of course. Impacts that accrue *gradually* over the post-intervention segment can be modeled as the first-order transfer function

$$X(I_t) = \frac{\omega_0}{1 - \delta_1 B} I_t$$

The rate of accrual—or "rate of gain"—is determined by the parameter δ_1. The absolute value of δ_1 is constrained to the bounds of system stability between zero and one. Our analysis of Australian traffic fatalities in Chapter 5.2.1 used the first-order transfer function model. In 1972, a mandatory seatbelt law took effect in Australia. Although the new law had no *immediate* impact on the level of the traffic fatality time series, small quarterly decrements began to accrue. After several years, the impact is visually apparent. Annual changes in the fatality time series are reported in Table 5.8. By the second quarter of 1982, 95 percent of the law's asymptotic impact was realized. The British traffic fatality time series analyzed in Chapter 5.2.2 used the same first-order transfer function model. Because the estimated value of the δ_1-parameter was negative, however, the results were difficult to interpret.

The results for the "talking out" analysis, reported in Table 5.11, are more typical. Following a classroom intervention, the number of daily incidents falls gradually throughout the post-intervention segment. Although the daily changes grow smaller and smaller, they continue to accrue, approaching the asymptotic impact reported in Table 5.12, -12.5 incidents per day. Persistent or permanent effects often accrue gradually, in our experience.

In contrast to impacts that persist throughout the post-intervention period, whether abrupt or gradual in onset, an important class of *temporary* phenomena decay throughout the post-intervention segment. Decaying effects can be represented by a first-order transfer function of a *pulse* function:

$$X(I_t) = \frac{\omega_0}{1 - \delta_1 B} \nabla I_t$$

Here the impact decays at a rate determined by the value of δ_1. Again, the absolute value of δ_1 is bounded by zero and one. As the value of δ_1 approaches zero, the rate of decay increases. As the absolute value of δ_1 approaches zero, the rate of decay decreases. When $\delta_1 = 1$, the first-order transfer function is identical to a zero-order transfer function.

The self-injurious behavior time series analyzed in Chapter 5.3.1 demonstrate the pratical use of this model. The treated and placebo patients react identically in the immediate aftermath of their interventions. For the treated patient, the effect persists throughout the post-intervention segment. For the placebo patient, however, the effect begins to wear off, decaying back to the pre-intervention level. For a short post-intervention segment, the treated and placebo effects are roughly equivalent and indistinguishable.

Decaying "spikes" would seem to be particularly useful models for single-subject research. The relatively short time series used in this literature limit their use, unfortunately. The placebo effects commonly enountered in evaluations of legal interventions and reforms are generated by analogous mechanisms. Even new laws that are expected to have no effects often produce temporary effects (Ross, McCleary, and LaFree, 1990). Placebo-like effects are found in the Australian Family Law Act (Chapter 5.4.1) and in the decriminalization of public drunkenness in Washington D.C. (Chapter 5.4.2). Both reforms had abrupt, permanent impacts, of course, but these changes were accompanied by dampened instability in the post-intervention period— by placebo effects. The complex impacts were modeled as the sum of two transfer functions. A slow, detailed reading of this chapter will pay dividends. Taken together, the zero-order and first-order transfer functions provide a rich menu of impact patterns.

6

Statistical Conclusion Validity

As long as we have a conception of how variation in results may be due to chance and regard it as applicable to our experience, we will have a need for significance tests

—MULAIK, RAJU AND HARSHMAN (1997, P. 81).

There is never a legitimate role for significance testing

—SCHMIDT AND HUNTER (1997, P. 49).

Despite these attacks, null hypothesis testing still dominates the social sciences. Its continued use is typically attributed to experimenters' ignorance, misunderstanding, laziness, or adherence to tradition. However, as an anonymous reviewer put it, "A way of thinking that has survived decades of ferocious attacks is likely to have some value."

—FRICK (1996, P. 379)

What to do? First, don't look for a magical alternative to null hypothesis significance testing, some other mechanical ritual to replace it. It doesn't exist.

—COHEN (1994, P. 1001)

Ignoring the apparent contradiction, we might agree with each of these statements. Significance testing *has* become a mindless ritual, taught and learned without reference to or appreciation of its roots. (If you doubt this, re-read Chapters 3 and 5, where we perform the mindless ritual again and again.) Significance testing has no place in an ideal scientific world. Misapplications and misuses abound. But significance testing *seems* to work and to the extent that it *does*, abundant misapplications and misuses may be an unavoidable, acceptable cost of knowledge. In any event, there appear to be no immediate alternatives to significance testing. The best that we can do is teach the logical foundations of significance testing and draw attention to the misapplications and misuses that commonly arise in time series designs. That is the purpose of this chapter.

When Campbell (1957) first wrote about the common threats to internal validity, computing resources were so scarce that most statistics textbooks included tables of random numbers. Experimental designs were preferred in those days not only for their internal validity but also for their computational tractability. To further complicate matters, the explicitly statistical threats to internal validity were difficult to understand and convenient to overlook. Indeed, Cohen (1992, p. 155) attributes the wholesale disregard of common statistical threats to the "meager and mathematically difficult literature." Compared to the nonstatistical threats to internal validity, the statistical threats played a minor role in that era.

Two decades later, when Cook and Campbell (1979) revisited internal validity, computers had become widely available. Due to the work of Cohen (1969, 1988) and others, moreover, the statistical threats to internal validity had become better understood and more difficult to ignore. Cook and Campbell (1979) addressed this development by creating a distinct subcategory of internal validity for the explicitly statistical threats. Continuing this tradition, Shadish et al. (2002, p. 38) define *statistical conclusion validity* as the "validity of inferences about the correlation (covariance) between treatment and outcome."

In principle, all nine of the common threats to statistical conclusion validity identified by Shadish et al. (Table 6.1) apply to time series designs. In practice, two of the nine are found regularly in the applied literature. Our analysis of statistical conclusion validity focuses then on two threats: *violated assumptions of statistical tests* and *low statistical power*. The threats posed by *violated assumptions* are controlled by making sure that the statistical assumptions underlying the *statistical tests* are warranted. If the significance test assumes a Normal time series, for example, use a Kologmorov-Smirnov statistic to make sure that the assumption is warranted. If Normality is unwarranted, transform the time series.

Table 6.1. THREATS TO STATISTICAL CONCLUSION VALIDITY (SHADISH ET AL., 2002)

> *Low statistical power*
> *Violated assumptions of statistical tests*
> *Fishing and the error rate problem*
> *Unreliability of measures*
> *Restriction of range*
> *Unreliability of treatment implementation*
> *Extraneous variance in the experimental setting*
> *Heterogeneity of units*
> *Inaccurate effect size estimation*

The threats posed by *low statistical power* are more difficult to analyze because they arise as a part of the modern significance test per se. Indeed, some critics argue that the surest way to control these particular threats to statistical conclusion validity is to replace the modern hypothesis test with Bayesian tests (Dienes, 2011). Though convinced that Bayesian methods are sensible and inevitable, we are naturally skeptical of Gordian-knot solutions to difficult epistemological problems. While Bayesian hypothesis tests have become the status quo in many fields, moreover, they are still relatively novel in other fields.

Our development of statistical conclusion validity begins with a survey of statistical inference. The modern significance test combines features of the tests proposed by Fisher (1925) and Neyman and Pearson (1928). Some criticisms of the modern test focus on shortcomings of the two "classic" tests. Fisher's test has no way to accept a null finding, for example, and says nothing about the truth of the theory being tested. Although the Neyman-Pearson test allows us to accept the truth of a null finding, it requires an unrealistic set of assumptions that, if strictly enforced, limit its use to a few experiments and virtually no quasi-experiments.

Despite the fact that the two classic approaches are fundamentally irreconcilable, they were merged forcibly at the start of the modern era into what Gigerenzer et al. (1989, p. 106) call the "hybrid null hypothesis significance test." Textbooks teach the modern test in cookbook fashion, paying little or no attention to the logical contradictions raised by the forced marriage. Virtually all of the parents' shortcomings are inherited by the offspring (Nickerson, 2000). While recognizing all these obstacles to validity, we note that somehow the modern test seems to work. Krueger (2001, p. 20) maintains that, despite its internal contradictions and shortcomings, the modern significance test "works in the long run." No matter how tempting a one-sentence Keynesian retort might be, and accepting Krueger's argument on its face, we still wonder whether there might not be a shorter, better-illuminated path to knowledge.

Edwards, Lindman, and Savage (1963) addressed this question 50 years ago, concluding that Bayesian inferential methods were the better-illuminated path for social science research. Resistance to Bayesian methods rests in part on Fisher's (1922b) rejection of Bayesian inference,[1] on the difficult task of computing posterior probabilities, and on cultural inertia. Fisher's (1935) alternative to

---

1. Fisher (1922b, p. 311): "It is this last confusion, in the writer's opinion, more than any other, which has led to the survival to the present day of the fundamental paradox of inverse probability, which like an impenetrable jungle arrests progress towards precision of statistical concepts. The criticisms of BOOLE, VENN, and CHRYSTAL have done something towards banishing the method, at least from the elementary text-books of Algebra; but though we may agree wholly with CHRYSTAL that inverse probability is a mistake (perhaps the only mistake to which the mathematical world has so deeply committed itself), there yet remains the feeling that such a

Bayesian inference has fallen out of favor in recent years, while the availability of powerful computers has removed the practical obstacles to Bayesian inference. Cultural inertia remains a formidable obstacle.

Bayesian methods have many advantages and solve many problems (Kruschke, Aguinis, and Joo, 2012). If we had to choose sides, we would probably be Bayesians. We are skeptics nevertheless. While Bayesian approaches would eliminate many of the misuses and abuses of hypothesis testing, we suspect that Bayesians would introduce their own misuses and abuses, creating new threats to statistical conclusion validity.

Since the most common threats to statistical conclusion validity are a direct consequence of the modern hybrid significance test, the threats will become uncommon as Bayesian methods predominate. In Chapter 6.1, we describe the early Fisher and Neyman-Pearson approaches to statistical inference. In Chapter 6.2, we describe the modern hybrid test. In Chapter 6.3, we describe a Bayesian alternative to the modern hybrid test. Readers who are familiar with this material may skip to Chapter 6.4, where we analyze five threats to statistical conclusion validity that affect time series designs.

6.1 THE CLASSICAL TESTS

The modern significance test is the synthetic product of two distinct inferential approaches developed in the 1920s and 1930s by Fisher (1925) and Neyman and Pearson (1928). Fisher's approach, described in *Statistical Methods for Research Workers*, was developed for the analysis of experiments. To test the hypothesis that a chemical facilitates crop growth, Fisher would randomly assign a sample of garden plots to be treated with the chemical or to go untreated. At the end of the growing season, Fisher would compare mean crop yields from the treated and untreated plots with the H_0,

$$H_0: \mu_{Treated} - \mu_{Untreated} = 0$$

If H_0 is true, the observed difference-in-means should be small. To assess the magnitude of the observed difference, Fisher would calculate the probability of observing an equal or larger difference under the assumption that H_0 is true. This

mistake would not have captivated the minds of LAPLACE and POISSON if there had been nothing in it but error."

conditional probability is the well-known p-value.[2]

$$p = \Pr(\widehat{\mu}_{Treated} - \widehat{\mu}_{Untreated} \mid H_0)$$

Fisher used p to measure the fit of the data to H_0. Though endorsing no universal threshold p-value for rejecting H_0, Fisher's *Statistical Methods for Research Workers* popularized the conventional $p < 0.05$ threshold that we used in Chapters 3 and 5 and that is used by modern social scientists. To Fisher, however, p "was not part of a formal inferential method" but rather "part of the fluid, non-quantifiable process of drawing conclusions from observations" (Goodman, 1999, p. 997). In that spirit, p was to be interpreted as evidence against H_0. If p was small, H_0 was probably false; the observed difference was probably due to the treatment.

Although it seems intuitively plausible to interpret a large p-value — say, $p > 0.75$—as evidence in favor of H_0, this intuition would be incorrect. No matter how large the p-value might be, it was calculated under the assumption that H_0 is true. Interpreting it as evidence that H_0 is true, then, would be a fallacy. In its orthodox form, Fisher's significance test had no way to "accept H_0." In Fisher's (1929, p. 191) words:

> The test of significance only tells [the practical investigator] what to ignore, namely all experiments in which significant results are not obtained. He should only claim that a phenomenon is experimentally demonstrable when he knows how to design an experiment so that it will rarely fail to give a significant result. Consequently, isolated significant results which he does not know how to reproduce are left in suspense pending further investigation.

This seems wasteful. If H_0 is true, we would expect to see a large p-value, say again $p > 0.75$. If this p-value cannot reject H_0, common sense might suggest that we can accept H_0. Unfortunately, failing to reject H_0 says *nothing* about the truth of H_0.

This lacuna precipitated a feud between Fisher and his critics. In a series of papers published between 1928 and 1933, Fisher's University College colleagues, Jerzy Neyman and Egon S. Pearson, proposed a method that, in their view, addressed this salient shortcoming of Fisher's significance test. Whereas Fisher's approach relied exclusively on a test of H_0, the Neyman-Pearson approach tested

---

2. See Appendix 6 for a brief review of probability concepts and a list of the notational conventions used in this chapter.

competing hypotheses H_0 and H_A.[3]

$$H_0: \textit{TestStatistic} = 0$$
$$H_A: \textit{TestStatistic} = \omega \neq 0$$

Written out this way, Neyman-Pearson hypothesis testing might seem to be an *extension* of—or an *improvement* on—Fisher's significance test. Although Fisher's significance test included no explicit H_A, for example, H_0 seems to imply the existence of an H_A. The superficial appearance of similarity is deceiving, however. Fisher's significance test had no way to connect H_A to the data and, hence, to H_0. A description of the Neyman-Pearson hypothesis testing process reveals other salient differences.

A Neyman-Pearson hypothesis test typically begins by specifying H_0 and H_A. Each hypothesis has an error rate. For H_0, the Type I error rate is defined as

$$\alpha = \Pr(H_0 \text{ rejected} \mid H_0 \text{true})$$

Type I errors are also known as "α-type" or "false-positive" errors. The complement of α is the "confidence level" for H_0.

$$1 - \alpha = \Pr(H_0 \text{ rejected} \mid H_0 \text{ false})$$

Fisher's p-value is not equivalent to α. Whereas a p-value can vary, the α-level must be fixed a priori at, say, $\alpha = 0.05$. As a consequence, in a Neyman-Pearson hypothesis test, there is no such thing as a "marginally significant" parameter estimate. Fixing the Type I error rate guarantees that the long-run frequency of false-positive decision errors will converge on α. If $N - x$ of N decisions are false-positive errors, in other words, then in the long run

$$\alpha = \lim_{N \to \infty} \frac{N - x}{N} \equiv \Pr(H_0 \text{ rejected} \mid H_0 \text{ true})$$

This fixed α-level assumes that we test the same H_0 again and again, of course, and that assumption has been controversial.

After fixing the Type I error rate, we must pay attention to the Type II error rate. For H_A, the Type II error rate is defined as

$$\beta = \Pr(H_0 \text{ accepted} \mid H_0 \text{ is false})$$

Type II errors are also known as "β-type" errors or "false-negative" errors. The complement of β is the level of "statistical power" for the Neyman-Pearson

---

3. We call the competing hypotheses H_0 and H_A as a matter of convenience. Some authors use H_1 and H_2. Neyman and Pearson (1928a) used "Hypothesis A" and "Hypothesis B." The errors associated with the two hypotheses were called "α" and "β" errors.

hypothesis test.

$$1 - \beta = \Pr(H_0 \text{ accepted} \mid H_0 \text{ is true})$$

With α fixed, we use the "most powerful" *Test Statistic* to test H_0. If the observed value of the *Test Statistic* falls below a threshold value, H_0 is rejected in favor of H_A. Otherwise, H_0 is accepted as true—which amounts to rejecting H_A.

We have not defined the "most powerful" *Test Statistic*, of course, and will not do so here.[4] We can describe its rationale, however. As its name suggests, the "most powerful" *Test Statistic* is the one for which β is smallest (and $1 - \beta$ is largest). With this statistic chosen, experimental design parameters, especially N, can be manipulated to ensure that β is no larger than some conventional level. In principle, the conventional β-error rate level reflects the realistic cost of a false-negative decision. Where this cost is unknown or difficult to calculate, convention sets β at no larger than four times the false-positive error rate, α. In the social, behavioral, and biomedical sciences this convention is $\beta = 0.2$ for $\alpha = 0.05$ (Cohen, 1988; Lipsey, 1990). The four-to-one β-to-α ratio implies that the cost of a false-positive error is four times the cost of a false-negative error.

The difference-in-means is not ordinarily the "most powerful" *Test Statistic* for a simple two-group experiment. Fisher used this test statistic for a purely pragmatic reason. Under H_0, the difference-in-means has a known distribution that allows calculation of a p-value with relatively little difficulty. In principle, however, any test statistic whose distribution is known under H_0 would do as well. Might another test statistic provide a "better" test of H_0? Along with their desire to accept H_0, when the data supported that decision, this question motivated Neyman and Pearson.

Their proposed answer, the Neyman-Pearson hypothesis test, provoked a feud that lasted until Fisher's death in 1962. The intensity and duration of the feud was due in part to Fisher's pugnacity. Although he was "a genius of the first rank, perhaps the most original mathematical scientist of the [20th] century" (Efron, 1976, p. 483), "he seemed to feel that his genius entitled him to more social indulgence than they were willing to concede; in short he could be, and not infrequently was, gratuitously rude" (Kendall, 1963, p. 6).

Even so, it would be a mistake to dismiss Fisher's (1955) critique of hypothesis testing. Fisher saw the Neyman-Pearson hypothesis test as better suited to industrial quality control than to science. The typical quality control application involved deciding to accept or reject a shipment of machine parts based on a sample of the shipment. Disease screening tests also seem well suited to the

---

4. Because the mathematics is beyond us. Mathematically prepared readers are directed to the source (Neyman and Pearson, 1967) or to Kendall and Stuart (1979, Chapter 22). Other readers are directed to Lenhard (2006, pp. 77-81). Spoiler alert: It's the likelihood ratio.

Neyman-Pearson approach. In these applications, one can imagine conducting identical hypothesis tests over and over. In the sort of scientific applications that interested Fisher, on the other hand, an unending sequence of identical hypothesis tests was unimaginable.

6.2   THE MODERN "HYBRID" TEST

The simple analogy to jury verdicts diagrammed in Table 6.2 is a useful way to introduce the significance testing procedures currently taught to and used by social scientists. Based on the evidence, juries convict or acquit defendants. Hopefully, most verdicts are true and correct. False, incorrect verdicts, which are presumably rare, fall into one of two categories. When the jury mistakenly convicts an innocent defendant, the verdict is a false-positive error or an α-error. When the jury mistakenly acquits a guilty defendant, the verdict is a false-negative error or a β-error. To complete the analogy, sometimes juries cannot reach a verdict. In cases where the jury hangs, no decision is made and no error is possible.

Null hypothesis significance tests and jury verdicts are analogous in that both lead to evidence-based decisions and, sometimes, to decision-making errors. There are important differences, of course. Whereas jury verdict error rates are unknown, for example, the error rates for null hypothesis significance tests are set a priori to 0.05 and 0.20 respectively for false-positive and false-negative errors. Whereas the cost of a jury verdict error is more or less a constant that can be ignored, moreover, the cost of a null hypothesis significance testing error is variable and is always of interest.

The distinction between the *substantive* and *statistical* magnitude of an effect parallels the cost of a decision-making error. To illustrate, imagine a $250,000 student loan debt, a 25-mile summer desert hike, or a 50-year prison sentence. No matter how *substantively* large (or small) these numbers might seem, each might be *statistically* small (or large) compared to their standard errors. Threats to statistical conclusion validity often involve unresolved discrepancies between the *substantive* and *statistical* size of an effect or between the a priori false-positive and false-negative error rates and the rates actually realized. Although we speak of these two aspects of the threats as if they were distinct and separable, they are ordinarily correlated and difficult to untangle.

Table 6.2. THE MODERN HYPOTHESIS TEST AS A JURY TRIAL

	Guilty Defendant	Innocent Defendant
Jury Convicts	*True-Positive*	*False-Positive*
Jury Hangs	*No Decision*	*No Decision*
Jury Acquits	*False-Negative*	*True-Negative*

The "modern" null hypothesis significance test consists of the set of procedures taught in the modern era, beginning about 75 years ago. There is no single reference authority for the modern hypothesis test. Our review of a nonrandom sample of statistics textbooks suggests that there are two distinct schools of thought. Both begin with a theoretically deduced null hypothesis, H_0, which ordinarily holds that the difference between the pre- and post-intervention levels of a time series is zero.[5]

$$H_0: \omega_0 = 0$$

When H_0 is false, there are two possible alternatives. The two-tailed H_A posits that H_0 is false and nothing more.

$$H_A: \omega_0 \neq 0$$

The one-tailed H_A posits not only that H_0 is false but also that the nonzero effect is either an increase,

$$H_A: \omega_0 > 0$$

or a decrease,

$$H_A: \omega_0 < 0$$

in the level of the time series. The choice between a two-tailed and a one-tailed alternative is based on conventional practice or, sometimes, on theory. The specific form of H_A has no bearing on the subsequent test of H_0.

Figure 6.1 plots test statistic distributions for the two-tailed and one-tailed alternatives. When H_0 is false, the test statistic

$$Z_{\hat{\omega}_0} = \frac{\hat{\omega}_0}{\sigma_{\hat{\omega}_0}}$$

is distributed as a standardized Normal variable. That is, when H_0 is true

$$Z_{\hat{\omega}_0} \sim \text{Normal}(0, 1)$$

The darkened regions in the distributions shown in Figure 6.1, which make up 5 percent of the areas under the curves, are called "rejection regions." If $Z_{\hat{\omega}_0}$ lies in

---

5. Since $P(\omega_0 = 0) = 0$, H_0 is false by definition. Though logically false, H_0 is a good approximation to the "nearly null" hypothesis (Rindskopf, 1997). For a substantively small number ϵ, H_ϵ holds that $-\epsilon < \omega_0 < +\epsilon$. Though not exactly equal to zero, however, the effect is so small that we can treat it as if it were zero. Approximating H_ϵ with H_0 avoids complicated mathematics while yielding similar results under realistic circumstances.

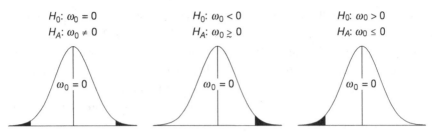

Figure 6.1 Critical Regions for Two-Tailed and One-Tailed Tests of H_0

these regions, H_0 is rejected as false with 95 percent confidence. There is nothing sacred about the conventional 95 percent confidence level. The rejection regions can be fixed at a lower or higher level—10 percent, say, or at 1 percent—defining 90 or 99 percent confidence levels. Whatever the confidence level, when $Z_{\hat{\omega}_0}$ lies in the rejection region, H_0 is rejected in favor of H_A.

The two modern schools draw similar inferences when $Z_{\hat{\omega}_0}$ lies in the rejection regions: H_0 is false and H_A is true. When $Z_{\hat{\omega}_0}$ lies *inside* the rejection regions, the two schools draw very different inferences that parallel the Fisher and Neyman-Pearson approaches. The first school, represented by Neter, Wasserman, and Whitmore (1993, p. 318), holds that H_0 must be *either* true *or* false and, hence, that if H_0 cannot be rejected as false, it can be accepted as true, subject to decision rules. The second school, represented by Agresti and Finlay (1997, p. 171), holds the opposite view: No matter the test result, H_0 should *never* be accepted.

Much of this disagreement reflects different motives. Whereas the first school views the statistical significance of $\hat{\omega}_0$ as a way to decide between H_0 and H_A, the second school views the statistical significance of $\hat{\omega}_0$ as a way to "nullify" a theory. Obviously, if we follow the first school, we must *either* reject H_0, thereby accepting H_A, *or* reject H_A, thereby accepting H_0. If we are focused narrowly on theory nullification, however, we might be reluctant to accept H_0. We know of no way to reconcile these two motives.

Using the statistical significance of $\hat{\omega}_0$ to decide between H_0 and H_A requires two decision rules. First, we must fix the long-run frequency of false-positive decision errors at α. This decision rule is inflexible, at least in theory, and assumes a long-run frequency definition of probability (see Dienes, 2011; or generally, Hájek, 2012). Absent a long-run sequence of identical H_0 tests, the rigidly fixed α-level makes little sense. Since tests of H_0 based on N_1 and N_2 observations are *not* identical, this decision rule, its underlying assumptions, and its implied payoffs are problematic for time series designs.

The problematic nature of the fixed-α decision rule might be resolved by assuming either that N_1 and N_2 are Platonic ideals or, else, that minor violations have minor consequences. One or the other of these alternatives seems to satisfy most critics. But some critics, especially Fisher (1955), would not be satisfied. We tend to agree with Fisher specifically and with critics of the "modern" H_0 test generally. Nevertheless, we agree with Cohen's (1994, p. 1001) pessimistic view that there is no alternative "mechanical ritual to replace" the modern H_0 test. One could argue that Bayesian H_0 tests are neither mechanical nor ritualistic, of course. We postpone that argument until we consider Bayesian alternatives in Chapter 6.3.

In a time series experiment, we would fix the α-level a priori at, say, $\alpha = 0.05$. Then for anticipated values of ω_0 and σ_a^2 divined from a review of prior research, we would select N_{pre} and N_{post} to guarantee $\beta \leq 0.2$. In a quasi-experiment, on the other hand, we often discover a time series with predetermined values of σ_a^2, N_{pre} and N_{post}. Instead of conducting the sort of power analysis that we would conduct to design an experiment, we pray that these values are sufficient to guarantee 80 percent statistical power. In most instances, our prayers are answered. But not always.

The time series in Figure 6.2, provided by Coleman and Wiggins (1996), represents the worst case scenario for a quasi-experiment. In January 1991, an investigative news report on a local television station questioned the business ethics of a Jacksonville, Florida, furniture rental company. Claiming that the report was inaccurate and that it had an adverse impact on sales, the company sued. In fact, mean monthly sales in the $N_{pre} = 25$ and $N_{post} = 11$ months were \$125,510 and \$121,994 respectively. Monthly means can be deceiving, of course, especially with time series as short as this one. Nor do we see an obvious

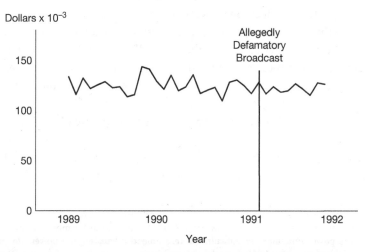

Figure 6.2 Monthly Sales Before and After a Broadcast (Coleman and Wiggins, 1996)

Table 6.3. MONTHLY SALES, ESTIMATION AND DIAGNOSIS

		Estimate	SE	t	Diagnosis
Model 1	$\hat{\theta}_0$	125490.10	1578.64	79.4954	$RSE = 5825.13$
	$\hat{\theta}_{12}$	$-.5368$	.1155	-4.65	$Q_{12} = 5.2$
	$\hat{\omega}_0$	-2679.97	2103.83	-1.27	$Z_{KS} = 0.81$

interruption in this time series. But visual impressions can also deceive, so we will address this question with a formal analysis.

The "best" *ARIMA* model for this time series—and, frankly, the best model is not very good—is

$$Sales_t = \theta_0 + (1 - \theta_{12}B^{12})a_t + \omega_0 I_t$$

Parameter estimates for this model are reported in Table 6.3. Prior to the intervention, the level of the time series was \$125,490.10 per month. After the intervention, the level was \$2,679.97 lower, consistent with the pre- and post-intervention means reported by the company. Unfortunately for the company, the value of $\hat{\omega}_0 = -2679.97$ is not statistically significant at the conventional 95 percent confidence level. We cannot reject H_0.

Should the fact that we cannot reject H_0 imply that we must accept H_0? In this particular instance, based on the design and evidence, we would not want to accept H_0. Common sense suggests that a post-intervenion time series of $N_{post} = 10$ months will not support valid inferences. Depending on our philosophy of hypothesis testing, however, we might not accept H_0 in any instance. Because the lawsuit forces us to either accept or reject H_0, however, we will try to make a reasonable, defensible decision between the two alternatives.

To make this decision, we fix the Type I error rate at some conventional level and then specify an alternative hypothesis, H_A. Fixing the Type I error rate is no problem. Per convention, we set the Type I error rate at $\alpha = 0.05$. Specifying H_A proves difficult. Prior research or legal precedent might ordinarily suggest a threshold value of ω_0 for our H_A. Lacking this sort of guidance, we must estimate the statistical power for the range of effect sizes plotted in Figure 6.3.[6] For $N_{pre} = 25$ and $N_{post} = 11$ observations, power crosses the 0.8 threshold at $\hat{\omega}_0 = -\$5,140$. This is the smallest effect size that we could hope to detect with this quasi-experimental design. Power for the observed effect size, $\hat{\omega}_0 = -\$2,680$, is

---

6. The power functions plotted in Figures 6.3 and 6.4 assume white noise. McLeod and Vingilis (2005) give the power functions for low-order *ARIMA* models, but for more realistic *ARIMA* models, the power functions are difficult. We recommend calculating the power functions of higher-order and seasonal *ARIMA* models by simulation. In our experience, given the same variance, white noise power functions are not a close approximation to the functions calculated with simulation methods.

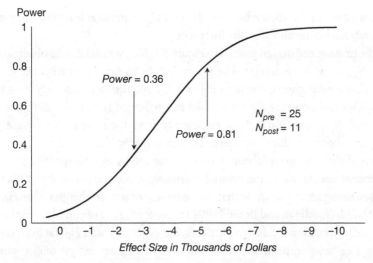

Figure 6.3 Statistical Power for a Time Series Experiment, Effect size

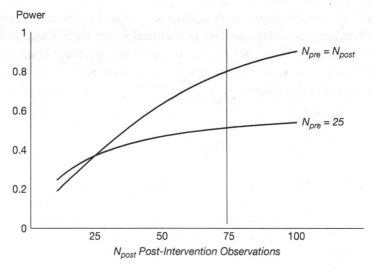

Figure 6.4 Statistical Power for a Time Series Experiment, Post-Intervention Observations

$1 - \hat{\beta} = 0.36$, but for reasons discussed below, this number must be interpreted cautiously.

The functions plotted in Figure 6.4 are more useful. Here power is calculated for values of N_{pre} and N_{post} given the observed effect size, $\hat{\omega}_0 = -\$2,680$. When the design is balanced with an equal number of pre- and post-intervention observations, the power function crosses the 0.8 threshold at $N_{pre} = N_{post} = 74$

observations. A valid choice between H_0 and H_A requires at least this number of observations before and after the intervention.

In the unbalanced design plotted in Figure 6.3, N_{pre} was fixed at 25 observations while N_{post} was made longer. The power functions for this unbalanced design show that a valid choice between H_0 and H_A requires an extremely long time series. Optimal power is always realized in a balanced time series design where N_{pre} and N_{post} are equal. In a sufficiently long time series, of course, the incremental power achieved through balance is negligible.

Beyond this egregious "abuse of power," the results of retrospective post hoc power analyses should be interpreted cautiously. Zumbo and Hubley (1998) use a Bayesian argument to show that the meaning of power changes after H_0 has been tested. Goodman and Berlin (1994) argue for the use of confidence intervals instead of power, even for design purposes, but especially after H_0 has been tested. Though agreeing in principle, there are reasons why an analyst might want to calculate $\beta_{\hat{\omega}_0}$, even after H_0 has been tested. The probability of replicating the test result under H_A is $1 - \beta_{\hat{\omega}_0}$ (see Gill, 1999, pp. 659-660). In that respect, $\beta_{\hat{\omega}_0}$ may be a more useful statistic than $p_{\hat{\omega}_0}$.

While descriptive analyses such as those summarized in Figure 6.3 may be helpful on occasion, valid questions of statistical power seldom arise in time series experiments. Statistical power is not a very useful concept in the design and analysis of time series experiments. There are many reasons why this is so. We return to this topic shortly.

6.3 BAYESIAN HYPOTHESIS TESTING

Having written about the past and the present, we now consider the future. Among the many shortcomings of the modern significance test, two are especially troubling. The first involves the dysfunctional influence of the sample size, N, on the decision to accept or reject H_0. When N is small, it is nearly impossible to reject H_0, no matter how preposterous it might be. When N is large, it is nearly impossible *not* to reject H_0, no matter how sensible it might be.[7] While the decision to accept or reject H_0 *should* be based on the magnitude and variability of a parameter estimate, in practice it is based largely on N (Kadane, 2011, p. 438).

The second shortcoming involves the interpretation of p. The most common misconception about p is that $1 - p$ can be interpreted as the probability that H_0 is true (Goodman, 2008). Too many of us believe that if $p < 0.05$, the probability that H_0 is true is less than 0.05. To see how mistaken this common belief is, recall

---

7. Another way to say this is that, as $N \to \infty$, $p \to 0$. This raises the Jeffreys-Lindley paradox (Spanos, 2013).

that p is defined as

$$p \equiv \Pr(\omega_0 = \hat{\omega}_0 \mid H_0)$$

Since p *assumes* that H_0 is true, it can hardly be used to measure the probable truth of H_0. The fact that so many of us think otherwise hints at the importance of knowing whether H_0 is true. Indeed, we conduct research in order to acquire that knowledge. This common misconception about p confuses p with its *inverse probability, p'*

$$p' \equiv \Pr(H_0 \mid \omega_0 = \hat{\omega}_0)$$

Although p says *virtually nothing* about the truth of H_0, it is relatively *easy* to calculate. In contrast, the inverse probability, p', tells us *exactly what we need to know* about H_0 but, unfortunately, is very *difficult* to calculate. Calculation of p' uses Bayes' Rule:[8]

$$\Pr(H_0 \mid \hat{\omega}_0) = \frac{\Pr(\hat{\omega}_0 \mid H_0) \times \Pr(H_0)}{\Pr(\hat{\omega}_0)}$$

Because it is calculated *after ω* has been estimated, $\Pr(H_0 \mid \hat{\omega}_0)$ on the left-hand side of Bayes' Rule is known as the *Posterior Probablity* of H_0. Because the p-value on the right-hand side of the expression, $\Pr(\hat{\omega}_0 \mid H_0)$, is the likelihood function for $\hat{\omega}_0$ under H_0, it is called the *Likelihood* of H_0.[9] $\Pr(H_0)$ and $\Pr(\hat{\omega}_0)$, also on the right-hand side, are called the *Prior Probablity* of H_0 and the *Evidence* for H_0 respectively. Using these new Bayesian terms and phrases, we express Bayes' Rule in words as

$$\text{Posterior Probability} = \frac{\text{Likelihood} \times \text{Prior Probability}}{\text{Evidence}}$$

Novel Bayesian terms and phrases, which we will use as needed in subsequent sections, are collected in Table 6.4.

The implied timeline for Bayes' Rule runs from right to left. On the right-hand side, the Prior Probability of H_0 reflects the strength of our belief in H_0 prior to the analysis. Based on everything that we know, that is, how strongly do we believe

---

8. Bayes' *Rule* is the formula that connects p and p'. Proofs of Bayes' *Theorem*—the source of Bayes' Rule—are found in most statistics textbooks. Fisher's (1970, pp. 8-17) discussion of Bayes' Theorem is interesting. Kruschke's (2013, pp. 52-74) treatment is accessible and readable. Howson and Urbach (1995) develop the philosophical issues and relate Bayesian thinking to inductive logic. Hacking (2001) is a truly excellent undergraduate textbook.

9. The simple Bayesian hypothesis test described in this section builds on our discussions of model selection and estimation in Chapter 3. Although this simplest test illustrates Bayesian thinking, the Bayesian t-test described by Kruschke (2011, 2012) parallels the modern hypothesis test.

Table 6.4. THE BAYESIAN VOCABULARY

$$\text{Posterior Probability of } H_0 = \frac{\text{Likelihood of } H_0 \times \text{Prior Probability of } H_0}{\text{Evidence for } H_0}$$

Posterior Probability of H_0	$\equiv$	$\Pr(H_0 \mid \hat{\omega}_0)$
Prior Probability of H_0	$\equiv$	$\Pr(H_0)$
Likelihood of H_0	$\equiv$	$\Pr(\hat{\omega}_0 \mid H_0)$
Evidence for H_0	$\equiv$	$\Pr(\hat{\omega}_0)$

Posterior Likelihood of $H_0 \propto \Pr(\hat{\omega}_0 \mid H_0) \times \Pr(H_0)$

Posterior Odds$(H_A{:}H_0)$ = Bayes Factor $\times$ Prior Odds$(H_A{:}H_0)$

Posterior Odds$(H_A{:}H_0)$	$\equiv$	$\dfrac{\Pr(H_A \text{ is true} \mid \hat{\omega}_0)}{\Pr(H_0 \text{ is true} \mid \hat{\omega}_0)}$
Prior Odds$(H_A{:}H_0)$	$\equiv$	$\dfrac{\Pr(H_A)}{\Pr(H_0)}$
Bayes Factor	$\equiv$	$\dfrac{\Pr(\hat{\omega}_0 \mid H_A \text{ is true})}{\Pr(\hat{\omega}_0 \mid H_0 \text{ is true})}$

in H_0? Depending on the strength of our belief, the Prior Probability of H_0 might be as large as, say, 0.95 or as small as, say, 0.05. If our prior belief in H_0 were larger than 0.95 or smaller than 0.05, testing H_0 would be a waste of time.

Within this practical range, depending on our circumstances and intentions, we might consider a single point-value, several point-values, or the entire practical range of $\Pr(H_0)$. Whatever set of point-values are considered, however, each must be weighted so that the set sums to unity. More on that shortly.

After the Prior Probability has been specified, the impact parameter, ω_0, is estimated. At this stage, the Prior Probability of H_0 and the Likelihood of H_0 yield a quantity known as the *Posterior Likelihood* of H_0. Specifically,

Posterior Likelihood of $H_0 \propto$ Likelihood of $H_0 \times$ Prior Probability of H_0

Because it does not necessarily lie in the closed $[0, 1]$ segment, the Posterior Likelihood is not a probability. To transform it into the more useful Posterior Probability of H_0, we divide the right-hand side by $\Pr(\hat{\omega}_0)$, the Evidence for H_0.

Conceptually, the Evidence for H_0 is the probability of observing $\hat{\omega}_0$ without regard to any particular theory. Since we do not ordinarily analyze time series in the absence of a motivating theory, $\Pr(\hat{\omega}_0)$ may strain our imaginations. Nevertheless, since the posterior probability on the left-hand side of the Bayes' Rule expression is a probability, we can think of $\Pr(\hat{\omega}_0)$ as a normalizing constant that constrains the value of $\Pr(\hat{\omega}_0)$ to the closed $[0, 1]$ segment where probabilities are defined.

But there is no immmediate need to evaluate $\Pr(\hat{\omega}_0)$. The simplest Bayesian hypothesis test compares two hypotheses about ω_0. For that, we deduce competing hypotheses, H_0 and H_A, from substantive theory. H_A posits that the impact of the intervention on a time series is ω_0.

$$H_A: \omega_0 \neq 0$$

We will test H_A against H_0 defined in the usual way.

$$H_0: \omega_0 = 0$$

Since Bayes' Rules for H_A and H_0 are

$$\Pr(H_A \mid \hat{\omega}_0) = \frac{\Pr(\hat{\omega}_0 \mid H_A) \times \Pr(H_A)}{\Pr(\hat{\omega}_0)}$$

$$\Pr(H_0 \mid \hat{\omega}_0) = \frac{\Pr(\hat{\omega}_0 \mid H_0) \times \Pr(H_0)}{\Pr(\hat{\omega}_0)}$$

We can construct the *odds* of H_A versus H_0— denoted $\Omega(H_A{:}H_0)$—by simple division:

$$\Omega(H_A{:}H_0) \equiv \frac{\Pr(H_A \mid \hat{\omega}_0)}{\Pr(H_0 \mid \hat{\omega}_0)} = \frac{\dfrac{\Pr(\hat{\omega}_0 \mid H_A) \times \Pr(H_A)}{\Pr(\hat{\omega}_0)}}{\dfrac{\Pr(\hat{\omega}_0 \mid H_0) \times \Pr(H_0)}{\Pr(\hat{\omega}_0)}}$$

The $\Pr(\hat{\omega}_0)$ terms in the numerator and denominator cancel. We rearrange terms and are left with

$$\Omega(H_A{:}H_0) \equiv \frac{\Pr(H_A \mid \hat{\omega}_0)}{\Pr(H_0 \mid \hat{\omega}_0)} = \frac{\Pr(H_A)}{\Pr(H_0)} \times \frac{\Pr(\hat{\omega}_0 \mid H_A)}{\Pr(\hat{\omega}_0 \mid H_0)}$$

The first two terms of this expression are known respectively as the *Posterior* and *Prior* odds of H_A versus H_0. The far right-hand-side term is known as the *Bayes Factor*. Using these new vocabulary terms, the odds-version of Bayes' Rule is

$$\text{Posterior } \Omega(H_A{:}H_0) = \text{Prior } \Omega(H_A{:}H_0) \times \text{Bayes Factor}$$

To illustrate the use of Bayes Factors, suppose that we conduct an experimental evaluation of a new treatment. Although the treatment itself is new, based on the results of prior research, the consensus opinion of experts is that this new treatment will work as well as—or even better than—the status quo treatment. Accordingly, we expect that our experiment will reject H_0 in favor of H_A. Before the experiment begins, then, we believe that the odds of rejecting H_0 are larger than unity. That is,

$$\text{Prior } \Omega\,(H_A{:}H_0) > 1$$

When we conduct the experiment, we calculate a Bayes Factor from the results and use it to update the strength of our belief in H_A. If the Bayes Factor is greater than unity, the experimental results *strengthen* our belief in H_A. If the Bayes Factor is less than unity, the results *weaken* our belief in H_A—or from the complementary perspective *strengthen* our belief in H_0.

The use of Bayes Factors to weigh H_A against H_0 originates with Jeffreys (1935). Table 6.5 shows a four-category scale suggested by Raftery (1995, Table 6)[10] that can be used to interpret Bayes Factors. In plain words, a Bayes Factor of three or less is "weak" evidence for H_A, while a Bayes Factor greater than 150 is "very strong" evidence for H_A. Between these two extremes, the evidence for H_A can be "positive" or "strong," depending on the magnitude of the Bayes Factor. The right-hand column of Table 6.5 translates the endpoints of the four categories from Bayes Factors into probabilities. The reader should note, however, that these probabilities are *not* the p-values used in Fisher and Neyman-Pearson tests of H_0 but, rather, the inverse probabilities that we have called p'.

To illustrate the use of Bayes Factors, we return to the U.K. traffic fatality time series analyzed in Chapter 5.2.2. Following the recommended algorithm, we modeled this time series as

$$H_A{:}UKFtl_t = \frac{(1 - .75B^{12})a_t}{\nabla^{12}(1 - .42B - .29B^2)}a_t - 312.26I_t$$

where I_t is a step function coded zero prior to a February 1983 mandatory seatbelt law and unity thereafter. The estimated effect of the new law is $\hat{\omega} = 312.3$. The value of $t = -3.82$ for this estimate has a very small p-value under H_0,

Table 6.5. INTERPRETING BAYES FACTORS (RAFTERY, 1995, TABLE 6)

Strength of Evidence	Bayes Factor	$p' \equiv \Pr(H_A\|Data)$
Weak	$0 \leq BF \leq 3$	$0.0 < p' \leq 0.75$
Positive	$3 < BF \leq 20$	$0.75 < p' \leq 0.95$
Strong	$20 < BF \leq 150$	$0.95 < p' \leq 0.99$
Very Strong	$BF > 150$	$p' > 0.99$

10. Raftery cites Jeffreys (1961, Appendix B) as the source of this idea but modifies Jeffreys' original scale slightly. Our Table 6.5 adopts Raftery's modification.

$p = 0.0000002$. Whether we test H_0 with the classic methods of Fisher or Neyman-Pearson or with the modern hypothesis test, this estimate rejects H_0 with a high degree of confidence.

Concurrence among the three approaches is not unusual, especially with an effect estimate as large as this one. A Bayesian hypothesis test will also reject H_0 under these circumstances, but the Bayesian test result will have a very a different character. To conduct a Bayesian hypothesis test, we re-estimate the model under H_0.

$$H_0 : UKFtl_t = \frac{-27.01 + (1 - .77B^{12})a_t}{\nabla^{12}(1 - .45B - .28B^2)}$$

In principle, a Bayes Factor can be calculated directly from the models estimated under H_A and H_0. A direct calculation is often difficult in practice, however. To circumvent the practical difficulty, we can use an approximation to the Bayes Factor based on the Bayesian Information Criterion (BIC) that we introduced in Chapter 3.7.1. Where BIC_0 and BIC_A are the BICs for models estimated under H_0 and H_A respectively,

$$BF \approx e^{\frac{1}{2}(BIC_0 - BIC_A)}$$

For this time series, the estimated Bayes Factor is[11]

$$\widehat{BF} = e^{\frac{1}{2}(2293.36 - 2286.67)} = 28.361$$

Using Raftery's (1995) four-category scale (Table 6.5), our analysis of the U.K. traffic fatality time series provides *strong* evidence for H_A—or in substantive terms, *strong* evidence for the hypothesis that the new law effected a large, significant reduction in traffic fatalities.

When we analyzed the impact of the 1983 U.K. seatbelt law in Chapter 5.2.2, the p-value for $\hat{\omega}_0$ was small enough to reject H_0 in favor of H_A. Since the status quo modern hypothesis test and the Bayesian hypothesis test lead to the same decision to reject H_0, skeptical readers might question the need for Bayesian methods. Krueger (2011) argues that, because Bayesian and non-Bayesian tests agree most of the time, the added value of Bayesian tests is questionable. Berger and Delampady (1987), Berger (2003), and Ghosh, Delampady, and Samanta (2006) cite instances where Bayesian and non-Bayesian tests produce contradictory results.

---

11. Since most time series software packages report the BIC, the reader can plug the reported numbers into the formulae as we have done here. Readers who want to understand the BIC approximation to the BF are directed to Masson (2011) for a tutorial on the use of BFs in Bayesian hypothesis testing.

Even when Bayesian and non-Bayesian tests arrive at similar outcomes, they follow different paths. Prior to our analysis of the U.K. traffic fatality time series, we pretended to be agnostic on the question of whether a mandatory seatbelt law would reduce the level of traffic fatalities. To express this feigned neutrality, we specified the prior odds as

$$\text{Prior } \Omega\,(H_A{:}H_0) = \frac{\text{Pr}(H_A)}{\text{Pr}(H_0)} = 1$$

After examining the evidence for H_A, our degree of belief changed drastically. Based on the results of our analysis,

$$\text{Posterior } \Omega\,(H_A : H_0) = 28.4$$

Our posterior belief in H_A was 28 times stronger than our prior belief in H_A. This assumed that we were entirely agnostic prior to our analysis, of course, and we were not. In Chapter 5.2.1, we analyzed the impact of a 1972 seatbelt law on an Australian traffic fatality time series. Using the parameter estimates from that analysis (Table 5.10) the estimated Bayes Factor for the Australian seatbelt law is

$$\widehat{BF} = e^{\frac{1}{2}(268.35-259.25)} = 94.6$$

Using Raftery's (1995) four-category scale again, this estimate constitutes *strong* evidence that the 1972 Australian law had a salutary impact on traffic fatalities. If the Australian and U.K. laws are comparable, we can use the Bayes Factor estimated for the 1972 Australian law as the prior odds for the 1983 U.K. law. In that case,

$$\text{Posterior } \Omega\,(H_A{:}H_0) = 94.6 \times 28.4 = 2686.6$$

Prior to our analysis of the 1983 U.K. law, based on our analysis of the 1972 Australian law, we had a *strong* belief in H_A. We then analyzed the 1983 U.K. law and, based on the results, the strength of our belief in H_A rose to *very strong*.

As the seatbelt law analyses demonstrate, Bayesian hypothesis testing provide a simple method of updating the strength of our belief in H_A. Bayesian test results apply directly to H_A, moreover, and are not unduly influenced by the length of a time series. Classic Fisher and Neyman-Pearson tests and the modern "hybrid" test suffer by comparison.

6.4   THREATS TO STATISTICAL CONCLUSION VALIDITY

Several of the threats to statistical conclusion validity identified by Shadish *et al.* (Table 6.1) are a product of the modern hypothesis test. If Bayesian hypothesis tests become more widely accepted and used, replacing the status quo modern hypothesis test, the plausibility of these common threats will diminish. The threat of *low statistical power* illustrates this point. A vestige of the classic Neyman-Pearson hypothesis test, statistical power will always make sense in the context of a Neyman-Pearson test. Since statistical power is a function of N, the threat seldom arises in sensibly designed time series experiments. The threat of *low statistical power* makes no sense at all in Bayesian hypothesis tests, however, and will vanish with the Bayesian revolution. Conceptually similar threats will take the place of *low statistical power* after the revolution, of course, but we cannot predict the future.

The threat to statistical conclusion validity that Shadish *et al.* call *violated assumptions of statistical tests* is another matter entirely. Since these common threats affect the likelihood function component of Bayes' Rule, they will survive the Bayesian revolution—though perhaps in a modified form. The common *violated assumptions* threats were discussed in Chapter 3, at least implicitly, when the *ARIMA* modeling strategy was developed. If the *ARIMA* noise model is not statistically adequate, the *violated assumptions* threats become plausible. The consequences of the uncontrolled threats are difficult to predict in general but "can lead to either overestimating or underestimating the size and significance of an effect" (Shadish *et al.*, 2002, p. 45). If the *ARIMA* model is statistically adequate, on the other hand, *violated assumptions* threats are implausible.

Table 6.6 lists five threats to construct validity that are particularly plausible in time series experiments. Each of the five is a variation of the threats that Shadish et al. call *violated assumptions* and *low statistical power*. Because these threats can affect the different stages of design and analysis differently, we discuss them as distinct threats to construct validity. They are not discussed in order of their relative plausibility or prevalence but, rather, in an order that faciliates their discussion and analysis.

Table 6.6. THREATS TO STATISTICAL CONCLUSION VALIDITY

Violated assumptions of statistical tests
1. *Normality*
2. *Outliers*

Low statistical power
3. *Short time series—small N*
4. *Forecasting abuses*
5. *Missing data*

6.4.1 Normality

Thirty years ago, McCleary *et al.* (1980) and McDowall *et al.* (1980) recommended "eyeball" inspections for verifying the Normality assumption. Most of the example time series in those prior works were Normal. One or two non-Normal time series were log-transformed. This present work recommends formal Normality tests prior to model identification (Chapter 3.2) and, for time series that fail, Box-Cox transformation analyses. The example time series in this present work include many non-Normal time series that require general power transformations. What happened in 30 years? With the growing popularity of time series designs, the body of example time series grew larger and longer time series—which often require transformation—became more common. More important, too many of the examples that appeared in the literature violated the Normality assumption. In light of this serious threat to construct validity—a special case of *violated assumptions of statistical tests*—we recommend formal Normality tests and power transformations as needed.

Although there are many examples of questionable Normality assumptions, the first to attract our attention was the time series plotted in Figure 6.5: Boston armed robberies from January 1966 through October 1975. A strict gun control law was enacted in April 1975. Analyzing the raw time series, Deutsch and Alt (1977) report a *marginally* significant 20 percent reduction in armed robberies. Analyzing the log-transformed time series plotted in Figure 6.6, Hay and McCleary (1979) report a smaller 10 percent reduction in armed robberies.

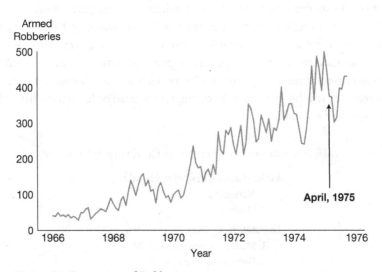

Figure 6.5 Boston Armed Robberies

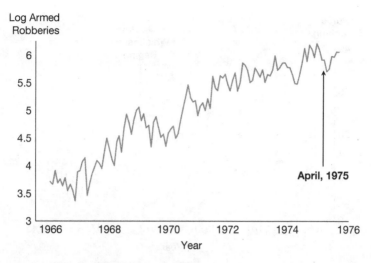

Figure 6.6 Logarithms, Boston Armed Robberies

Their estimate is *not* statistically significant, however, and that result reinforces the importance of the Normality assumption.

While the 1975 Massachusetts gun control law may have had an impact on gun deaths, the consensus opinion is that it had little or no effect on armed robberies (e.g., Rivara and Kellermann, 2007). The contrary view, associated with Deutsch and Alt, is due only in part to a violation of the Normality assumption. A more important factor is the relatively short post-intervention time series. In general, $N_{post} = 7$ monthly observations will not support a reliable estimate of ω_0. We revisit this problem when we discuss forecasting abuses.

6.4.2 Outliers as a Violation of Normality

Some time series fail Normality tests because the underlying generating process is systemically non-Normal. The Boston armed robbery time series plotted in Figure 6.5 is an example. General power transformations are required for this non-Normal class. Another class of time series fail Normality tests because of an outlier or two. The Normality assumption can be ensured for these time series by a pragmatic adjustment of the outliers.

The time series plotted in Figure 6.7 might fail on both grounds. These data are purse snatchings in the Hyde Park neighborhood of Chicago, aggregated by lunar month, from January 1969 to September 1973. Reed (1978) collected these data to evaluate *Operation Whistlestop*, a community crime prevention program. Arriving at nonsensical analytic results, Reed suspected that one of the monthly totals was a recording error. Returning to the primary data records,

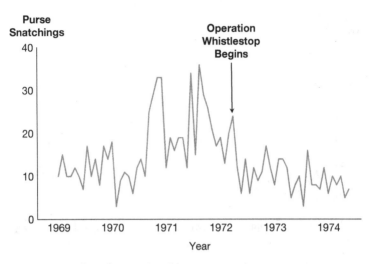

Figure 6.7 Hyde Park Purse Snatchings

Reed arrived at a more reasonable, correct number for the anomalously large observation. McCleary *et al.* (1980) used this time series to illustrate the effects of an anomalous outlier on the identification and estimation of an *ARIMA* model. Harvey and Fernandes (1989), Fruhwirth-Schnatter (1995), and Brandt and Williams (2001) used it to propose and illustrate Poisson time series models. We touch on both issues here but focus largely on the threat to statistical conclusion validity posed by outliers.

The Normal (or Gaussian) probability model maps a time series observation onto the real line. Since most social and behavioral time series are counts, the Normal distribution is almost always the "wrong"—but nevertheless "useful"—model. The simplest probability model for time series of counts is the Poisson process. Where Y_t is an observation and μ is the Poisson mean, estimated in the ordinary way, the Poisson probability function is

$$\Pr(Y_t = m) = \mu^m e^{-m}/m! \qquad m = 0, 1, 2, \ldots$$

The Poisson probability function assumes that time series observations are independent. That is,

$$\Pr(Y_t = m|Y_{t-k}) = \Pr(Y_t = m) = \mu^m e^{-m}/m!$$

So long as the independence assumption holds, μ is both the mean and the variance of the Poisson distribution.

$$E(Y_t) = E[Y_t - E(Y_t)]^2 = \mu$$

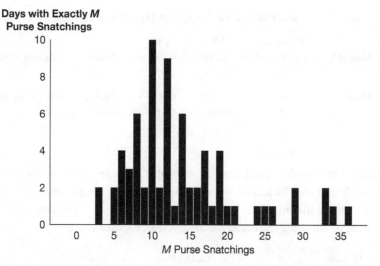

Figure 6.8 Histogram: Days with Exactly M Purse Snatchings

When the independence assumption fails, Y_t behaves as if it were generated by what Coleman (1964) calls a "contagious cousin" of the Poisson process. Contagion can arise through any of several empirically indistinguishable mechanisms, but whatever the mechanism, contagion destroys the equality of variance and mean. If contagion arises through positive autoregression, the process variance is inflated, leaving apparent "outliers" in the time series.

The Hyde Park purse snatchings time series is a typical example. Figure 6.8 shows a histogram of the time series. Ignoring a half-dozen of the most extreme values makes the distribution appear approximately Normal. This time series could then be modeled either as a Poisson process, probably contagious, or relying on the Normal approximation to the Poisson, as an *ARIMA* model. Both the simple and contagious Poisson models can be written as

$$Ln(\mu_t) = \theta_0 + \omega_0 I_t \quad \text{or} \quad \mu_t = e^{\theta_0 + \omega_0 I_t}$$

Parameter estimates for the simple and contagious models are reported in Table 6.7 as Model 1 and Model 2.[12] The only structural difference between the models is the parameter ζ, which accounts for "extra-Poisson dispersion." To explain that phrase, the variance of a simple Poisson process is μ. The variance of a contagious Poisson process is a function of μ/ζ, which, based on our experience, will usually be larger than μ.

12. We used the Stata 12 **poisson** and **nbreg (mean)** routines to estimate these parameters. There are several ways to model contagious Poisson time series. Interested readers are directed

Table 6.7. Poisson Parameter Estimates, Hyde Park Purse Snatchings

		Estimate	SE	*t*	
Model 1	θ_0	2.780	0.038	72.68	$LR_1 = 45.79$
	ω_0	−.451	0.068	−6.61	
Model 2	θ_0	2.780	0.070	39.87	$LR_2 = 114.40$
	ω_0	−0.451	0.113	−3.99	
	ζ	0.141	0.035		

Model 1 and Model 2 yield identical estimates of the pre- and post-intervention means, θ_0 and ω_0. That is as it should be, of course; the parameter ζ models the *variance* of the time series, *not* the mean. When $\zeta = 1$, the two models are identical, so choosing the better model amounts to testing

$$H_0: \zeta \neq 1$$

Since Model 1 is nested in Model 2, the *LR*s reported in Table 6.7 can be used for this test. Under H_0, the difference in *LR*s is distributed as χ_1^2. For Model 2 and Model 1,

$$LR_2 - LR_1 = 114.40 - 45.79 = 68.61$$

Since values of $\chi_1^2 \geq 68.61$ occur with probability $p < 0.0001$, we reject the simple Poisson Model 1 in favor of the contagious Poisson Model 2.

Not unexpectedly, the simple and contagious Poisson models agree that *Operation Whistlestop* had a large impact but disagree on the level of significance; and to the extent that Poisson contagion exaggerates the significance level of parameter estimates, contagion is analogous to autoregression. In Model 2, which accounts for contagion, the value of $t = -3.99$ for $\hat{\omega}_0 = -0.451$ is large enough to reject H_0. We conclude then that *Operation Whistlestop* worked.

Since the values of $\hat{\theta}_0$ and $\hat{\omega}_0$ are reported in the natural logarithm metric, we exponentiate the model to facilitate interpretion of the results.

$$\hat{\mu}_t = e^{2.780 - 0.451 I_t}$$

Prior to the onset of *Whistlestop*, $I_t = 0$, so

$$\hat{\mu}_t = e^{2.780} = 16.119$$

Thereafter, $I_t = 1$, so

$$\hat{\mu}_t = e^{2.780 - 0.451} = e^{2.329} = 10.268$$

to Cameron and Trivedi (1998) or to Barron (1992) for surveys. For this particular analysis, the alternative models support the same inference.

The one-time reduction of $(16.119 - 10.268 =) \, 5.851$ purse snatchings per lunar month amounts to a 36.3 percent reduction. This impact estimate is both large and statistically significant.

Though the contagious Poisson Model 2 provides a better fit than the simple Poisson Model 1, neither model has the flexibility of an *ARIMA* model. Should we let the tail (outliers) wag the dog (seasonality, autocorrelation, drift, and other dynamic behaviors)? Sometimes the advantages of an explicit count model outweigh the disadvantages. Other times, the disadvantages demand an *ARIMA* model. If an *ARIMA* model is used to represent a discrete count time series, extreme values must be accommodated. If the extreme values are part of an underlying non-Normal distribution, a transformation might accomplish this. When a few outliers are the exception to another otherwise approximately Normal distribtution, however—and the Hyde Park purse snatching time series is a good example—even the "best" Box-Cox transformation will fail. In that case, pulse functions can be incorporated in an *ARIMA* model to account for outliers.

To demonstrate this approach, we estimated *ARIMA* impact models for the Hyde Park purse snatching time series with pulse functions incorporated for each set of outliers. Specifying an abrupt, permanent impact for *Operation Whistlestop*, the model is

$$Y_t = N(a_t) + \omega_0 I_t + \sum_{j=1}^{6} \omega_j P_{j,t}$$

The results of our analyses are reported in Table 6.8. Since the $N(a_t)$ components of the models change slightly as pulse functions are incorporated, we do not report noise parameter estimates. In every case, the time series was modeled as the most parsimonious, statistically adequate model.

The columns of Table 6.8 correspond to *ARIMA* models with as many as five outliers fit with pulse functions. The first column reports an *ARIMA* model

Table 6.8. ARIMA MODELS, HYDE PARK PURSE SNATCHINGS

N	71	70	69	67	65
$Y_t \leq$	36	34	33	29	26
$\hat{\mu}$	13.92	13.60	13.30	12.72	12.22
$\hat{\sigma}^2$	56.51	50.16	44.68	33.93	26.45
p_{Normal}	0.044	0.054	0.066	0.115	0.207
$p_{Poisson}$	0.001	0.004	0.011	0.077	0.296
$\hat{\omega}_0$	−2.42	−2.28	−1.81	−2.03	−4.18
$t_{\hat{\omega}_0}$	−0.86	−0.81	−0.79	−0.93	−1.95

estimated with one outlier fit, for example. The second column reports a model estimated with two outliers fit, and so forth. The table's first two rows report the number of observations (N) and the value of the largest observation $(Y \leq)$. The third and fourth rows report means $(\hat{\mu})$ and variances $(\hat{\sigma}^2)$. The fifth and sixth rows report p-values for the Kolomogorov-Smirnov goodness-of-fit tests for Normal (p_{Normal}) and simple Poisson $(p_{Poisson})$ distributions. Finally, the seventh and eighth rows report effect estimates $(\hat{\omega}_0$ and $t_{\hat{\omega}_0})$ for *Whistlestop*.

Most of the statistics reported in Table 6.8 are expected. As more outliers are controlled, means and variances of the time series grow smaller while goodness-of-fit to the Normal and Poisson distributions improves. With the four most extreme values controlled, the distribution of time series observations is only marginally different than Normal or simple Poisson. With the five most extreme values controlled, the estimated impact of *Whistlestop* is large $(\hat{\omega}_0 = -4.18)$ and statistically significant $(t_{\hat{\omega}_0} = -1.95)$.

Readers should not be surprised that the contagious Poisson and *ARIMA* models lead to similar conclusions about the effectiveness of *Operation Whistlestop*. Comparing contagious Poisson and *ARIMA* impact models in a variety of substantive areas, Thompson et al. (2009), Kuhn, Davidson, and Durkin (1994), Tobías et al. (2001), and others report the same experience.

For discrete count time series, the choice between contagious Poisson and *ARIMA* models should reflect theoretical and practical considerations.

More generally, outliers strain the Normal approximation and distort the sample statistics used to build *ARIMA* models (Tsay, 1986; Chen and Liu, 1993). Some characteristics of an outlier are not controversial. Determining whether the magnitude of an observation exceeds the threshold is a straightforward exercise in the construction of confidence intervals. Other defining characteristics are more problematic. How many outliers can we observe before concluding that the cluster is something more than an isolated departure from Normality?

Outliers are a sample phenomenon, not a population phenomenon. In a cross-sectional sample of five people, it would be unusual to find a seven-foot-tall person. Relying on our understanding of the population and sampling process, the seven-footer would be an outlier. We could assume safely that the anomalous seven-footer was due to sampling error. Finding *two* seven-footers in a sample of 10 would challenge this sampling error explanation, however: It would be more likely that we were not sampling from the general population or that our samples deviated in some bizarre way from the random model. This same line of reasoning applies to longitudinal analyses. Whereas one or two isolated extreme values can always be rationalized away, a cluster of extreme values are probably *not* random deviations from Normality.

6.4.3 Short Time Series

We know of no way to control the threats to statistical conclusion validity that arise in the analysis of a single short time series. How short is "short"? Conventional wisdom sets the threshold at $N < 50$ observations, but this convention ignores the role of variance in statistical conclusion validity. If the time series is a smooth realization of a white noise process, $N = 30$ observations may be sufficient for many inferences. If the time series is an unruly realization of a high-order *ARIMA* process, on the other hand, $N = 100$ observations may be insufficient for even the simplest inferences. Deciding whether a particular time series is too short requires a knowledge of the mean and variance of the time series and the proposed inference.

With all that said, the time series plotted in Figure 6.9 is too short for a meaningful statistical analysis. These data are nightly bedtime disruptions—crying, leaving the bedroom, and so forth—for a three-year-old boy (Friman et al., 1999). During the two baseline phases of 15 and seven nights each, the boy's parents handled the disruptions as they normally would. During the two treatment phases of eight and six nights each, the parents gave the boy a token that could be exchanged for an out-of-bedroom visit to get a glass of water or a hug or to go to the bathroom.

Visual inspections of the time series are ambiguous; some might see an effect, others might not. We might ordinarily resolve this ambiguity with a formal

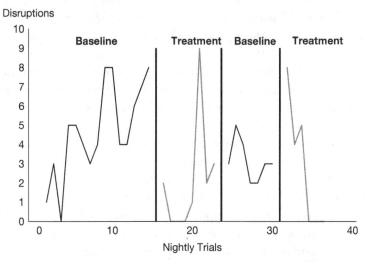

Figure 6.9 Bedtime Disruptions for a Three-Year-Old Boy (Friman et al., 1999)

statistical analysis, but in this case the analytic results are equally ambiguous. Entertaining the null hypothesis that the treatment had no effect or that the effect is zero,

$$H_0: \omega_0 = 0$$

Regressing the nightly disruption time series on I_t with an $AR1$ noise component, the estimated model is

$$Disruption_t = \frac{4.05}{1 - 0.27B} a_t - 1.55 I_t$$

The t-statistic for $\hat{\omega}_0 = -1.55$ is $t_{\hat{\omega}_0} = -1.36$. Since this value of $t_{\hat{\omega}_0}$ has a one-tailed probability of $p = 0.09$, we cannot reject H_0, at least not at the conventional $p < 0.05$ level. Still, $\hat{\omega}_0$ amounts to nearly a 40 percent reduction in nightly disruptions, and given the large *substantive* size of this effect, it would be imprudent to interpret the *statistical* size of $\hat{\omega}_0$ to mean that the treatment is *ineffective*.

There are several ways to convey the ambiguity of this (or any other) analytic result. We might report that $\hat{\omega}_0$ is "marginally" significant, for example; or that "$\hat{\omega}_0$ occurs with probability $p = 0.09$ under H_0" and allow readers to draw their own conclusions. These compromises ignore the *real* problem: *This time series is too short for any meaningful statistical analysis.*

A step-by-step review of the *ARIMA* modeling strategy (Figure 3.1) for the disturbance time series reinforces that point. As always, we began by rejecting a white noise model because its residuals failed a Q-test. We next considered $AR1$ and $MA1$ models. Although the residuals of both models were not different than white noise, their $AR1$ and $MA1$ parameter estimates were not statistically significant. What a dilemma: A Q-test *rejects* the white noise model while t-tests reject any model *except* white noise! Since Q-tests and t-tests assume a long time series, there is no real dilemma, of course. The time series is just too short.

The fields of applied psychology, where short single-subject time series abound, have been preoccupied with this false dilemma. Since single-subject time series tend to be too short for formal *ARIMA* modeling, Crosbie (1993), Edgington (1996), and others have proposed alternative approaches. Huitema (2004) reviews this literature and the implied threats to statistical conclusion validity. Ultimately, there are no simple design structures that can control the threats to statistical conclusion validity posed by short time series. This should not deter single-subject researchers, however, but rather should reinforce the value of patience. The evolutionary process by which true knowledge accumulates works slowly.

6.4.4 Forcasting and Intervention Discovery Methods

An alternative to standard intervention methods is to build an *ARIMA* model for only the pre-intervention segment of a time series and then use this model to forecast the post-intervention segment. The differences between the forecasts and the actual series observations—the forecast errors—should be trivially small if the intervention impact is zero. A large and statistically significant difference between the forecasts and the actual values is evidence that the intervention influenced the series.

Using forecasting to estimate intervention impacts can be intuitively appealing on its surface. This is especially so for short post-intervention segments, such as a time series with only five or six observations after the intervention. In these cases it seems natural to forecast the post-intervention segment and then compare the forecasts with actuality. Box and Tiao (1976) show that this approach provides reasonable results, but they also point out that it offers no advantages over standard intervention methods.

Substituting forecasting for other approaches to intervention analysis does have a large potential disadvantage, however, in that it cannot feasibly distinguish between abrupt-permanent impact patterns and other possibilities. Models of dynamic impacts usually require a long post-intervention period to obtain stable estimates, and this is a reason to avoid short post-intervention series in the first place. Hay and McCleary (1977), for example, re-analyzed the data from an evaluation that relied on forecasting and six post-intervention observations. They found that gradual-temporary models fit the series as adequately as did the abrupt model that the original author favored. Given the similar model fits, the only satisfactory way to distinguish between the possibilities would be to collect more data.

Besides estimating intervention impacts, forecasting also has a second and more problematic use in locating intervention points. The logic here is that, if an intervention affects a series, model forecasts should begin to diverge from the actual values at the moment of impact. One might then work backward to find the time point at which the change most likely began. Deutsch (1978; Deutsch and Alt, 1977), for example, developed an *ARIMA* model on a long pre-intervention time series and then used it to forecast a short post-intervention segment. To identify the point at which the intervention began to take hold, Deutsch selected the first observation that significantly deviated from its forecasted value.

In the simple form in which Deutsch used it, intervention discovery methods suffer from obvious "fishing" threats to statistical conclusion validity. By successively applying null hypothesis tests with a constant α-level, the nominal probability of a Type I error is much higher than the stated α. Andrews (1993) addressed this multiple testing problem by deriving the sampling distribution for time series with unknown change points. The Andrews distribution requires much stronger evidence of a change than do the methods that we have discussed for known change points and so have greater statistical power. The power of tests using the Andrews distribution also breaks down completely near the beginning or end of a series, making it unappealing for situations with short post-intervention segments.

A slight variation on using forecasting to find a change point is to estimate a set of intervention models that cover all dates between a fixed lower and upper bound. Instead of looking for the first potential breakpoint, this strategy considers a range of possible points and selects the largest as the most likely instant of change. Quandt (1960) originally proposed the general approach, and more recent work combines it with the Andrews sampling distribution. See Hansen (2001) for a useful introduction. The Quandt-Andrews method shares the statistical power problems that are inherent in the sequential estimation strategy, and it has an obvious disadvantage compared to estimates that assume a known intervention date.

More generally, searches for an intervention point undermine the internal validity of the research design. History is an especially serious threat, for example, because the number of plausible alternative explanations of a post-intervention change increases with the number of intervention points. The nature of the intervention itself also becomes ill defined in these situations and can present the problems inherent in the "fuzzy" responses to an intervention that will be described in Chapter 8.

6.4.5 Missing Data

Missing data threats come in *simple* and *complex* varieties. The overlapping time series plotted in Figure 6.10 illustrate the complex threat. Meltzer et al. (1980; Shumway and Stoffer, 1980, Table I) report annual physician expenditures from the Social Security Administration (1949–73) and the Health Care Financing Administration (1965–76). Since each year has at least one observation, the missing data threat is not immediately apparent. On the contrary, if anything, we have too much data. That can be a problem too. A potential threat arises in the nine-year segment (1965–73) where the time series overlap. If the two time series measure the same phenomenon, discrepancies must be small enough to pass for rounding errors and, hence, small enough to be ignored. The largest discrepancies occur in the first and last years, however, 1965 and 1973, so a rounding error explanation is implausible.

Even if the discrepancies between these two time series were uniform in magnitude and randomly distributed, their relatively short histories and common accelerating trends argue against simple, obvious solutions. If complex missing

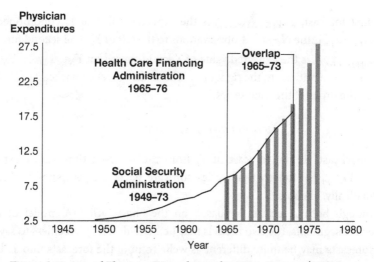

Figure 6.10 Annual Physician Expenditures from Two Sources (Meltzer et al., 1980)

data pose a threat to statistical conclusion validity, the threat must be controlled by filling in gaps with maximum likelihood estimates. R-language software for that purpose is widely available. Since complex missing data are rarely found in the time series experiments at the core of this book, we will not work through a solution for complex missing data. Interested readers are directed to Shumway and Stoffer (2011).

Simple missing data are commonly encountered in time series experiments. Control of the threats posed by simple missing data require three conditions. First, the data are missing from a single time series. Second, the missing data are contiguous. Third, the missing data cannot occur near the intervention. Although we typically do not think in these terms, when we forecast a time series of N observations, $Y_{N+\ell}$ is a missing value. If for some reason we needed an estimate of $Y_{N+\ell}$, we could use the conditional expected value, $E(Y_{N+\ell}|Y_1, \ldots, Y_N)$. The maximum likelihood estimate of $Y_{N+\ell}$ requires the "best" ARIMA model, of course, and due to missing data, this model is unavailable. In a nutshell, that is the threat to statistical conclusion validity posed by simple missing data.

In lieu of the "best" ARIMA model, we use the "best" models estimated from the time series segments on either side of the gap. The simplest nontrivial situation where the three conditions hold occurs when the time series has one missing observation and no intervention. If Y_j is the missing observation, we have two possible forecasts:

$$\hat{Y}_{j|Y_1,\ldots,Y_{N-j-1}} = E(Y_j|Y_1,\ldots,Y_{N-j-1}) \text{ and}$$
$$\hat{Y}_{j|Y_{N-j+1},\ldots,Y_N} = E(Y_j|Y_{N-j+1},\ldots,Y_N)$$

The first forecast, $\hat{Y}_{j|Y_1,\ldots,Y_{N-j-1}}$, is the expected value of Y_j conditioned on $Y_1,\ldots,Y_{N-j-1}$, the $N-j-1$ observations to the left of Y_j. The second forecast, $\hat{Y}_{j|Y_{N-j+1},\ldots,Y_N}$, is the expected value of Y_j conditioned on $Y_{N-j+1},\ldots,Y_N$, the $N-j+1$ observations to the right of Y_j. This is the so-called backcast of Y_j. If we reverse the order of the time series,

$$Y_N,\ldots,Y_{N-j+1},Y_j,Y_{N-j-1},\ldots,Y_1$$

The "backcast" is the forecast of Y_j from the reversed time series segment $Y_N,\ldots,Y_{N-j+1}$. Modern time series software packages compute "backcasts" automatically, of course.

Although both forecasts are based on the "best" *ARIMA* model of their respective segments, the two models may be quite different. Needless to say, the two forecasts may be quite different as well. To pool the forecasts into a "best" estimate of Y_j, we recommend a variation of the weights proposed by Abraham (1981). For forecast variances σ^2_{N-j-1} and σ^2_{N-j+1}, as defined in Chapter 4.2, the "best" estimate of Y_j is

$$\hat{Y}_j = \frac{\hat{Y}_{j|Y_1,\ldots,Y_{N-j-1}}\sigma^2_{N-j-1} + \hat{Y}_{j|Y_{N-j+1},\ldots,Y_N}\sigma^2_{N-j+1}}{\sigma^2_{N-j-1} + \sigma^2_{N-j+1}}$$

We must now combine $\hat{Y}_{N-j-1}$ and $\hat{Y}_{N-j+1}$ into a pooled estimate of the missing observation, Y_j.

6.5 CONCLUSION

The common threats to statistical conclusion validity can arise—or can become plausible—either through model misspecification or through hypothesis testing. These two threat sources overlap to some degree. The risk of a serious model misspecification is inversely proportional to the length of the time series, for example, and so is the risk of mistating the Type I and Type II error rates. The two threat sources are distinct for the most part, however, and can be discussed as non-overlapping categories. We begin with the potential model misspecification threats discussed in Chapter 6.4.

The most common threats to statistical conclusion validity involve violations of the Normality assumption. When the departure from Normality reveals itself through a heavily skewed unimodal distribution, the threat can *usually* be controlled by a Box-Cox transformation. In the relatively few instances where Box-Cox transformations fail, a more complicated control strategy may be required. But since these instances are rare, we will not discuss them here.

When the departure from Normality can be traced to a few "outliers," the threat can be controlled by using pulse functions to represent the anomalous observations. Widely used computer software packages have built-in routines for that purpose. In instances where the Normal distribution is used to approximate a Poisson distribution, the threat can be traced to the approximation itself. If the approximation is weak, parametric Poisson regression models are recommended. Pulse functions can be used to represent seasonality; nonstationary behavior can be represented by contagious models.

The threats to statistical conclusion validity that arise through hypothesis testing are less commonly encountered, in our experience, but are more vexing. We begin our introduction to this topic with two general recommendations. First, *the threats associated with low statistical power are almost never plausible in a well-designed time series experiment.* Indeed, orthodox Neyman-Pearson hypothesis tests are poorly suited to time series experiments. Neyman-Pearson hypothesis tests make sense in fields where virtually all research uses the same design. In biomedical trials, for example, the results of successive trials might be viewed as a sequence of samples that, in the long run, converge on a planned level of power. This argument is problematic in fields where time series experiments are found. Ultimately, a sequence of time series experiments must be viewed as a sequence of "case study" results that do not satisfy the fundamental Neyman-Pearson strategy.

Second recommendation: *Avoid radical solutions to common problems.* We are convinced that Bayesian statistical tests will prevail—but only eventually. One obstacle to the inevitable triumph of Bayesianism is that time series designs are scattered across a wide range of disciplines—criminology, economics, education, epidemiology, political science, policy analysis, program evaluation, public health, psychology, sociology and so forth. The thought of coordinating a revolution across these diverse disciplinary boundaries is daunting to say the least. But then, patience is always rewarded.

To illustrate the contrary argument, in early 2015, the editors of *Basic and Applied Social Psychology*, a peer-reviewed scientific journal, actually banned null hypothesis significance testing procedures. Under the new editorial policy, manuscripts that reported null hypothesis significance tests would still be sent out for peer-review but then

> prior to publication, authors will have to remove all vestiges of the null hypothesis significance testing procedure (p-values, t-values, F-values, statements about "significant" differences or lack thereof, and so on) ... [C]onfidence intervals also are banned ... [W]ith respect to Bayesian procedures, we reserve the right to make case-by-case judgments, and thus Bayesian procedures are neither required nor banned. (Trafimow and Marks, 2015, pp. 1–2)

Though agreeing that null hypothesis significance testing could be abused and misused, most critics question the usefulness of an outright ban on any procedure (Tarran, 2015). Leek and Peng (2015, p. 612–13) are skeptical that the validity of a research finding depends crucially on one particular step of a multistep research protocol:

> The last step [in a successful study] is the calculation of an inferential statistic such as a P-value, and the application of a "decision rule" to it (for example, $P < 0.05$). In practice, decisions that are made earlier in data analysis have a much greater impact on results—from experimental design to batch effects, lack of adjustment for confounding factors, or simple measurement error. Arbitrary levels of statistical significance can be achieved by changing the ways in which data are cleaned, summarized or modelled. P-values are an easy target: being widely used, they are widely abused. But, in practice, deregulating statistical significance opens the door to even more ways to game statistics— intentionally or unintentionally—to get a result. Replacing P-values with Bayes factors or another statistic is ultimately about choosing a different trade-off of true positives and false positives. Arguing about the P-value is like focusing on a single misspelling, rather than on the faulty logic of a sentence.

We agree with Leek and Peng. Although the common threats to statistical conclusion validity listed in Table 6.6 are closely tied to the modern null hypothesis significance test, eliminating the modern test will not eliminate threats to statistical conclusion validity. Any inferential strategy that replaces the modern test will introduce exotic new threats. If deducing and evaluating hypotheses is inherent to the scientific method—and in our view, it is—then so is statistical conclusion validity.

Nevertheless, we resolve to do a better job of teaching the epistemological foundations of significance testing. The debate between Fisher (1925) and Neyman-Pearson (1928) is a convenient place to start. Fisher proposed the p-value to measure the fit between the data and H_0. A small p-value—say, $p < 0.05$—meant that H_0 is probably false. Though it seems natural to interpret a large p-value— say, $p > 0.75$—to mean that H_0 is probably true, this symmetry was not part of Fisher's significance test. The alternative strategy proposed by Neyman and Pearson addressed this apparent shortcoming by defining two logically complementary hypotheses—which we have called H_0 and H_A — and then devising a test that would support one and reject the other.

The Neyman-Pearson test was not a mere "improvement" on Fisher's test. Foundations of the two tests have little overlap and, indeed, are contradictory in some respects. To emphasize their differences, Gigerenzer et al. (1989) call the

Fisher and Neyman-Pearson approaches "significance testing" and "hypothesis testing" respectively. These distinctive names are not widely used, of course, and the differences between the two approaches are obscure.

Over many years, the Fisher and Neyman-Pearson approaches were merged into a unitary modern hybrid test. Since it borrows from both approaches, it has the look and feel of the Neyman-Pearson test—more so when a jury verdict analogy (Table 6.2) is used. This superficial resemblance is deceiving, however. When the Neyman-Pearson test is appropriate—say, in biomedical trials—the modern hybrid test is no substitute.

Critics fault Fisher's test, the Neyman-Pearson test and the modern hybrid test for their common reliance on p-values. One problem with these tests is that, if N is "too large," every H_0 is rejected. If N is "too small," no H_0 is ever rejected. Another problem involves a common misconception about p. Contrary to popular belief, p says *nothing* about the credibility of H_0. This popular misconception confuses p with the inverse probability, p'. Since Bayesian tests rely on inverse probabilities, they are immune to both problems. This is not to say that Bayesian tests have no problems. But the serious problems that weigh so heavily in p-value tests are undefined in Bayesian tests.

In preparation for this chapter, we reviewed more than one thousand peer-reviewed applications from public health, criminology, education, program evaluation, and other fields where time series experiments are used. Only a few of these articles tested hypotheses with methods that could be construed as "Bayesian." A majority used p-values, confidence intervals, or some other non-Bayesian method. That is the state of the art. There are many reasons to believe that Bayesian methods will prevail eventually, but that is in the future. Meanwhile, we urge students to begin learning about Bayesianism, starting with inductive logic and epistemology.

Hacking's (2001) *Introduction to Probability and Inductive Logic* provides a solid foundation for neophytes. (We read and recommend anything by this author.) Skyrms' (2000) *Choice and Chance* covers the same material at a slightly higher level. Howson and Upchurch (1989) is a readable description of the Bayesian approach to scientific reasoning. Fisher's (1970, pp. 8-17) short discussion of Bayes' Theorem is worthwhile for many reasons. Pawitan's (2013, pp. 9-19) short history of the the frequentist-Bayesian debate, and Fisher's "third way"—likelihood—is exceptional.

As powerful computers have become widely available, "Bayesian statistical analysis" has become synonymous with "Markov-chain Monte Carlo (MCMC)" methods. Kruschke's (2010) *Doing Bayesian Data Analysis* and *Bayesian Data Analysis* by Gelman et al. (2004) are both recommended for their accessibility and readability. Both require a background knowledge of the R programming language, however.

APPENDIX 6 PROBABILITY AND ODDS

For most readers, this is a review. To facilitate the review, the fundamental probability concepts are in bold typeface. Let J and K be the numbers realized on the first and second rolls of a fair die. The probability space of the two dice consists of 36 (J, K) pairs, each represented as a rectangle.

	$J=1$	$J=2$	$J=3$	$J=4$	$J=5$	$J=6$
$K=1$	(1,1)	(2,1)	(3,1)	(4,1)	(5,1)	(6,1)
$K=2$	(1,2)	(2,2)	(3,2)	(4,2)	(5,2)	(6,2)
$K=3$	(1,3)	(2,3)	(3,3)	(4,3)	(5,3)	(6,3)
$K=4$	(1,4)	(2,4)	(3,4)	(4,4)	(5,4)	(6,4)
$K=5$	(1,5)	(2,5)	(3,5)	(4,5)	(5.5)	(6,5)
$K=6$	(1,6)	(2,6)	(3,6)	(4,6)	(5,6)	(6,6)

Assuming that the dice are fair, each of the 36 (J, K) pairs is equally likely. To acknowledge this fact, the 36 rectangles are constructed so that they have equal areas. A **random variable** is a rule that assigns the outcomes of a probability space to a set of numbers. If the random variable X is the sum of J and K, for example, X is distributed over the integers $2 \leq X \leq 12$ as

					(6,1)					
				(5,1)	(5,2)	(5,3)				
			(4,1)	(4,2)	(4,3)	(4,4)	(4,5)			
		(3,1)	(3,2)	(3,3)	(3,4)	(3,5)	(3,6)	(6,4)		
	(2,1	(2,2)	(2,3)	(2,4)	(2,5)	(2,6)	(6,3)	(5,5)	(6,5)	
(1,1)	(1,2)	(1,3)	(1,4)	(1,5)	(1,6)	(6,2)	(5,4)	(4,6)	(5,6)	(6,6)
2	3	4	5	6	7	8	9	10	11	12

Since each of the 36 (J, K) pairs is equally likely, the probability that X is equal to any integer is proportional to the number of rectangles stacked above the integer. To make these numbers conform to our notions of probability, we standardize each by the total number of rectangles in the space. Since $X = 7$ has six of the 36 rectangles, for example, $\Pr(X = 7) = 6/36$. $X = 3$ has two of the 36 rectangles, so $\Pr(X = 2) = 2/36$, and so forth.

Each of the 11 possible values of X is a **simple event**. If M is a specific value of X and $\neg M$ is some other value, M and $\neg M$ are logically **exclusive**, so the conjunction of two simple events is an impossibility.

$$\Pr[(X = M) \ AND \ (X = \neg M)] = 0$$

This generalizes to any set of the 11 simple events. The set of simple events is also logically **exhaustive**, so the disjunction of M and $\neg M$ is a sure thing. Thus,

$$\Pr[(X = M) \ OR \ (X = \neg M)] = 1$$

This generalizes to the disjunction of all 11 simple events,

$$\Pr[(X = 2) \ OR \ (X = 3) \ OR \ \ldots \ OR \ (X = 11) \ OR \ (X = 12)] = 1$$

Compound events are defined by disjoining or conjoining the 11 simple events. To illustrate, let the compound events A and B be

$$A : X \text{ is prime}$$
$$B : X \text{ is even}$$

The probabilities of A and B are calculated by summing the probabilities of their component simple events. Thus,

$$\Pr(A) = \Pr(X = 2,3,5,7,11) = \frac{1}{36} + \frac{2}{36} + \frac{4}{36} + \frac{6}{36} + \frac{2}{36} = \frac{15}{36}$$

$$\Pr(B) = \Pr(X = 2,4,6,8,10,12) = \frac{1}{36} + \frac{3}{36} + \frac{5}{36} + \frac{5}{36} + \frac{3}{36} + \frac{1}{36} = \frac{18}{36}$$

Unlike the simple events, $X = \{2,3,4,5,6,7,8,9,10,11\}$, compound events A and B are *not* exclusive. This means that A and B can be simultaneously true. The **conditional probability** that A is true (or that A will occur) given that B is true (or that B has already occured) is defined as

$$\Pr(A \mid B) = \frac{\Pr(A \ AND \ B)}{\Pr(B)} = \frac{\Pr(X = 2)}{\Pr(X = 2,4,6,8,10,12)} = \frac{\frac{2}{36}}{\frac{18}{36}} = \frac{1}{9}$$

The conditional probability that B is true (or that B will occur) given that A is true (or that A has already occurred) is

$$\Pr(B \mid A) = \frac{\Pr(B \ AND \ A)}{\Pr(A)} = \frac{\Pr(X = 2)}{\Pr(X = 2,3,5,7,11)} = \frac{\frac{2}{36}}{\frac{15}{36}} = \frac{2}{15}$$

So although it can happen that $Pr(A \mid B) = Pr(B \mid A)$, in this particular case,

$$Pr(A \mid B) \neq Pr(B \mid A)$$

Bayes' Rule gives the relationship between the two conditional probabilities for events A and B,

$$Pr(B \mid A) = \frac{Pr(A \mid B) Pr(B)}{Pr(A)} = \frac{\left(\frac{1}{9}\right)\left(\frac{1}{2}\right)}{\left(\frac{5}{12}\right)} = \frac{2}{15}$$

and

$$Pr(A \mid B) = \frac{Pr(B \mid A) Pr(A)}{Pr(B)} = \frac{\left(\frac{2}{15}\right)\left(\frac{5}{12}\right)}{\left(\frac{1}{2}\right)} = \frac{1}{9}$$

which are the correct conditional probabilities.

Another manipulation of the conditional probabilities gives the probability of the conjunction of events A and B. The probability that both A and B are true (or that both A and B have occurred) is given by the **multiplication rule**:

$$Pr(A \ AND \ B) = Pr(A \mid B) \times Pr(B) = \frac{15}{36} \times \frac{2}{15} = \frac{1}{18}$$

The conjunction of B and A has the same probability:

$$Pr(B \ AND \ A) = Pr(A \ AND \ B) = \frac{1}{18}$$

The probability that either A or B is true (or that either A or B has occurred) is given by the **addition rule**:

$$Pr(A \ OR \ B) = Pr(A) + Pr(B) - Pr(A \ AND \ B) = \frac{15}{36} + \frac{18}{36} - \frac{2}{36} = \frac{31}{36}$$

When A and B are exclusive events, of course, $Pr(A \ AND \ B) = 0$.

Each of the probability concepts has an **odds** analog. For the complementary events M and $\neg M$,

$$Pr(M) = 1 - Pr(\neg M)$$

The **odds** of M are defined as

$$\Omega(M) = \frac{Pr(M)}{Pr(\neg M)} = \frac{Pr(M)}{1 - Pr(M)}$$

Table 6.9. Useful Facts and Formulae

Odds (Ω)	Probability (Pr)
$\Omega(M) = \dfrac{\mathrm{Pr}(M)}{1 - \mathrm{Pr}(M)}$	$\mathrm{Pr}(M) = \dfrac{\Omega(M)}{1 + \Omega(M)}$
$0 \le \Omega(M) < \infty$	$0 \le \mathrm{Pr}(M) \le 1$
$\Omega(M) \times \Omega(\neg M) = 1$	$\mathrm{Pr}(M) + \mathrm{Pr}(\neg M) = 1$
$\Omega(\neg M) = \dfrac{1}{\Omega(M)}$	$\mathrm{Pr}(\neg M) = \dfrac{\Omega(\neg M)}{1 + \Omega(\neg M)}$
$\Omega(\neg M) = \dfrac{\mathrm{Pr}(\neg M)}{1 - \mathrm{Pr}(\neg M)}$	$\mathrm{Pr}(\neg M) = 1 - \mathrm{Pr}(M)$

Whereas $\mathrm{Pr}(M)$ lies in the closed $[0, 1]$ interval, $\Omega(M)$ lies in the half-open $[0, \infty)$ interval with no upper bound. Otherwise, $\mathrm{Pr}(M)$ and $\Omega(M)$ convey the same information.

Table 6.9 collects some useful formulae for translating between odds and probabilities. In Chapter 6.3, for example, a Bayesian analysis of the impact of a 1983 U.K. seatbelt law on traffic fatalities gave the posterior odds of H_A as

$$\text{Posterior } \Omega(H_A{:}H_0) = 28.361$$

The posterior probability of H_A is then

$$\mathrm{Pr}(H_A \mid \hat{\omega}_0) = \frac{28.361}{1 + 28.361} = 0.9659$$

Independent investigations of the same phenomenon using probabilities and odds cannot arrive at contradictory conclusions. Since probabilities and odds differ only in format, a choice between the two measures can be arbitrary. Many readers feel comfortable with probabilities but not odds. Odds seem foreign. Nevertheless, for some purposes—*especially* Bayesian thinking—it is easier and more practical to think and speak in the language of odds.

In Appendix 3A, we ended our treatment of maximum likelihood estimation with a cautionary note on the difference between likelihoods and probabilities. Repeating that note, likelihoods are *not* probabilities. Since odds are just another way to express the fundamental meaning of probabilities, it follows as well that likelihoods are *not* odds. Now crude analogies between likelihoods and probabilities or odds are sometimes useful. But like all arguments-by-analogy, this one is limited, and more so because of its crudeness. Ultimately, scrupulous attention should be paid to the *differences* between likelihoods and probabilities or odds.

So what are these differences? Modern statistical significance tests define prob-abliity as the long-run limit of a sequence of observed probabilities. Although this so-called frequentist definition works reasonably well in fields where long sequences of identical trials (or repeated samples) are the norm, long sequences are rare—or even nonexistent— in most fields. Since Bayesian significance tests define probability in terms of subjective belief, they seem more appropriate. Bayesian tests have their own shortcomings, of course. In light of the shortcom-ings of the Bayesian and frequentist approaches, Fisher proposed what Pawitan (2013, p. 15) calls the "third way." Likelihoods are *not* probabilities or odds and, thus, are immune to the problems of frequentist and Bayesian tests.

7

Internal Validity

We have knowledge of a thing only when we have grasped its cause.
—ARISTOTLE (1984, P. 121)

All philosophers imagine that causation is one of the fundamental axioms of science, yet, oddly enough, in advanced sciences such as gravitational astronomy, the word "cause" never occurs ... The reason why physics has ceased to look for causes is that, in fact, there are no such things. The law of causality, I believe, like much that passes muster among philosophers, is a relic of a bygone age, surviving, like the monarchy, only because it is erroneously supposed to do no harm.
—RUSSELL (1918, P. 180)

Our position on causality falls midway between Aristotle's mystical reverence and Russell's ribald skepticism. Although Russell's strong objection to the use of causal explanations in scientific theories might seem odd and out of place today, it was typical of the logical positivists who dominated the early 20th century. Since the causal connection between X and Y could not be empirically verified, Russell and his logical positivist peers believed that statements like "X causes Y" must be rooted out of science. We will have more to say about this in Chapter 8 when we discuss construct validity. Chapter 7 focuses on the relationship between causality and internal validity. These two concepts are not synonymous. Ruling out the common threats to internal validity establishes a correlation between intervention and impact, but demonstrating that the "correlation implies causality" requires more work.

With that said, internal validity is surely the most satisfying of the four natural validities. Ruling out a threat to internal validity leaves one with a feeling of accomplishment—the feeling that "in this specific experimental instance" the treatment did indeed "make a difference" (Campbell and Stanley, 1966). While no less important, ruling out a threat to the other validities does not offer the same psychic reward. Campbell's earliest writings seemed to share this relative view of the validities. Of the two validities that were recognized in the 1950s and 1960s, internal validity was the sine qua non. That view changed subtly in 1970s and 1980s.

Campbell's (1957) early interest in the character of empirical inferences was motivated by two related problems. While the results of non-laboratory research seemed unreliable, they were easily generalized to other situations. While the results of laboratory research seemed reliable, on the other hand, they were difficult to generalize. Empirical results could be *either* reliable *or* generalizable but not both. Causal validity requires both.

Borrowing conceptual terms from ANOVA models, Campbell named these two problems "internal" and "external" validity. Although the terms soon entered the social science vocabulary, their meanings were changed drastically. Whereas Campbell intended the validities to refer to causes and effects as they were operationalized in a specific research milieu, most social scientists had simpler, broader understandings.

The semantic gap between the validities as originally intended by Campbell and as subsequently understood by social scientists is more apparent in the case of internal validity. We have already noted that some years later, Campbell (1986) proposed alternative terms that emphasized his original meanings. Campbell's alternative terms never entered the social science vocabulary, unfortunately. We will spend no more time on this issue. Campbell's concerns are addressed to some extent in the rigorous development of construct validity by Shadish et al. (2002). We follow that same path, hoping to convey the proper meaning of internal validity.

At a more concrete level, internal validity is typically taught and learned as a list of discrete threats. The nine threats to internal validity listed in Table 7.1

Table 7.1. THREATS TO INTERNAL VALIDITY (SHADISH ET AL., 2002)

  Ambiguous temporal precedence
  Selection
  History
  Maturation
  Regression
  Attrition
  Testing
  Instrumentation
  Additive and interactive effects of threats to internal validity

differ little from the list of eight threats identified by Campbell (1957; Campbell and Stanley, 1966). The threat of *ambiguous temporal precedence* is plausible only for the designs that Campbell and Stanley (1966) called "pre-scientific." Of the remaining threats, only five are plausible for time series designs. Our development of internal validity focuses on these threats.

7.1 FIVE COMMON THREATS – THE USUAL SUSPECTS

The Directory Assistance time series (Figure 5.2) is atypical in several respects, most notably in the size and nature of its impact. Few reasonable critics would doubt our interpretation of "what happened." Impacts are more typically less dramatic, however, and in the more typical cases, threats to internal validity are plausible. We define a threat to internal validity, loosely, as a natural phenomenon, possibly unrelated to the intervention, which can impact a time series. The dilemma posed by uncontrolled threats to internal validity is that, given a rejected null hypothesis, the impact may be due to the intervention or to an uncontrolled threat to internal validity. Campbell and Stanley (1966) list eight common threats to internal validity; Cook and Campbell (1979) expand the list to 13. We will deal only with those threats that frequently arise in time series experiments.

7.1.1 History

History as a threat to internal validity refers to the possibility that an impact may be due not to I_t but to some coincidental historical event. Figure 7.1 shows annual U.S. motorcycle fatality rates from 1959 to 1979. From 1966 to 1969, 47 states enacted mandatory helmet laws for motorcyclists. The time series declines sharply over the three-year period. From 1976 to 1979, 27 states repealed their mandatory helmet laws and the time series increases sharply. The National Highway Traffic Safety Administration interprets this impact causally: Mandatory helmet laws reduce motorcycle fatalities. Now the time series obviously supports this interpretation, but it supports another interpretation as well: history as an uncontrolled threat to internal validity.

The 1966–69 reduction, to some extent, might be a continuation of the downward trend exhibited throughout the 1960s. The three-year reduction is visually striking, of course, but we cannot forget that this period coincides almost exactly with the onset of the Vietnam War. The impact might simply reflect the removal of young men from our highways by the Selective Service. The 1976–79 increase might easily reflect the end of the Vietnam War.

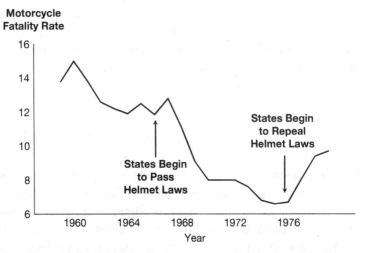

Figure 7.1 Annual U.S. Motocycle Fatality Rates (Ross and McCleary, 1983)

We do not endorse this alternative explanation; we *do* endorse the use of helmets by motorcyclists. But it is an eminently plausible alternative hypothesis and, until it is ruled out, the time series does not unambiguously support the inference that mandatory helmet laws cause reductions in motorcycle fatalities.

7.1.2 Maturation

Maturation as a threat to internal validity refers to the possibility that an impact may be due only to some natural change process. In the context of a time series experiment, the drift and trend associated with integrated processes raise potent maturation threats. The time series plotted in Figure 7.2 is undoubtedly the best-known social science example. These data are 270 weekly productivity means for five workers in the first relay assembly room of the Hawthorn Western Electric plant near Chicago. From 1927 to 1932, a group of social scientists conducted experiments to evaluate the impact of rest breaks, eight-hour work days, and wage incentives on productivity. In Chapter 5, we analyzed an 80-week segment of this time series during which workers' daily rest breaks were eliminated and reinstated. We estimated the impact of this intervention on productivity with the *IMA* model

$$P_t = \frac{\theta_0 + (1 - \theta_1)B}{\nabla} a_t + \omega_0 I_t$$

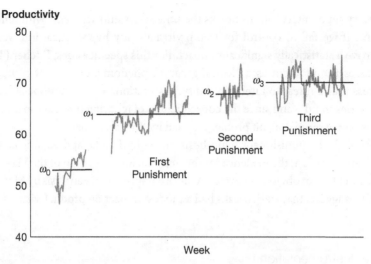

Figure 7.2 Weekly Productivity in the Bank Wiring Room (Franke and Kaul, 1978)

The estimated impact of the intervention, I_t, on productivity, P_t, was statistically significant. Though conducting no formal statistical analyses, the Hawthorn experimenters interpreted this impact as evidence that rest breaks had a salutary impact on productivity (Schlaifer, 1980). Franke and Kaul (1978; Franke, 1980) offer a more cynical interpretation. Noting that the machine operators were "punished" for inadequate performance at three specific points in time, Franke and Kaul argue that productivity increases resulted not from improved social relations, but from threats of punishment.

The time series is plotted in Figure 7.2 to emphasize the four distinct segments hypothesized by Franke and Kaul: the baseline period ($1 \leq t \leq 38$ weeks), the first punishment regime ($39 \leq t \leq 130$ weeks), the second punishment regime ($131 \leq t \leq 157$ weeks), and the third punishment regime ($158 \leq t \leq 270$ weeks). To test the punishment hypothesis, Franke and Kaul regressed a step function coded for the three punishment regimes on the weekly productivity measures. Assuming a white noise disturbance, this model is

$$P_t = \theta_0 + \omega_1 Punishment_{1t} + \omega_2 Punishment_{2t} + \omega_3 Punishment_{3t} + a_t$$

The parameter estimates from this regression are superimposed on the productivity measures in Figure 7.2. Since $\hat{\theta}_0 < \hat{\omega}_1 < \hat{\omega}_2 < \hat{\omega}_3$, Franke and Kaul interpreted their results to mean that productivity rose with the onset of a punishment regime. Ignoring the implausibility of their white noise assumption, the uncontrolled threat of maturation poses a fundamental obstacle to this interpretation. Whenever a time series follows a trend, as in this instance, any arbitrary set of interventions breaks the time series into segments with different means. If we fail to control for trend, virtually any hypothetical intervention will have a statistically significant impact. For this specific series, Pitcher (1981) discusses the problem as a "learning curve" phenomenon, but of course, we address it as a threat to internal validity: maturation. Since many social science time series trend – and since the consequences of ignoring trend are so serious – this is one of more difficult problems posed by time series data.

Although the punishment hypothesis posed by Franke and Kaul is clearly a maturation artifact, the evidence for the nominal interpretation of the Hawthorn experiment is not obviously correct. A more comprehensive analysis by McCleary (2000) suggests that work breaks had a modest impact on productivity.

7.1.3 Instrumentation

Instrumentation as a threat to internal validity refers to the possibility that an impact may be due to some change in the measuring process. The time series shown in Figure 7.3 illustrates this rather common threat. These data are Uniform Crime Report (UCR) burglaries for Tucson, Arizona, from January 1975 to June 1981 (McCleary et al., 1981, 1982). Prior to 1979, burglary complaints were investigated by patrol officers. Thereafter, burglary complaints were investigated by detectives; UCR burglaries drop immediately. Two years later, the program was canceled due to budget cutbacks and the time series returns immediately to its pre-intervention level.

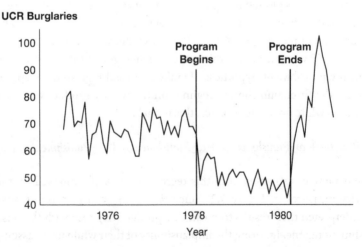

Figure 7.3 Tucson UCR Burglaries (McCleary, Nienstedt, and Erven, 1981)

Since the time series responded consistently to both onset and termination of the intervention, history and maturation are implausible. If some coincidental historical event had caused the first impact, one would not expect to see a mirror-image impact when the intervention was terminated. Maturation threats are ruled out for the same reason. Manipulation of the intervention, in this sense, plays the same role as a control series.

The more obvious causal explanation is also implausible, however. If the intervention had improved the quality of burglary investigations, leading to more arrests, one might expect an eventual impact but not the immediate impact in Figure 7.3. McCleary et al. show that this impact was due to changes in the way burglaries were counted. Patrol officers typically counted crimes such as criminal trespass and vandalism as burglaries even though these crimes do not meet the technical definition of UCR burglaries. Since detectives have a better understanding of the technical definition, they were better able to classify crimes. Crimes that patrolmen had incorrectly recorded as UCR burglaries were instead recorded as the correct crime. The intervention did not reduce the level of burglaries in Tucson, then, but, rather, displaced a portion of these crimes to other UCR categories.

Instrumentation artifacts are also commonly encountered in public health time series. Figure 7.4 shows an annual time series of U.S. diabetes mortality rates for men aged 55–64 years (Mausner and Kramer, 1985, p. 74). Diabetes mortality declines gradually from 1930 to 1948 until 1949, when the time series drops abruptly to a new level. This sudden change reflects a revision of the International

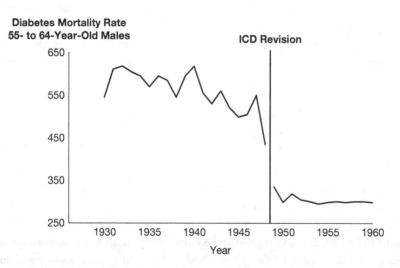

Figure 7.4 Diabetes Mortality Rates (Mausner and Kramer, 1985)

Statistical Classification of Diseases, Injuries and Causes of Death. The "ICD," as it is commonly called, plays the analogous role in public health statistics as the UCR plays in crime statistics, providing rigorous definitions of diseases and causes of death. The ICD is revised every decade to reflect emerging public health problems and changes in medical knowledge. Although many definitions do not vary across ICD revisions, some definitions change abruptly.

This diabetes example represents a type of instrumentation artifact that few researchers would miss. Other types of instrumentation artifact may be subtler, however, and not so easily recognized. Prior to the 1980s, when sudden infant death syndrome (SIDS) was given a unique ICD code, for example, SIDS deaths had been misclassified under other causes. As medical examiners began to use SIDS as a cause of death, infant deaths from other causes declined slowly.

7.1.4 Regression

Regression as a threat to internal validity refers to the expected change in a naturally varying process from an abnormally high or low value. Campbell (1957) analyzed this threat in the context of a "one-group pretest-posttest" design.

$$O_{pre} \qquad X \qquad O_{post}$$

When subjects are selected on the basis of extreme values of O_{pre}, the pretest-posttest change score, $O_{post} - O_{pre}$, is spuriously correlated with the value O_{pre}. The more extreme the value of O_{pre}, that is, the larger the absolute value of the change score.

As we noted in Chapter 1, of course, examples of this design are difficult to find. A more pernicious regression artifact arises in the more common "pretest-posttest control-group" design.

$$\begin{array}{llll} \text{Treated Group} & O_{pre} & X & O_{post} \\ \text{Control Group} & O_{pre} & . & O_{post} \end{array}$$

When treatment and control subjects are assigned on the basis of their extreme O_{pre} scores, the two groups regress to their respective pretest means. In a worst-case scenario, the control group changes from "very bad" to "not so bad" while the treated group changes from "very good" to "not so good" (Campbell and Erlebacher, 1970; Campbell and Kenny, 1999). Matched treatment-control designs (Rubin, 2006) offered a method of controlling these most pernicious regression threats. Campbell's experience with antipoverty programs had nevertheless left him with a distrust of matching. Rubin's (2010, p. 39) description of his first meeting with Campbell conveys the depth of this distrust:

> Because my doctoral thesis was on matched sampling in observational studies under Cochran, I thought that I understood the general context fairly well, and so I was asked by the Educational Testing Service to visit Campbell at Northwestern University in Evanston, Illinois, which is, incidentally, where I grew up. I remember sitting in his office with, I believe, one or two current students or perhaps junior faculty. The topic of matching arose, and my memory is that Campbell referred to it as "sin itself" because of "regression to the mean issues" ... I was flabbergasted! However, I recently realized that I misunderstood the context for Campbell's comment, which is accurately expressed in Campbell and Erlebacher (1970).

Campbell's students heard his negative opinions of matching on a daily basis. In retrospect, Campbell's negative opinions appear to have exaggerated the problem. We consider a specific use of matching in Section 7.4.

In theory, time series regression artifacts can be expected whenever an intervention or reform is implemented in reaction to exceptionally high or low levels of some target phenomenon. Reactive interventions are common. Anticrime programs are often precipitated by abnormally high crime rates, for example. Public health initiatives are precipitated by epidemics and, presumably, wars are precipitated by arms races or by abnormally high levels of international tension. Although reactive interventions are common, our experience suggests that regression artifacts are a relatively uncommon occurrence in well-designed time series experiments.

The "Connecticut crackdown on speeding" is the most widely cited example of a regression artifact precipitated by a reactive intervention (Campbell and Ross, 1968; Glass, 1968). Figures 7.5 and 7.6 show the annual and monthly Connecticut traffic fatality time series for 1952–59. The highest number of annual fatalities during the eight-year period was 214 in 1955. In response to this abnormally high number, the governor ordered a crackdown on speeding. Though acknowledging that there were 36 fewer fatalities in 1956—a reduction of nearly 17 percent— Campbell and Ross could not rule out regression as a threat to internal validity.

Analyzing a monthly fatality time series, Glass (1968) found a modest effect of the crackdown. Failing to find similar effects in monthly fatality time series of nearby states, on the other hand, Glass concluded that regression was not a plausible threat to internal validity. The results of our analyses with annual time series data agree with these results in general. Since the annual time series available in 2014 is shorter than the monthly time series available in 1968, however, the statistical significance of the effect estimate is debatable.

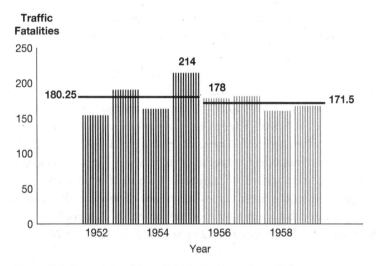

Figure 7.5 Connecticut Motor Vehicle Fatalities, Annual Means

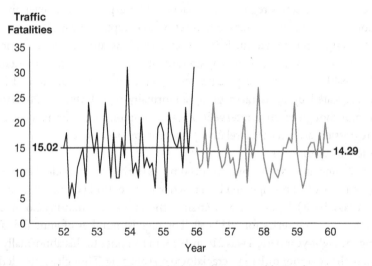

Figure 7.6 Connecticut Motor Vehicle Fatalities, Monthly Totals

Impact parameter estimates for our reanalysis are reported Table 7.2. The effect estimate for Model 2, $\hat{\omega}_{56-59} = -.73$, amounts to a 5 percent reduction in fatalities, but the estimate is not statistically significant. Allowing each of the post-intervention years to have individual effects, as in Model 3, does not improve the fit of the model to the time series. The question of whether the modest effect could be a regression artifact must wait until we discuss design.

Table 7.2. MODEL SELECTION, CONNECTICUT CRACKDOWN ON SPEEDING

		Estimate	SE	t	Diagnosis
Model 1	$\hat{\theta}_0$	14.6563	0.5332	27.49	$BIC = 598.98$
Model 2	$\hat{\theta}_0$	15.0208	0.7522	19.97	$BIC = 603.08$
	$\hat{\omega}_{56-59}$	−.7292	1.0637	−.69	
Model 3	$\hat{\theta}_0$	15.0208	0.7487	20.06	$BIC = 615.89$
	$\hat{\omega}_{56}$	−.1875	1.6742	−.11	
	$\hat{\omega}_{57}$	.0625	1.6742	0.04	
	$\hat{\omega}_{58}$	−1.6875	1.6742	−1.01	
	$\hat{\omega}_{59}$	−1.1042	1.6742	−.66	

7.1.5 Selection

In a two-group design, the threat of selection becomes plausible when the experimental and control time series differ significantly on some theoretical dimension. A cynical methodologist might suggest ruling out this threat by discarding the control time series. The *truly* cynical might even cite Campbell and Stanley (1966, p. 37) as the authority:

> If a bar of iron which has remained unchanged in weight for many months is dipped in a nitric acid bath and then removed, the inference tying together the nitric acid bath and the loss of weight by the iron bar would follow some such experimental logic. There may well have been "control groups" of iron bars remaining on the shelf that lost no weight, but the measurement and reporting of these weights would typically not be thought necessary or relevant.

This argument is not entirely meritless. The impact in the Directory Assistance time series (Figure 1.5) is per se large enough to rule out all of the common threats to internal validity. Looking for and failing to find an equally large impact in a well-chosen control time series would not enhance the validity of this inference. Few impacts are large enough to support this argument, of course. More important, the argument ignores another important role of control time series.

In addition to rendering plausible threats to internal validity implausible, a control time series demonstrates that the impact was *caused* by the intervention. For that purpose, control time series must be chosen carefully from available candidates. The appropriateness of the control time series is dictated not only by theory but also by empirical considerations related to the threat of selection. When appropriate control time series are not available, it is sometimes possible to *construct* one. We will return to this issue after a short, necessary digression.

7.2 DESIGN

As we use the term, "design" has three slightly different meanings. In experimental contexts, "design" refers to assignment or allocation schemes that optimize the statistical power and efficiency of experiments. We addressed the issues associated with that meaning in Chapters 6.1 and 6.2. In quasi-experimental contexts, "design" refers to the structures and procedures used to rule out threats to internal validity. Time series designs are unique in that some of these structures and procedures are part of the statistical model. Strong design necessarily begins, then, with a properly specified statistical model, especially the impact component. A third meaning of "design" refers to the logic and empirical procedures used to demonstrate that an observed effect is a *causal* effect. We develop this third meaning of "design" in Chapters 7.3 to 7.5. In preparation, we elaborate on the design issues associated with ruling out threats to internal validity.

To introduce the design structures and procedures that are not part of the statistical model, imagine a hypothetical polygraph test. As the subject responds verbally to an examiner's questions, the subject's autonomic functions are recorded. From time to time, the smooth record will change, presumably as a *latent* response to the examiner's questions. The examiner would like to interpret each change as a sign of deception, but that inference is flawed. The changes may not reflect conscious guilt but, instead, may be a natural reaction to the stressful situation. To rule out this threat, the subject is instructed to give a false response to a "control" question. If the subject's deceptive response to "What is your name?" or "How old are you?" produces a change in the subject's autonomic functions, other changes can be interpreted as signs of deception.

There are many other plausible threats to internal validity, of course. Noise in the room may have coincided with the test question (history), for example, or the subject may have been fatigued by the time the test question was asked (maturation). The polygraph record itself may have been affected by power surges and internal heat (instrumentation). In this case, a simple design strategy might rule out all threats to internal validity. If the test and control questions are asked in random order, any threat might explain a single response, but it is unlikely that any threat could explain a pattern of responses. More to the point, if test and control questions are randomly ordered, it is quite unlikely that a threat could cause a response coinciding only with test questions.

Turning an intervention "on" and "off" achieves a degree of internal validity unmatched in the most powerful quasi-experiment. Manipulating I_t optimizes internal validity at the expense of external validity, of course, and this may be too dear a price to pay. Many interventions, moreover, are not easily manipulated. In either case, by choice or of necessity, in quasi-experimental designs, no inference is valid until all threats to internal validity are ruled out.

Threats to internal validity may be ruled out, or rendered implausible, at least, by quasi-experimental contrasts. Rejecting the null hypothesis, we infer that I_t caused an impact in Y_t. To test the internal validity of this inference, however, alternative explanations must be ruled out. Toward that end, we must find a "control" series, Z_t, that resembles Y_t in every respect but one: I_t could not possibly have impacted Z_t. If the null hypothesis cannot be rejected for Z_t, we have ruled out the alternatives.

Readers are no doubt familiar with this fundamental principle of the normal scientific method. Familiarity ignores the more important question, however: Where does one find such a perfect Z_t? Perfect control series are an ideal, of course, and the appropriateness of any series as a control rests on how well the series approximates the ideal. Consider some examples.

Figure 7.7 shows two monthly time series of British highway fatalities reported by Ross et al. (1971). The intervention is a law enacted in October 1967 designed to deter drunk drivers. Instrumentation is a plausible threat to internal validity in this case. New laws seldom change sanctions without simultaneously changing bureaucratic recordkeeping. To rule out this threat, Ross *et al.* disaggregate the fatality series by time of day. If the new law were effective, one would expect to see the largest impact on weekend nights when drinking houses are traditionally busiest; the impact in the nighttime series is visually striking. If the impact were due largely to instrumentation, on the other hand, one would expect a similar impact in a control series. As a control, Ross et al. used a time series of traffic fatalities occurring after legal "closing time." For the same reason that the law would be expected to have a large impact on weekend nights, it would be expected

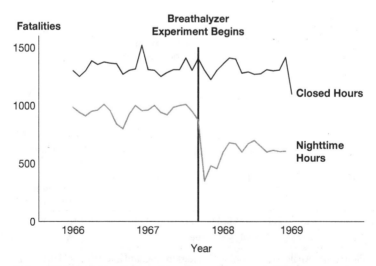

Figure 7.7 British Breathalyzer Experiment (Ross et al., 1971)

to have a small impact when drinking establishments are closed. With no impact in the control series, the threat to internal validity is ruled out.

Quasi-experimental contrasts of disaggregated series often provide compelling evidence of an impact. Disaggregating the time series by theoretical dimensions such as time of day, target population, and so forth produces a range of expected effects, from "large" to "small" to "none," and consistent findings across a range of expected effects support the strongest possible causal inferences.

The time series plotted in Figure 7.8 show another example of how control time series can be created by disaggregation. Co-proxamol was widely used to treat arthritis pain in the U.K. until January 2005. At that time, responding to the concerns of suicide researchers, the U.K. Committee on Safety of Medicines announced that co-proxamol would be withdrawn from general use. Co-proxamol prescriptions dropped abruptly (Figure 1.10). Suicides by co-proxamol poisoning dropped abruptly at the same time. While the visual evidence (Figure 7.8) is compelling, the threat of instrumentation remains plausible. To control this threat, Hawton et al. (2009) use suicides by other analgesics as a control time series. Finding no effect in the control time series, instrumentation as a threat to internal validity is rendered implausible.

Where disaggregation is unfeasible, other jurisdictions may be used as controls. Figure 7.9 shows abortion-related death series from Romania, Yugoslavia, and Poland reported by Legge (1985). The intervention is a 1966 Romanian anti-abortion law that, Legge argues, had an unintended impact on abortion-related deaths. The data are consistent with this interpretation, but the Yugoslavian and Polish series fail to control the most plausible threat to internal validity. Since the 1966 Romanian law was motivated by concerns over low birth rates, the

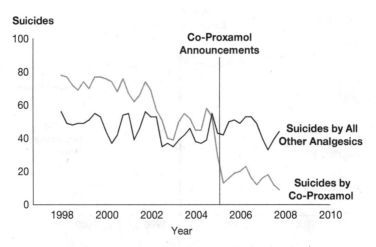

Figure 7.8 Analgesic Poisoning Suicides in England and Wales (Hawton et al., 2009)

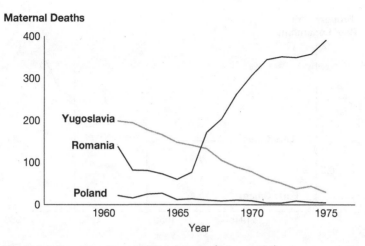

Figure 7.9 European Puerperal Death Rates (Legge, 1985)

law may have coincidentally impacted maternal health care statistics: *instrumenta-tion*. We do not challenge Legge's interpretation, but internal validity would have been stronger if Romanian health statistics were used as control time series.

Data availability and, hence, design potential vary across substantive areas. The potential for design will ordinarily be greater in the U.S. and western Europe than in eastern Europe and the Third World. We do not argue that eastern Europe and Third World interventions should not be analyzed. They should be analyzed. The analyst must ultimately use the best possible design to make the strongest possible inferences.

Although design potential is necessarily a function of available control series, idiosyncratic properties of the intervention sometimes lend themselves to design. Figure 7.10 shows two time series of UCR property crime reported by Hennigan et al. (1981) for 34 cities where TV was introduced in 1951 and for 34 cities where TV was not introduced until 1955. Hennigan *et al.* argue that the introduction of TV led to an increase in property crime, and analyses of the two series finds impacts beginning in 1951 and 1955 respectively.

Since many coincidental events could account for these impacts, history is a plausible threat to internal validity. The Korean War began in 1951, for example, and mobilization changed routine activity structures. Husbands were called away to military service and wives left their homes to work. If homes were left unattended as a consequence of the Korean War, burglaries could have increased beginning in 1951. In 1955, furthermore, the economy went into a deep recession, which, for different reasons, could also have impacted property crime rates. While history is a plausible threat to the internal validity of either impact, however, it is implausible for both impacts. If the impact in the first series were due to the Korean War, a similar impact is expected in the second series; none was found.

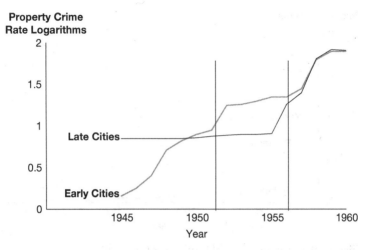

Figure 7.10 UCR Property Crimes in 80 Cities (Hennigan *et al.*, 1981)

If the impact in the second series were due to economic recession, a similar impact is expected in the second series; none was found. The threat of history is implausible because the finding is replicated in two distinct sets of cities at two distinct times.

7.3 CAUSALITY

There are two competing—apparently contradictory—themes in Campbell's early work. First, in terms of internal validity, the results of a well-designed quasi-experiment are roughly comparable to the results of a true experiment. Second, however, knowledge of cause and effects can be acquired only through true experimentation. According to Campell, this preference for true experiments is an evolutionary product:

> From among all the observable correlations in the environment, man and his predecessors focused upon those few which were, for him, manipulable correlations. From this emerged man's predilection for discovering "causes," rather than mere correlations. In laboratory science, this search is represented in the experiment, with its willful, deliberate intrusion into ongoing processes. Similarly for the ameliorative social scientist: Of all of the correlations observable in the social environment, we are interested in those few which represent manipulable relationships, in which by intervening and changing one variable we can affect another. No amount of passive description of the correlations in the social environment can sort out which

are "causal" in this sense. To learn about the manipulability of relationships one must try out manipulation. (Campbell, 1991[1971], p. 231)

Campbell's views on experimentation were more complicated and nuanced than this quotation might suggest. Although he urged the use of experimental designs in large-scale program evaluations, given his roots in evolutionary epistemology (Campbell, 1974), Campbell believed that *valid* causal knowledge emerged slowly, as well-tested evidence accumulated from diverse sources. Obviously, some of this evidence would involve the use of nonexperimental or observational designs.

Statements like "X caused Y" or "Y occurred because of X" are meant to explain why something happened. We were late to class (Y) because traffic (X) was heavier than usual, for example; or a funny joke (X) made us laugh (Y). X and Y can be concrete things or abstract ideas and words. But whatever X and Y might be, the causal relationship implies predictability. If we know the status or value of X, that is, we can predict the status or value of Y. Given the fundamental role of prediction in the modern scientific method, scientific hypotheses are necessarily causal. "Validity" necessarily refers then to the strength of our causal explanations.

Although social and behavioral scientists deal with causal statements routinely, the concepts are often misunderstood. Part of the misunderstanding arises from the fact that "causality" has multiple distinct meanings. Bunge (1959, p. 3) notes three. First, "causality" might refer to the special empirical relationship between, say, lightning (X) and thunder (Y). Second, "causality" might refer to formal, logical statements like "Y will occur *if and only if* X has occurred." Third, "causality" might refer to phenomena where some X reproduces itself as a Y. A larger part of the misunderstanding, however, stems from a mixing of philosophical, empirical, and commonsensical definitions and concepts.

Philosophical discussions of causality typically begin with The Philosopher, Aristotle.[1] Aristotle recognized four distinct categories or types of cause: *material, formal, efficient,* and *final* causes. Aristotle's four causes make little sense to modern readers and do not seem well suited to describing mundane experience. If we agree that stubbing a toe causes pain, for example, we might still disagree on which of the four causes is involved. Bunge (1959, pp. 32–33) could argue that the act of toe-stubbing is an *efficient* cause of the ensuing pain; but in light of the coincident inflammation, others might argue that the act was a *formal* cause. Aristotle's four causes make good sense in the context of Aristotelean physics.

---

1. See Falcon (2014) for a concise, readable introduction to Aristotelian causality. Most of the social scientists who discuss Aristotle's ideas—including us—have either not read the original source or else have misunderstood the context. Kuhn (2000) argues persuasively that Aristotle's definition of causality included *changes* in the position, state, and composition of things. The four causalities are sensible in that broader context.

Readers who doubt this are directed to Kuhn (2000, pp. 15-20). But outside this narrow context, Aristotelian casuality seems quaint and not at all useful.

Hume's discussion of causality seems modern and useful, in contrast, and on first examination, particularly well suited to describing mundane experience.[2] In laying out the Induction Problem, Hume argued that we recognize a causal relationship between X and Y when three conditions are satisfied:

Priority: X occurs prior to Y.

Contiguity: X and Y occur in more or less the same place and time.

Necessary Connection: Y occurs if X occurs; if X has occurred, Y will occur.

Since Hume's three criteria are amenable to empirical verification, Humean causality seems at least consistent with the modern scientific method. This impression is misleading, however, and for many phenomena probably incorrect. Hume's third criterion would reject a causal relationship between smoking (X) and lung cancer (Y), for example. This nonsensical result can be eliminated by redefining Hume's *necessary connection* in probabilistic terms. Probabilistic causality, usually attributed to Suppes (1970), holds that if

$$Pr(Y|X) > Pr(Y)$$

then the XY relationship is causal. If smoking and lung cancer are caused by some third variable, of course—say, a genetic factor—the causal relationship is spurious (Skyrms, 2000, p. 134).

But even if the obstacle posed by Hume's *necessary connection* criterion is circumvented, in practice, the first and second criteria pose even greater obstacles. The relationship between the lunar orbit (X) and earthly tides (Y) illustrates their practical shortcomings. Although this XY relationship is certainly causal, X and Y occur simultaneously and at a vast distance, thereby violating Hume's *priority* and *contiguity* criteria. The fact that this particular example was well known in 1740 does not detract from the brilliance and importance of Hume's *Treatise*. Hume proposed his definition of causality not as a scientific tool but, rather, as a thought experiment aimed at demonstrating the Induction Problem.

The best-known workable "scientific" definition of causality is due to John Stuart Mill (2009[1843]), who proposed a definition organized around five methods. Two of the five are sufficient to illustrate Mill's theories. Mill's *method of*

---

2. Although Hume's theory appears in several places and times, the versions are consistent. We rely on his 1739–40 *A Treatise of Human Nature* (Norton and Norton, 2000).

agreement infers a relationship between an effect and its *necessary* cause. Suppose that A and B arrive at an emergency room with food poisoning symptoms. A few hours earlier, A and B had been at a picnic where crab salad, smoked turkey, and lemon mousse had been served. C also attended the picnic but showed no food poisoning symptoms. A public health investigator interviews A, B, and C with the following results:

	A	B	C
Ate the crab salad?	**Yes**	**Yes**	No
Ate the smoked turkey?	No	Yes	Yes
Ate the lemon mousse?	Yes	No	No
Food poisoning symptoms?	**Yes**	**Yes**	No

Because A and B, who ate the crab salad, were poisoned while C, who abstained, was not, we can infer that this particular batch of crab salad was the *necessary* cause of the food poisoning outbreak. No crab salad (X), in other words, no food poisoning (Y).

Mill's *method of difference* infers a relationship between an effect and its *sufficient* cause. Suppose that A, B, C, D, and E are involved in a high-speed head-on collision and that D and E did not survive the crash. An investigation reveals the following facts:

	A	B	C	D	E
Legally intoxicated?	Yes	Yes	Yes	Yes	Yes
Older than 25?	No	Yes	Yes	Yes	No
Wearing a seatbelt?	Yes	Yes	Yes	**No**	**No**
Survived the crash?	Yes	Yes	Yes	**No**	**No**

Since A, B, C, D, and E were all legally intoxicated, that variable is ruled out as a *sufficient* cause of death in a high-speed, head-on collision. And since survivor A and non-survivor E were both under age 25, the facts eliminate that variable too. Because survivors A, B, and C wore seatbelts, on the other hand, while non-survivors D and E did not, we infer that *not* wearing a seatbelt is a *sufficient* cause of death in a high-speed, head-on collision.

Mill's methods parallel Francis Bacon's list-driven inductive logic (Jardine and Silverthorn, 2000). Sociologists may also recognize Becker's (1953; Znaniecki, 1934) analytic induction in Mill's methods. Skyrms (2000, pp. 69–108) develops the logic of Mill's methods in greater detail and Lieberson (1991) discusses the practical limitations of Mill's methods in comparative social science. Campbell's (1975) discussion of comparative case studies is also particularly relevant.

7.4 COUNTERFACTUAL CAUSALITY

The causalities of Aristotle, Hume, and Mill represent the *philosophical, natural,* and *empirical* traditions. Modern causality draws from all three traditions, as well as from the experimental work of Fisher (1925, 1935) and Neyman (1990[1923], 1934). Recognizing the seminal contributions of Donald B. Rubin, Holland (1986) calls modern causality *Rubin's model.* In recognition of the early contributions of Neyman (1990[1923], 1934), the model is also called the *Neyman-Rubin model.* To emphasize the modern model's logical foundation, some writers (e.g., Glymour, 1986; Winship and Morgan, 2007) refer to the modern *counterfactual* causal model. Rubin himself (1990) refers to the *potential outcomes* model, and there are reasons to prefer that name. We will use that term when appropriate and the more general term *Rubin causality.*

Empirical causal models, exemplified by Mill's methods, define causality in terms of observable events. Counterfactual models define causality in terms of observable *and* unobservable events. A *counterfactual* is a conditional statement predicated on something that *could* have happened but did not. For example, "If we had purchased Apple stock in the late 1970s, we would be fabulously wealthy today." Since many of the people who purchased Apple stock in the late 1970s are *not* fabulously wealthy today, there is no reason to assume that this counterfactual is true. Nor is there any obvious way to confirm it empirically. Likewise, in a two-group design, there is no way to know how the control subjects would have responded to the treatment. Had the control subjects been treated, one might naturally expect their responses to be similar to the treated subjects' responses. But since this counterfactual is unobservable, there is no way to confirm the natural expectations. Holland (1986) calls this the "fundamental problem of causal inference."

But now suppose that the two-group design is a *true experiment.* Using a modified version of Campbell's (1957; Campbell and Stanley, 1966) notation, we diagram this design as

$$\begin{array}{llll} \text{Random Assignment to Treatment} & O_{1,i} & X_i & O_{2,i} \\ \text{Random Assignment to Control} & O_{1,i} & X_i & O_{2,i} \end{array}$$

Subjects are first randomly assignment to treatment or control and are then indexed, starting with the treatment group. The binary variable X_i indicates the *i*th subject's group membership. For the first N_T subjects who belong to the treatment group

$$X_i = 1 \qquad \text{for } i = 1, N_T$$

The next N_C subjects belong to the control group:

$$X_i = 0 \qquad \text{for } i = N_{T+1}, N$$

If the treatment effect for the ith subject is given by the difference score Y_i

$$Y_i = O_{2,i} - O_{1,i}$$

Then the average effect of the treatment is

$$E(Y_i | X_i = 1) - E(Y_i | X_i = 0) = \omega$$

The fact that most scientists interpret ω *causally* raises what might be called—apologies to Holland (1986)—the "fundamental question of causal inference." *Why* do experimental scientists interpret their results in causal terms?

Causal interpretations of ω have been embedded in the working scientist's common sense – part of the *scientific method*, that is – for at least four centuries. Nearly all working scientists accept the scientific method without thinking, so most would be puzzled by the fundamental question. The minority who choose to answer the question would cite the *manipulability* of X_i. It was, after all, the experimenter who assigned the ith subject to treatment or control, and since the experimenter used a random assignment mechanism, the ith subject's response to assignment, Y_i, must be the causal effect of X_i. That is what we mean when we say "cause."

Like most commonsense answers, this one has latent assumptions, loopholes, and flaws. The answer implies that X_i and Y_i are independent, and this is arguable. Independence implies that for the ith subject,

$$E[(Y_i | X_i = 1)(Y_i | X_i = 0)] = 0$$

If $(Y_i | X_i = 1)$ is observed, however, then $(Y_i | X_i = 0)$ is *not* observed. Since both $(Y_i | X_i = 1)$ and $(Y_i | X_i = 0)$ can never be observed at the same time, their product cannot be observed. This is not a mere philosophical quibble. Rubin (1974, p. 690) cites practical obstacles to inferring a treatment effect from the observed results:

> We may have the same unit measured on both treatments in two trials (a repeated measure design) but since there may exist carryover effects (e.g., the effect of the first treatment wears off slowly) or general time trends (e.g., as the child ages, his learning ability increases), we cannot be certain that the unit's responses would be identical at both times.

Readers will recognize Rubin's (1974) "carryover effects" and "general time trends" as examples of Campbell's (1957; Campbell and Stanley, 1966) threats to internal validity. Indeed, there are many similarities between Campbell (1957) and Rubin (1974). Both recognize the potential trade-off between the threats to internal and external validity,[3] for example, and that quasi-experimental results can be interpreted causally. Though using different terms, both recognize the obstacle posed by uncontrolled threats to internal validity.[4] And in a two-group design, both link internal validity to the similarity of treatment and control units.

We discuss one important disagreement shortly. With that exception, differences between the Campbell and Rubin models reflect different focuses and emphases. Although there is no explicit treatment of causality in Campbell (1957) or in Campbell and Stanley (1966), Cook and Campbell (1979; Shadish et al., 2002) devote their first chapter to the causal traditions. Subsequent chapters describe statistical models for estimating unbiased causal effects. Because Campbell and his collaborators balance internal validity against the other validities, however, their treatment of causality is not comprehensive.

Focused narrowly on the "fundamental problem of causal inference," Rubin's (1974) model is *explicitly* causal. The model provides a framework for estimating causal effects under a range of theories and assumptions about the data and about the design. It is particularly relevant to the interrupted time series designs that concern us in this book.

7.4.1 The Fundamental Problem of Causal Inference

Rubin's model (1974) defines the observed treatment effect, Y_i, as a realization of two potential outcomes, Y_{i1} and Y_{i0}. Subscripts on these potential outcomes refer to the ith unit, or subject, and to the value of the binary assignment variable, X_i. In terms of X_i and the potential outcomes,

$$Y_i = (X_i)Y_{i1} + (1 - X_i)Y_{i0}$$

When $X_i=1$,

$$Y_i = (1)Y_{i1} + (0)Y_{i0} = Y_{i1} = (Y_i|X_i = 1)$$

And when $X_i=0$,

$$Y_i = (0)Y_{i1} + (1)Y_{i0} = Y_{i0} = (Y_i|X_i = 0)$$

3. Rubin (1974, p. 690): "Of course, in order for the results of a study to be of much interest, we must be able to generalize to units and associated times other than those in the study."

4. Rubin (1974, p. 700): "In both randomized and nonrandomized studies, the investigator should think hard about variables besides the treatment that may causally affect Y and plan in advance how to control for the important ones."

The workhorse "statistic" of Rubin's causal model is the *Average Causal Effect* (*ACE*), defined as

$$ACE = E(Y_{i1} - Y_{i0})$$

Distributing the expectation operator across the right-hand side,

$$ACE = E(Y_{i1}) - E(Y_{i0}) = E(Y_i|X_i = 1) - E(Y_i|X_i = 0)$$

The *ACE* is averaged over all N subjects. It is more useful to break the *ACE* down into *ACEs* for the N_T treated and N_C control subjects. For the N_T treated subjects,

$$ACE_{X_i=1} = E(Y_i|X_i = 1) = E(Y_{i1} - Y_{i0}|X_i = 1)$$

Following the same steps for the N_C control subjects,

$$ACE_{X_i=0} = E(Y_i|X_i = 0) = E(Y_{i1} - Y_{i0}|X_i = 0)$$

Adding the *ACEs* for the two groups,

$$ACE = ACE_{X_i=1} + ACE_{X_i=0}$$

Or by substitution,

$$ACE = E(Y_{i1}|X_i = 1) - E(Y_{i0}|X_i = 1) + E(Y_{i1}|X_i = 0) - E(Y_{i0}|X_i = 0)$$

This expression shows that the *ACE* is the sum of two *observed* terms and two *unobserved* terms. To emphasize this important point, we array the four component terms of the *ACE* in a two-by-two contingency table:

	Treatment	Control
Observed	$E(Y_{i1}|X_i = 1)$	$E(Y_{i0}|X_i = 0)$
Unobserved	$E(Y_{i0}|X_i = 1)$	$E(Y_{i1}|X_i = 0)$

The rows of this contingency table suggest that the *ACE* can be written as

$$ACE = ACE_{Observed} + ACE_{Unobserved} \quad \text{where}$$
$$ACE_{Observed} = E(Y_{i1}|X_i = 1) - E(Y_{i0}|X_i = 0) \quad \text{and}$$
$$ACE_{Unobserved} = E(Y_{i1}|X_i = 1) - E(Y_{i0}|X_i = 0)$$

The *ACE* cannot be estimated from data because it has an unobserved component, $ACE_{Unobserved}$, and *that* is what Holland (1986) calls the "fundamental problem of causal inference."

Rubin's causal model solves the fundamental problem by making some reasonable assumptions about the data collection process. To illustrate, consider the normal scientist's faith in random assignment. Is our faith justified? We begin with the observed part of the ACE:

$$ACE_{\text{Observed}} = E(Y_{i1}|X_i = 1) - E(Y_{i0}|X_i = 0)$$

If we assume that subjects were randomly assigned to the treatment and control groups, then Y_i and X_i are independent. Since independence implies that

$$E(Y_{i1}|X_i = 1) = E(Y_{i1}) \qquad \text{and} \qquad E(Y_{i0}|X_i = 0) = E(Y_{i0})$$

By substitution,

$$ACE_{\text{Observed}} = E(Y_{i1}) - E(Y_{i0}) = E(Y_{i1} - Y_{i0}) = ACE$$

Rubin's causal model, along with an assumption about the data collection process – random assignment in this instance – allows us to estimate the *unobserved* causal parameter from *observed* data.

The implications for time series designs should be intuititively clear. When the design includes random assignment to treatment and control groups, the parameter ω has a *causal* interpretation. If the units are randomly assigned to treatment and control regimes, causal interpretation depends on controlling the potential threat to internal validity posed by "carryover" from one regime to the next (Rubin, 1974, p. 690). In either case, random assignment to treatment and control is sufficient for a valid causal interpretation of ω.

What about nonrandom assignment? Sometimes unanticipated events can approximate the effects of random assignment, ensuring the independence of the ith unit's treatment status, X_i, and response to treatment, Y_i. The internal validity of these "natural experiments" (Campbell, 1969) is proportional to how well the effects of unanticipated events approximate the effects of random assignment. Strong approximation, strong internal validity. Weak approximation, weak internal validity. What could be simpler?

Though agreeing with Campbell (1969) on the internal validity of natural experiments, Holland (1986) cites an obvious shortcoming. Natural experiments occur routinely in a range of substantive areas, presenting opportunities to learn nature's secrets. "Normal" scientists cannot wait around for a specific natural experiment to occur, however. Bacon cited this same shortcoming as a rationale for experimental manipulation, so it is an important consideration. Nevertheless, when a natural experiment does occur, the parameter ω has a valid *causal* interpretation.

7.4.2 Causality for Nonexperimental Data

Ironically, Campbell played a significant role in the formulation of Rubin's model. Criticizing a quasi-experimental evaluation of *Operation Head Start*, Campbell and Erlebacher (1970) argued that the evaluation was biased by a regression artifact inherent to the quasi-experimental design. Citing this fatal flaw, Campbell and Erlebacher argued that politically sensitive programs should be evaluated with experimental designs. Campbell's views on the relative validity of experimental and quasi-experimental designs are summarized in the Manifesto for his "Experimenting Society":

> True experiments involving randomization are undoubtedly the most efficient and valid. While I have been an advocate of some quasi-experimental designs where randomization is not possible, detailed consideration of specific cases again and again reinforces my belief in the superiority of true experiments. As advisors to the experimenting society we will often recommend such research designs. (Campbell, 1991[1971], p. 232.)

Campbell was an early advocate of strong quasi-experiments, particularly the interrupted time series and regression discontinuity designs. Strong quasi-experimental designs were acceptable when random assignment was unfeasible. Campbell believed that there were few situations where random assignment was categorically unfeasible, however, and that given their "druthers," cynical policymakers would always choose weak quasi-experimental designs.

Because he had more experience with observational data—and perhaps because he had less experience with cynical policymakers—Rubin rejected Campbell's distrust of quasi-experimental designs and observational data:

> Recent psychological and educational literature has included extensive criticism of the use of nonrandomized studies to estimate causal effects of treatments (e.g., Campbell and Erlebacher, 1970). The implication in much of this literature is that only properly randomized experiments can lead to useful estimates of causal effects. If taken as applying to all fields of study, this position is untenable. Since the extensive use of randomized experiments is limited to the last half century, and in fact is not used in much scientific investigation today, one is led to the conclusion that most scientific "truths" have been established without using randomized experiments. In addition, most of us successfully determine the causal effects of many of our everyday actions, even interpersonal behaviors, without the benefit of randomization. (Rubin, 1974, p. 688.)

Following this initial essay, Rubin devised methods for causal analyses of nonexperimental data. One of these methods, "matched" sampling (Rubin, 2006), is particularly relevant to the design and analysis of time series quasi-experiments. Constructing a control group by matching is counterintuitive. The matching algorithm may discard or ignore data, for example. If the data are a random sample of a population, moreover, matching seems to defeat the rationale for random sampling. As Rubin explains, however, both intuitions are incorrect:

> Now suppose that the two units are very similar in the way they respond . . . By this we mean that on the basis of "extra information," we know that the two trials are closely "matched" . . . [I]f the two units react identically in their trials, . . . randomization is absolutely irrevelant. Clearly, having closely "matched" trials increases the closeness of the calculated experimental minus control difference to the typical causal effect for the two trials, while random assignment of treatments does not improve that estimate.

> Although two-trial studies are almost unheard of in the behavioral sciences, they are not uncommon in the physical sciences. For example, when comparing the heat expansion rates (per hour) of a metal alloy in oxygen and nitrogen, an investigator might use two one-foot lengths of the alloy. Because the lengths of alloy are so closely matched before being exposed to the treatment (almost identical compositions and dimensions), the units should respond almost identically to the treatments even when initiated at different times, and thus the calculated experimental (oxygen) minus control (nitrogen) difference should be an excellent estimate of the typical causal effect. (Rubin, 1974, p. 691)

Proper matching can reduce the bias and imprecision of a causal effect estimate in both experimental and nonexperimental designs. Nevertheless, Campbell remained convinced that effect estimates based on matched control comparisons were biased. Students who tried to convince him otherwise eventually gave up.

7.5 SYNTHETIC CONTROL TIME SERIES

In principle, control time series are chosen so as to render *plausible* threats to internal validity *im*plausible. This assumes a theoretical understanding of the plausible threats and the availability of appropriate control time series. A literature review often suggests the most plausible threats, thereby satisfying the first assumption. A literature review may also suggest the whereabouts of appropriate control time series, but that is less likely. Sometimes, appropriate control time series do not exist. If a set of somewhat-less-than-appropriate control series can be found, however, it might be possible to construct an *ideal* control time series.

In November 1988, California voters passed Proposition 99, the *Tobacco Tax and Health Protection Act*. Proposition 99 was a complex law (see, e.g., Glantz and Balbach, 2004). Some provisions were aimed at making tobacco products less available. Cigarette taxes rose by $0.25 per pack, for example, cigarette vending machines were removed from public places, and sales of single cigarettes were banned. Proposition 99 also funded anti-tobacco media campaigns and treatment programs. Taken as a whole, Proposition 99 would be expected to *reduce* cigarette sales in California, and most experts concluded that it did (Burns et al., 1991; Glantz, 1993; Hu, Sung, and Keeler, 1995). Our concern is more narrowly focused on designing a time series experiment to test the effectiveness of Proposition 99.

Figure 7.11 shows an annual time series of per capita cigarette sales in California plotted against the mean sales of the other 49 states. The visual impression of this contrast is intriguing but not convincing. The sort of abrupt drop that Campbell and Stanley would find compelling is absent. California cigarette sales decline after 1988, to be sure, but sales were in decline prior to 1988. This control time series only adds to visual ambiguity. Although California cigarette sales begin to decrease in the mid-1970s, similar sales reductions are observed in the other 49 states. The downward trend is steeper in California, of course, but even accepting this difference, the visual evidence might suggest that the 1988 act had at best a small impact on California cigarette sales. That dismal conclusion assumes that the other 49 states are an appropropriate control for California, of course, and that assumption is not necessarily warranted. Indeed, we can think of no sound theoretical rationale for equating California to any single state or to any group of states. Nevertheless, it may be possible to construct an *ideal* control time series.

Figure 7.12 shows the same annual California time series plotted against an *ideal* control time series. Using the weights reported by Abadie, Diamond, and

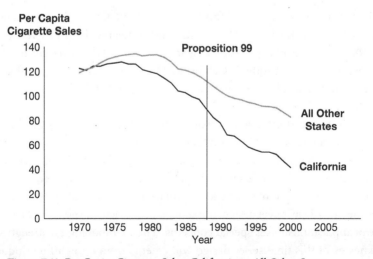

Figure 7.11 Per Capita Cigarette Sales, California vs. All Other States

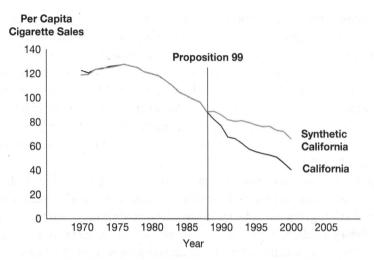

Figure 7.12 Per Capita Cigarette Sales,California vs. Synthetic California

Hainmueller (2010), this so-called Synthetic California time series is

$$Synthetic\ California_t = 0.334 \times Utah_t +$$
$$0.234 \times Nevada_t +$$
$$0.199 \times Montana_t +$$
$$0.164 \times Colorado_t +$$
$$0.069 \times Connecticut_t$$

Pre-intervention trends for California and Synthetic California time series are practically indistinguishable. The two time series diverge sharply thereafter after the 1988 act. By 2000, per capita cigarette sales in California are nearly 40 percent lower than in Synthetic California. The visual evidence is unambiguous. Proposition 99 had a large, salutary impact on cigarette sales, and, under Rubin causality, the effect is *causal*.

Causal interpretation assumes that Synthetic California is an *ideal* control time series, of course, and in our opinion, it is. Skeptical methodologists might disagree, especially as it relates to causal interpretation. Some skeptics might reject synthetic control inferences altogether. In our view, however, that would be a mistake. The rigor of synthetic control designs varies widely. Although this might be said of *any* novel design, the sudden unregulated explosion of synthetic control applications raises special concerns. The methodological strengths and weaknesses of this time series design will emerge from thoughtful critiques of these applications.

In Chapter 3.7.3, we introduced the idea of co-integration. Due originally to Granger (1981; Granger and Engle, 1987), a co-integrated pair of time series shares a set of driving forces that keep them on a common path. In addition to their shared forces, each of the time series has its own unique random forces that nudge it off their common path. This defines the *ideal* control time series. Prior to the intervention, the treated and ideal control time series are a co-integrated pair. The intervention destroys the co-integrated relationship, sending the treated time series on a new path. Divorced, the formerly co-integrated time series pair follow divergent paths. The distance between their new paths is interpreted as the causal effect of the intervention.

7.5.1 Legalization of Medical Marijuana

In November 1996, California voters approved Proposition 215, which legalized the use of marijuana for medical purposes. Campaigns for and against the proposition focused largely on the medical need for and effectiveness of marijuana. Although the debate emphasized cancer, AIDS, and spinal cord injuries, however, the proposition's language included virtually all chronic conditions, thereby effectively decriminalizing most marijuana use (Vitiello, 1998). Cultural values played a smaller role in the campaign. Opponents argued that legalization would "send the wrong message" to youth, for example, and this fear was realized to some extent. Public opinion surveys conducted before and after the election found increased acceptance of marijuana by Californians but no change in actual use (Khatapoush and Hallfors, 2004).

The potential collateral consequences of legalization played no role in the public debate over Proposition 215. Would easier access to marijuana lead to an increase in driving under the influence, for example, and if so, would the higher prevalence of driving under the influence lead to an increase in traffic fatalities? To test this hypothesis, Anderson et al. (2013) compared traffic fatality rates before and after legalization of medical marijuana in 14 states and the District of Columbia. Their surprise finding: Traffic fatality rates *decreased* in medical marijuana states. How is that possible? Anderson et al. speculate that, unlike alcohol, which is consumed in public places, marijuana is consumed at home:

> If marijuana consumption typically takes place at home, then designating a driver for the trip back from a restaurant or bar becomes unnecessary, and legalization could reduce traffic fatalities even if driving under the influence of marijuana is every bit as dangerous as driving under the influence of alcohol. (Anderson et al., 2013, p. 360)

Though one should view all post facto explanations with some skepticism, this one makes some sense. Another possibility, of course, is that Anderson et al. failed to control plausible threats to internal validity. To investigate this possibility, we devise a time series experiment for California's Proposition 215 using a Synthetic California time series to control the common threats to internal validity.

7.5.2 Timeframe and Donor Pool

The first step in any time series experiment consists of selecting a motor vehicle fatality measure. Anderson et al. use annual fatality counts reported by the National Highway Traffic Safety Administration (NHTSA). We will use annual fatality counts reported by the National Center for Health Statistics (NCHS). In principle, annual fatality counts from these two sources should be similar, but in practice NHTSA and NCHS annual counts may differ by as much as 20 percent. Some part of this discrepancy is attributed to the difference between complete and sample censuses.[5] Another part reflects the differences between the worldviews of medical examiners and traffic engineers. Each NCHS death record originates with a medical examiner (or coroner/medical examiner) who is concerned primarily with determining the *proximal* cause of death. Granting that the proximal cause of death was a motor vehicle crash, on the other hand, traffic engineers are concerned primarily with determining the *distal* causes of the death—the road conditions, mechanical failures, and driver behaviors that caused the crash.

Time and place are probably the best-known differences between the two worldviews. The time and place of death are relatively unimportant to the medical examiner's determination of the proximal cause. If a fatal motor vehicle crash occurs in Maryland but the victims are transported to a District of Columbia hospital, a medical examiner counts the fatalities in the jurisdiction where the death certificates were signed—in Washington D.C. Concerned primarily with the causes of the crash, on other other hand, a traffic engineer counts the fatalities in the place where the adverse road conditions existed or where the mechanical failures and driver behaviors occurred—in Maryland. If a victim survives the crash but dies within a year, a medical examiner counts the death as a motor vehicle fatality. The traffic engineer waits only 30 days. Crash victims who survive

---

5. It appears that the NHTSA counts for large states are a sample census. Colleagues who work with these data tell us that the NHTSA counts are a complete census. We continue to investigate this issue.

beyond the 30-day threshold are presumed to have died from causes other than road conditions, mechanical failures, or behaviors.

The cumulative effects of time and place differences are small enough to be ignored in some instances. Differences in the privacy rules recognized by medical examiners and traffic engineers are another matter. Whereas the NHTSA reported traffic fatalities by state without interruption between 1977 and 2014, the NCHS began masking the states of residence and occurrence in 2005. For that reason, our analysis begins in 1970 and ends in 2004. This 35-year time series constructed from the NCHS database includes eight post-intervention years, and that will be sufficient for our immediate purposes. When our analyses require longer post-intervention segments, we will construct time series from the NHTSA database.

Table 7.3 lists the states that enacted medical marijuana laws during five-year segments beginning in 1996 when California enacted the first law. By 2014, 22 states and the District of Columbia had followed California's lead. Two of those states, Colorado and Washington, subsequently legalized all marijuana use. It makes little sense to use as controls the nine states that had enacted medical marijuana laws during the 1996–2004 post-intervention period, so Washington (December 1998), Oregon (January 1999), Alaska (March 1999), Maine (January 2000), Hawaii (January 2001), Colorado (July 2001), Nevada (October 2001), Vermont (July 2004), and Montana (November 2004) are excluded from the synthetic control "donor pool."[6]

Figure 7.13 plots the annual motor vehicle fatality rates for California and an average of the rates for 41 donor states. Although short segments of the two time series follow the same path—1979 through 1983, for example—they diverge during most of the 35-year history. Both time series trend downward from 1987

Table 7.3. MEDICAL MARIJUANA LAWS BY STATE AND FIVE-YEAR PERIOD

1996–2000	2001–2005	2006–2010	2011–Present
California	Colorado	Rhode Island	Delaware
Oregon	Nevada	New Mexico	Connecticut
Washington	Montana	Michigan	Massachusetts
Alaska	Vermont	D.C.	Illinois
Maine		Arizona	New Hampshire
Hawaii		New Jersey	Maryland
			Minnesota
			New York

6. We use the dates reported in Anderson et al., Table 1, p. 336.

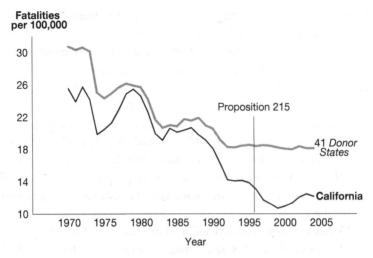

Figure 7.13 Motor Vehicle Fatality Rates, California vs. 41 Donor States

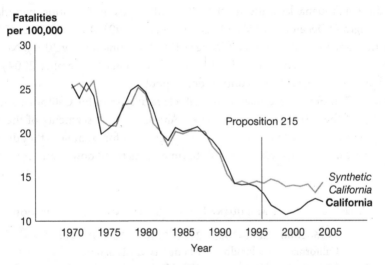

Figure 7.14 Motor Vehicle Fatality Rates, California vs. Synthetic California

through 1992. California continues to drop after 1992, however, while the average donor state time series levels off. Although the difference between the two time series in the first post-intervention year is large, this difference might be a simple extrapolation or continuation of the pre-intervention trends.

Figure 7.14 plots the annual motor vehicle fatality rates for California and a synthetic control time series composed of an weighted average of six donor states.[7] Specifically,

$$Synthetic\ California_t = 0.245 \times Connecticut_t +$$
$$0.202 \times Rhode\ Island_t +$$
$$0.173 \times Arizona_t +$$
$$0.138 \times Texas_t +$$
$$0.105 \times New\ Hampshire_t +$$
$$0.060 \times West\ Virginia_t$$

$California_t$ and $Synthetic\ California_t$ follow the same path throughout most of the pre-intervention segment and then begin to diverge. Divergence is visually apparent in the few months preceding the intervention, and that poses a minor obstacle to interpretation. Otherwise, to the extent that the pre-intervention segments of $California_t$ and $Synthetic\ California_t$ are comparable, the difference in their post-intervention segments can be interpreted as the causal effect of legalized medical marijuana on motor vehicle fatalities. Consistent with Anderson et al., the effect is a large decrease in motor vehicle fatalities.

$Synthetic\ California_t$ is constructed by finding a set of weights that can be applied to the donor states to yield the "best" match to $California_t$. The set of weights satisfy two constraints. First, the weights must be non-negative:

$$W_i \geq 0$$

Second, the weights must sum to unity:

$$\sum_{i=1}^{41} W_i = 1$$

Within these constraints, the W_i are selected so that $Synthetic\ California_t$ matches $California_t$ observation for observation between 1970 and 1976. If $California_t$ and $Synthetic\ California_t$ diverge after 1976, the difference between the two time series is taken as the effect on motor vehicle fatalities of legalizing medical marijuana in California.

The matching algorithm minimizes the Mean Square Prediction Error ($MSPE$) conditioned on several predictor variables. Although the predictor variables are generally suggested by theory and dicated by practical availability, the choice

7. We used the *synth* routine in Stata 14.0 to construct our synthetic control time series. See Abadie, Diamond, and Hainmueller (2011) for the formulae and details of the algorithm.

of predictor variables is arbitrary. In this example, we minimized the MSPE on pre-intervention values of $California_t$ and its first difference, $\nabla\ California_t$. Thus,

$$MSPE = f(W_i \mid California_t, \nabla California_t)$$

Other analysts might prefer to use predictor variables that are presumed to *cause* motor vehicle fatalities in a state—the size of the motor vehicle fleet, the number of 15- to 35-year-old drivers, per capita alcohol consumption, and so forth. Indeed, judging from the literature, that seems to be the convention. Even if annual time series of theoretically relevant predictor variables were available, however, fitting them into the MSPE minimization function is always difficult. In many instances, for example, the causal nexus between predictor variables and motor vehicle fatalities is known only crudely. If the effect of a particular cause varies from state to state, moreover, or from year to year—or if several causal variables interact—plugging those predictor time series into an MSPE minimization function requires guesswork. Then too, if the predictor time series are nonstationary, their complex patterns of trend or drift will probably not match the pattern observed in $California_t$. This problem can be addressed to some extent by using short, trendless segments of the predictor variable time series. But that too involves guesswork.

The alternative approach that we recommend requires little guesswork and is relatively noncontroversial. Suppose that both the level and change in a state's motor vehicle fatality rate are unknown functions of the causal variables. That is, if

$$California_t = f(\text{motor vehicles, 15- to 35-year-olds, alcohol consumption, etc.})$$
$$\nabla California_t = g(\text{motor vehicles, 15- to 35-year-olds, alcohol consumption, etc.})$$

Then $California_t$ and $\nabla California_t$ capture the causal effects of $f(.)$ and $g(.)$ on motor vehicle fatalities. In our experience, furthermore, constructing the synthetic control time series from the treated time series and its first differences invariably produces the "best"-fitting synthetic control time series. That is certainly true in this case.

7.5.3 Placebo Tests

The post-intervention difference between $California_t$ and $Synthetic\ California_t$ amounts to a reduction of 3.27 motor vehicle fatalities per 100,000 residents per year during 1997 through 2004. The obvious follow-up question asks whether this 22 percent reduction in motor vehicle fatalities might be due to chance. Unfortunately, the statistical tests used in Chapter 5 assume long time series of white noise observations. Since these assumptions are seldom warranted in synthetic control group designs, conventional significance tests are not available. In light of this obstacle, the *exact* significance of the post-intervention difference between a treated time series and its synthetic control must be calculated from a permutation test model. Although the basic concepts are due to Fisher (1922a), the application of permutation tests and exact significance to synthetic control designs is due to Abadie and Gardeazabal (2003; Abadie, Diamond, and Hainmueller, 2010). In the synthetic control context, permutation tests have come to be called "placebo" tests. Since placebo effects are often thought to be threats to external validity, this name may be confusing. The implied threats belong to statistical conclusion validity or, perhaps, to internal validity.

There are generally two types of placebo tests that can be used to calculate the exact significance of the post-intervention difference. Figures 7.15 and 7.16 plot the results of two in-sample placebo tests. In both instances, the test result was calculated by assigning California's treatment status to each of the 41 donor states. If the post-intervention difference between $California_t$ and $Synthetic\ California_t$ were due to chance, we would expect comparable post-intervention differences for the other states. Figure 7.15 plots the mean post-intervention difference between a state and its synthetic control. Since only New Mexico and Georgia have higher differences, the exact probability for a no-difference null hypothesis is

$$Pr(California_t = Synthetic\ California_t) = 2/42 \approx 0.048$$

Figure 7.16 plots the post-intervention *MSPEs* for the same in-sample placebo test. If the post-intervention difference between $California_t$ and $Synthetic\ California_t$ is due to chance, we might expect a relatively small post-intervention

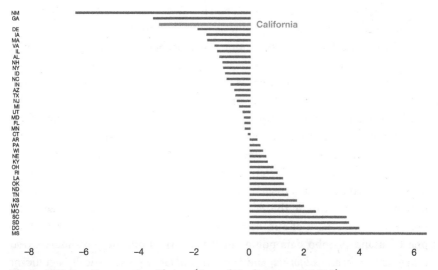

Figure 7.15 Post-Intervention Change (Annual Fatalities per 100,000)

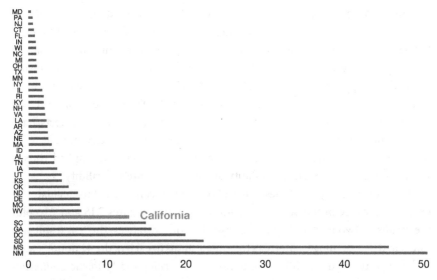

Figure 7.16 Post-Intervention *MSPE*

fit statistic. In this instance, however, the post-intervention *MSPE* is relatively large, indicating that the gap between the California time series and its synthetic control widens after 1996. Since six states have smaller *MSPEs*,

$$Pr(California_t = Synthetic\ California_t) = 6/42 \approx 0.143$$

By analogy, the placebo test results plotted in Figures 7.15 and 7.16 are interpreted as one-tailed and two-tailed hypothesis tests respectively. The one-tailed null hypotheis is rejected at the conventional significance level. The two-tailed null hypothesis is not.

An in-time placebo test is based on the distribution of post-intervention differences and *MSPEs* estimated for each year between 1971 and 2003. If the 1997–2004 effect is due to chance, we would expect to see comparable effects from other post-intervention segments. In-time placebo tests are useful when in-sample placebo tests are limited by the size of the donor pool. And that is why analysts should be reluctant to discard pre-intervention observations to improve the fit between a treated time series and its synthetic control. But that problem does not arise in this example analysis. In this example, the size of the donor pool and length of our time series provides a distribution of more than one thousand placebo data points. In that distribution, the post-intervention difference between *California_t* and *Synthetic California_t* is statistically significant well beyond the conventional level.

7.5.4 Robustness Tests

Rejecting the chance null hypothesis, we entertain the hypothesis that the results are a spurious artifact of the model used to construct the synthetic control time series. Constructing a synthetic control time series involves a series of artful, educated decisions and it is possible that a questionable downstream modeling decision could have generated a biased result. Just as modeling decisions vary from analysis to analysis, the appropriate robustness tests will vary from result to result. Nevertheless, two robustness tests are recommended in every analysis.

The first test assesses the relative influence of individual donor states in the construction of a synthetic control time series. The first column of numbers in Table 7.4 reports the state weights, pre-intervention fit, and post-intervention effect estimate for the baseline model. The subsequent columns report the weights and statistics for the synthetic control time series constructed after states are excluded from the donor pool. After excluding Connecticut, the fit between $California_t$ and $Synthetic\ California_t$ is looser—$MSPE = 0.702$ versus 0.647. The post-intervention difference is still large and negative, however, suggesting that Connecticut does not exert an undue influence on the construction.

The subsequent columns of Table 7.4 exclude from the donor pool Connecticut and Rhode Island, Connecticut, Rhode Island, and Massachusetts, Connecticut, Rhode Island, Massachusetts, and New York, and finally, Connecticut, Rhode Island, Massachusetts, New York and Ohio. As more states are excluded from the donor pool, the pre-intervention fit deteriorates slightly but the large, negative post-intervention differences persist. Since the results are roughly comparable, the test suggests that the baseline results were not unduly influenced by any single state.

The second recommended robustness test applies the same general logic to the pre-intervention segment. Table 7.5 reports the state weights, pre-intervention fits, and post-intervention differences for synthetic control time series constructed by discarding the first 5, 10, 15, and 20 years from the pre-intervention segment. As the pre-intervention segment grows shorter, the fit between $California_t$ and $Synthetic\ California_t$ improves in gradual increments. That should come as no surprise. Regardless of how long or short the pre-intervention segment, however, large, negative post-intervention differences persist. The baseline result is not sensitive to the choice of pre-intervention segments.

Table 7.5 raises the interesting possibility of improving the fit between a treated time series and its synthetic control by discarding pre-intervention observations. In experiments where a short time series has an "outlier," depending on practical considerations, dropping the anomalous observation may be a reasonable modeling decision. Otherwise, this method is not generally recommended. The weights

Table 7.4. RESULTS OF A "DISCARD-A-STATE" TEST

States Discarded		1	2	3	4	5
Arizona	0.173	0.154	0.121	0.159	0.105	0.118
Connecticut	0.245	Out	Out	Out	Out	Out
Delaware	—	—	0.114	0.117	0.115	0.078
Florida	—	0.044	—	—	—	—
Illinois	—	—	—	—	—	0.132
Massachusetts	—	0.123	0.336	Out	Out	Out
Maryland	—	—	—	—	0.139	0.158
New Hampshire	0.105	0.084	—	0.079	0.097	0.158
New Jersey	—	—	—	—	0.099	0.142
New York	—	—	0.113	0.408	Out	Out
Ohio	—	—	—	—	0.239	Out
Oklahoma	—	0.052	—	—	—	—
Rhode Island	0.202	0.321	Out	Out	Out	Out
Texas	0.138	0.089	0.197	0.200	0.207	0.149
West Virginia	0.137	0.133	0.120	0.036	—	0.065
Pre-Intervention *MSPE*	0.647	0.702	0.746	0.831	0.865	0.856
Post-Intervention *Difference*	−3.273	−3.394	−2.841	−2.538	−2.975	−2.962

Table 7.5. RESULTS OF "DISCARD-A-SEGMENT" TEST

Years Discarded		5	10	15	20
Arizona	0.173	0.162	0.132	—	—
Connecticut	0.245	0.014	—	—	—
Delaware	—	—	—	—	0.050
D.C.	—	—	—	—	0.041
Florida	—	0.019	—	—	—
Illinois	—	—	—	—	0.326
Massachusetts	—	0.385	0.653	0.686	0.004
Michigan	—	—	—	—	0.008
New Hampshire	0.105	0.049	—	—	0.039
New Mexico	—	0.130	0.181	0.263	—
New York	—	0.241	0.034	0.052	0.182
Rhode Island	0.202	—	—	—	—
Texas	0.138	—	—	—	—
Virginia	—	—	—	—	0.231
West Virginia	0.060	—	—	—	0.119
Pre-Intervention *MSPE*	0.774	0.462	0.344	0.200	0.090
Post-Intervention *Difference*	−3.273	−2.978	−2.955	−2.538	−3.387

and statistics in Table 7.5 illustrate the dilemma. Based on *MSPE* statistics, the *Synthetic California$_t$* constructed from the 1990–96 pre-intervention segment is relatively attractive. Although the synthetic control time series with shorter pre-intervention segments have lower *MSPEs*, however, their constructions are dominated by Massachusetts.

Now if we were forced to choose a single state to use as a control for California, it would probably not be Massachusetts. Beyond this very specific consideration, however, in general, single-state dominance challenges the implicit rationale for sythetic control designs. As a rule, synthetic control time series should be constructed from the widest practicable donor pools. Furthermore, the ideal synthetic control time series should tap a diverse range of states. The synthetic control time series with the lowest *MSPE* is not necessarily "best."

The circumstances of this particular experiment suggest the need for another robustness test. Recall that our *Synthetic California$_t$* was conditioned on observations of *California$_t$* and ∇ *California$_t$*. Although these two time series proved to be reasonable proxies for the underlying causes of motor vehicle fatalities, we noted that other analysts might prefer to condition *Synthetic California$_t$* directly on the causal variable time series. Although direct representation of the causal variables introduces modeling decisions that we have characterized as "guesswork," the alternative view is eminently reasonable, if nothing else.

The only relevant methodological question asks whether either approach is associated with bias. To investigate the potential biasing effects of this modeling decision, we constructed *Synthetic California$_t$* conditioned on the predictor variable time series listed in Table 7.6. The fit between the treated time series and its synthetic control is somewhat weaker—pre-intervention *MSPE* = 1.117 versus 0.774—but acceptable. The post-intervention difference inferred from this alternative model is roughly comparable to the difference inferred

Table 7.6. SYNTHETIC CALIFORNIA CONSTRUCTED FROM PREDICTORS

	California	Synthetic California
Alcohol Consumption per capita	2.996	2.814
Beer Consumption per capita	1.281	1.432
Percent 15–44 Years Old	47.961	46.921
Percent 65 and older	10.162	10.213
Percent Poverty	13.111	13.121
Automobile Registration per capita	0.500	0.504
Motorcycle Registration per capita	0.026	0.018
Pre-Intervention *MSPE*	1.117	
Post-intervention *Difference*	−2.947	

from the baseline model, however. Since the two models support the same inference—that motor vehicle fatalities in California dropped after medical marijuana was legalized—there is no difference between the two approaches to constructing the synthetic control time series.

7.6 CONCLUSION

As this chapter opened, we used the polar extremes of Aristotle and Russell to reveal ourselves as middle-of-road moderates on questions of causality. Following Shadish et al., we believe that valid causal inference necessarily involves all four validities. Nevertheless, due largely to its historical association with random assignment, internal validity remains the sine qua non of validity. Throughout the social and behavioral sciences, internal validity has become synonymous with the "validity of causes." Although that word association may be unfortunate, it emphasizes the fact that methodologists should know *exactly* what it means to say that "X causes Y." Without an explicit definition on the table, internal validity becomess a meaningless buzzword.

An acceptable definition must rest on a philosophical foundation. As we understand it, Aristotelian causality addresses the overly broad concept of *change*. To Aristotle, for example, water causes steam. The "X causes Y" statements of modern normal science need a narrower, empirically driven definition. Though empirically driven, Hume's causality suffers from a similar defect. Since Hume invented his causality for the limited purpose of illustrating the Induction Problem, many of the causal phenomena that interested mid-18th-century scientists were excluded. Finally, though self-consciously philosophical, Mill's causality satisfies our need for a *narrow, empirically driven* definition. We resolve in the future to assign excerpts from Mill's *System of Logic* to students who want to—or who *need* to— understand internal validity.

We do not want to suggest that nothing happened in the 150 years after Mill's *System*. For time series designs specifically, however, the development of internal validity jumps from Mill (1843) to Campbell (1957) to Rubin (1974). If the post-intervention gap plotted in Figure 7.14 has a causal interpretation, it relies on *Rubin* causality.

The strict assumptions of Rubin causality may limit its appeal or utility. Although virtually all Y's can be *effects*, for example, not all X's can be *causes* in the conventional Rubin causal model. Rubin's (1986) widely quoted aphorism that there can be "no causation without manipulation" does not imply that variables like race and gender do not cause things. Obviously, they do. But since these variables cannot be manipulated, their effects cannot be interpreted causally in the conventional Rubin causal model.

Another set of strict assumptions arises from the experimental *milieu*. To introduce these assumptions, recall that the observed treatment effect for the *i*th subject, Y_i, is the realization of two potential outcomes, Y_{i1} and Y_{i0}, only one of which can be observed. If X_i is a binary variable indicating assignment to treatment, when $X_i = 1$, or to control, when $X_i = 0$, the conventional Rubin causal model is

$$Y_i = (X_i)Y_{i1} + (1 - X_i)Y_{i0}$$

In the case of an uncomplicated random assignment, the expected value of the Rubin causal model equates the observed factual on the left-hand side and the observed part of the right-hand side counterfactual. This interpretation of the expected value assumes that there is no interference or interaction between subjects, however. Rubin (1980) calls this the "stable unit treatment value assumption" (SUTVA). When the SUTVA fails, the expected value of the Rubin causal model fails and cannot be interpreted.

Although definitions of the SUTVA are technically demanding, hypothetical violations convey the general idea. Manski (2013) offers several hypothetical examples. A job skills training program is evaluated by randomly assigning eligible subjects either to a treatment group, where they receive job skills training, or to a control group. During the program's training phase, subjects in the treatment group are taken out of the labor force, making it easier for control subjects to find good jobs. After the training phase, treatment subjects return to the labor force with their new skills, making it more difficult for control subjects to find jobs. In either phase, the treatment affects subjects in both groups, thereby violating the SUTVA. Evaluations of vaccination and school-based tutoring programs provide other hypothetical examples:

> Vaccination of person j may reduce the chance that this person will become ill, and vaccination of other persons may also reduce his probability of illness, reinforcing the effect of their own vaccination. Or consider provision of tutoring to a class of students. Tutoring student j may increase her achievement, and tutoring other students in the class may help her achieve as well. (Manski, 2013, p. S10)

In all of these hypotheticals, the treatment (or nontreatment) of one subject affects the treatment (or non-treatment) outcome of other subjects. We usually think of these SUTVA violations as between-group interference or contamination, but within-group interference or contamination also violates the SUTVA.

The remaining relevant question concerns the plausibility of SUTVA violations in our statewide synthetic control time series designs. The SUTVA requires both well-defined units and an instantaneous treatment that does not affect the nontreated units. Taking California's 1996 legalization of medical marijuana, the SUTVA would be violated if California's reform affected marijuana use in neighboring states such as Arizona. If there were reason to believe that California's medical marijuana laws did in fact affect marijuana use in neighboring states, these states must be dropped from the donor pool.

8

Construct Validity

There are two perspectives in test validation. From the viewpoint of the psychological practitioner, the burden of proof is on the test. A test should not be used to measure a trait until its proponent establishes that predictions made from such measures are consistent with the best available theory of the trait. In the view of the test developer, however, both the test and the theory are under scrutiny. She is free to say to herself privately, "If my test disagrees with the theory, so much the worse for the theory." This way lies delusion, unless she continues her research using a better theory.

— CRONBACH AND MEEHL (1955, P. 296)

It can still be liberating suddenly to realize that something is constructed and is not part of the nature of things, of people, or human society.

—HACKING (1999, P. 36)

Construct validity has its roots in logical positivism, an empirical doctrine that reached its zenith in the early 20th century. Logical positivists argued that knowledge acquired through scientific methods could be trusted because it could be empirically *verified*. Knowledge acquired through mathematics or logic could also be trusted, though for other reasons. But knowledge acquired through any other method could not be trusted. The logical positivist view of scientific theory was summarized in Russell's (1918, p. 155) widely quoted maxim: "Wherever possible logical constructions are to be substituted for inferred entities." A scientific theory could use unobserved or unobservable constructs, but only temporarily. As the theory evolved, its "inferred entities" would be discarded.[1]

---

1. The vocabulary has changed since 1910 when Russell wrote this maxim. What Russell called an "inferred entity" modern social scientists would call a "construct" (Beck, 1950, p. 74).

Though focused on physics, Russell's brand of logical positivism had a strong influence on American psychology. To comply with Russell's maxim, Mac-Corquodale and Meehl (1948, p. 97) proposed that psychological theories be rewritten to distinguish between *empirical* and *hypothetical* constructs. Empirical constructs could be observed and, hence, used to test hypotheses deduced from a theory. Empirical verification of a theory did not entail the existence of its hypothetical constructs, however. To claim otherwise would be to accept an ontological fallacy.

The influence of logical positivism is apparent in a 1954 American Psychological Association report on test standards. Endorsing the report, Cronbach and Meehl (1955) coined the term "construct validity" to describe the correlation between a test score and the criterion attribute that it purports to measure.[2]

The definition and the validation procedures described by Cronbach and Meehl provoked a reaction. When Bechtold (1959, p. 622) faulted construct validity because its "'constructs' . . . appear to be 'vague,' open, and 'not explicitly defined,'" Campbell (1960, p. 546) responded that "it would seem inappropriate if the eloquence of Bechtold's attack led to the removal of the category of construct validity." Campbell's view prevailed, of course, not only in the fields of psychology where variables were measured with paper-and-pencil tests, but in the social and behavioral sciences generally.

In their attempt to generalize construct validity from psychological testing to other social scientific measures, Cook and Campbell (1979, p. 59) characterized it as "what experimental psychologists are concerned with when they worry about 'confounding'." Compared to the external validity threats of Campbell and Stanley (1966), the threats to construct validity assumed an explicit *causal* theory. Nevertheless, Cook and Campbell (1979, p. 63) cautioned that "it would be a mistake to think that construct validity should only be a concern of the theoretician." On the contrary, construct validity was to be used in the same way that the other validities were used. It was a *practical* validity, one whose threats could be controlled by careful attention to theoretical constructs.

Although the concept of construct validity translated neatly from physics to psychological tests, translation to other disciplines and applications proved more difficult. Reichardt (2011) goes so far as to question the need for a distinction between construct and external validity. Though not endorsing this argument completely, it is difficult to ignore the fuzzy boundary between these two validities. Setting a sharp demarcation line between construct and external validity leaves us open to a charge of arbitrariness. Since we have no choice, we use this distinction: External validity includes questions of whether an effect generalizes to other populations, settings, and timeframes. Construct validity

2. Replace "test" with "construct" in the Cronbach-Meehl quotation that introduced this chapter and reread.

Table 8.1. THREATS TO CONSTRUCT VALIDITY (SHADISH ET AL., 2002)

Inadequate explication of constructs
Construct confounding
Mono-operation bias
Mono-method bias
Confounding constructs with levels of constructs
Treatment-ensitive factorial structure
Reactive self-report changes
Reactivity to the experimental situation
Experimenter expectancies
Novelty and disruption effects
Compensatory equalization
Compensatory rivalry
Resentful demoralization
Treatment diffusion

includes questions of whether the effect generalizes to alternative measures of hypothetical causes and effects.

In the first attempt to develop a list of threats to construct validity, Cook and Campbell (1979) proposed 10 threats. Two decades later, Shadish et al. (2002) kept the same scope and emphasis but expanded the original list to the 14 threats to construct validity listed in Table 8.1. The system of threats that we describe in the next section will focus more narrowly on practical methods for controlling the threats to construct validity commonly encountered in time series designs.

Although each of the Shadish et al. threats to construct validity might plausibly affect the results of a time series experiment, some seem to fall outside our arbitrary definition of construct validity. For example, the last four threats — *compensatory equalization, compensatory rivalry, resentful demoralization,* and *treatment diffusion*—are violations of the SUTVA and, as such, might be analyzed as threats to internal validity. Along with other listed threats, on the other hand, these four might be analyzed as pure threats to external validity. This minor point has no simple, obvious resolution.

Though concurring with the list of 14 threats identified by Shadish et al. (Table 8.1), many of these threats are either implausible in a time series design or else apply to all designs equally. We will focus on a narrowly defined subset of the 14 that arise uniquely and frequently in time series designs. To highlight the methods aimed at controlling these common threats, we write the *ARIMA* impact model in its most abstract form:

$$Y_t = N(a_t) + X(I_t) \qquad \text{or}$$
$$[Y_t - N(a_t)] = X(I_t)$$

Table 8.2. THREATS TO CONSTRUCT VALIDITY FOR TIME SERIES DESIGNS

Left-Hand Side	*Timeframe definition*
	Period definition
Right-Hand Side	*"Fuzzy" onset*
	"Fuzzy" response
	Detection modeling

This representation divides the plausible threats to the construct validity into those that affect the left-hand side of the model and those that affect the right-hand side of the model.

Table 8.2 lists five threats to contruct validity that are plausible in time series designs. Two of the threats are found on the left-hand side of the model, three on the right-hand side. Although the names of these threats are ours, all five are elaborations of the 14 Shadish et al. threats. In principle, each is controlled by proper specification of the statistical model and by conservative interpretation of the results. One might argue then that these five threats could be better analyzed as threats to statistical conclusion validity. We appreciate that argument. In addition to wholly stochastic aspects of the phenomenon, however, the statistical model must also represent grounded aspects of the phenomenon. If the representation is inadequate or weak, the resulting inferential problems are best analyzed as threats to construct validity.

8.1 THREATS ON THE LEFT-HAND SIDE

For primary data, researchers ordinarily address plausible threats to construct validity prior to data collection. Secondary data do not afford this luxury. Plausible threats to construct validity are addressed, if at all, only after data collection. The fit between the data *as collected* and the construct *as defined* is never perfect. Common threats to construct validity are always plausible. Minor discrepancies between data and constructs are unavoidable. Although these discrepancies need not pose fatal threats to construct validity, however, the inferential limitations posed by these threats must be reported and discussed.

At the other extreme, the discrepancy between data and constructs may be so large as to pose a fatal threat to construct validity. Lacking suitable secondary data, threats to construct validity can only be controlled by collecting suitable primary data. That advice may be obvious and impractical, of course, and hence worthless.

Two *nonobvious* threats to construct validity involve the construction of the time series Y_t. Both threats are controlled by reconstructing Y_t. Although this solution might seem obvious, in our experience it is not. We often see time series that have been constructed with little attention to the theoretical generating process. Analysts seem to believe that a statistically adequate noise component on the right-hand side corrects any shortcomings on the left-hand side of the model. Assuming a well-behaved generating process and a large N, this belief is correct. It is unwise to put too much faith in the noise component, however, especially when attention paid to construction of the time series can mitigate the most common problems.

8.1.1 Timeframe Definitions

Selecting a timeframe is the first nontrivial consideration in the design of a time series experiment. To control plausible threats to statistical conclusion validity, the time series must be as long as possible. Yet in light of a common threat to construct validity, a time series can be too long. The time series in Figure 8.1 illustrates the dilemma. These are monthly admissions to California prisons. The $N = 348$ monthly observations of this time series are sufficient to detect most impacts and, hence, to control the most common threats to statistical conclusion validity. Shorter timeframes—say, $N = 120$ monthly observations—would also yield sufficient power, however, and in this instance, shorter might be "better."

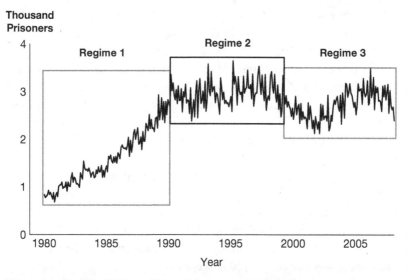

Figure 8.1 Monthly California Prison Admissions, 1980–2007

The longer timeframe is not free but comes at the expense of construct validity. Visual inspection of Figure 8.1 suggests that the 28-year time series consists of at least two, possibly three distinct regimes. From 1980 through 1990, the time series level rises at a nearly linear rate. Variance increases proportionately, suggesting an *IMA* model of natural logarithms. Exponentiating both sides, we write the Regime 1 model as[3]

$$\text{Regime 1:} \qquad Prisoners_t = \nabla^{-d} e^{N(a_t)}$$

Variance stabilizes after 1990, eliminating the need for natural logarithms. The linear trend in level also ends abruptly in about 1990, giving way to a relatively "flat" segment of the time series:

$$\text{Regime 2:} \qquad Prisoners_t = N(a_t)$$

Finally, the time series begins to drift in a pattern that suggests an *IMA* model:

$$\text{Regime 3:} \qquad Prisoners_t = \nabla^{-d} N(a_t)$$

In principle, the entire 28-year history of this time series could be accommodated by combining the three models into a single model. But we endorse a more practical solution: The threat to construct validity arises because this time series evolves in distinct regimes. The threat is controlled by acknowledging the regimes and taking appropriate steps to represent them.

When a time series is long enough to effectively control plausible threats to statistical conclusion validity, as in this example, plausible threats to constuct validity can be controlled by truncating the time series. For most time series, statistical power crosses a threshold at $N = 120$ observations. Given a stable generating process, statistical conclusion validity grows stronger with each additional observation. But power increments grow smaller and smaller, even in the best-case scenario. If the additional observations introduce a new regime, the incremental power is bought at the expense of a potent, plausible threat to construct validity.

Because they often acquire an authoritative status that was not intended, we are reluctant to introduce new rules of thumb. Nevertheless, faced with visual evidence of multiple regimes, such as that shown in Figure 8.1, we recommend truncating the time series to eliminate all but one secular regime. The potential threat to statistical conclusion validity raised by truncation will be implausible if the remaining segment is $N > 120$ observations.

---

3. Remember that $e[Ln(Y_t)] = Y_t$

8.1.2 Period Definition

Seasonality (or periodicity) poses a threat to construct validity that can sometimes be minimized or even avoided. The time series plotted in Figures 8.2 and
8.3 demonstrate this point. Both time series were constructed from a database of
7,042 patients who were treated at a level-one trauma center for gunshot or knife
wounds. Although the two time series reflect the same underlying phenomenon,

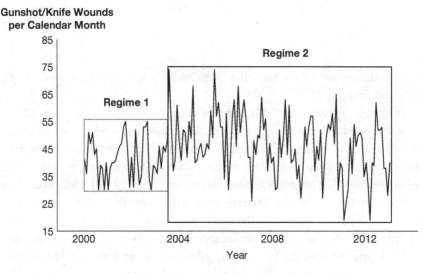

Figure 8.2 Patients Treated for Gunshot or Knife Wounds, Calendar Months

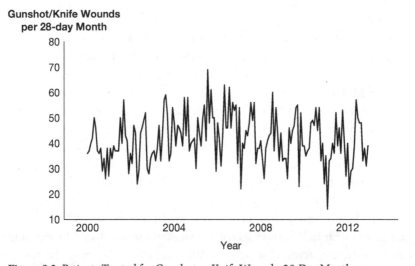

Figure 8.3 Patients Treated for Gunshot or Knife Wounds, 28-Day Months

Table 8.3. PATIENTS TREATED FOR GUNSHOT OR KNIFE WOUNDS, VARIOUS
AGGREGATIONS

	Days	Weeks	28 Days	Months	Quarters
N	4749	678	169	156	52
Mean	1.48	10.39	41.59	45.14	135.42
Median	1.0	10.0	40.0	45.0	134.5
Variance	1.77	15.68	90.90	108.01	604.17
Minimum	0	1	14	19	74
Maximum	8	24	69	74	193
Z_{KS}	15.50	2.21	0.90	0.84	0.43

due to differences in the way they were constructed, they have qualitatively different properties.

Table 8.3 aggregates the 7,042 patients into time series of days, weeks, 28-day months, calendar months, and quarters. The daily and weekly time series are significantly non-Normal. That would not ordinarily pose an obstacle. When the time series can be constructed from individual records, however, choosing a level of aggregation that produces a Normal time series is preferred. Unlike the daily and weekly time series, the quarterly time series is approximately Normal. It is too short, however. Dismissing the daily, weekly, and quarterly time series leaves the two monthly time series. Both are approximately Normal and relatively long.

To decide between the two monthly time series, we build *ARIMA* models. Parameter estimates for the "best" *ARIMA* models are reported in Table 8.4. The calendar month model has one less parameter and, hence, might be the more parsimonious representation. The model for the 28-day months has a smaller *Q*-statistic and *RSE*, on the other hand, so its extra parameter is not wasted.

Unfortunately, there is no obvious way to compare the two competing models. Since the two models have different dependent variables, the information criteria methods described in Chapter 3.7.1 are no help. Although *RSEs* favor the time series of 28-day months model, the difference in *RSEs* may reflect the difference in *N*s. The two monthly time series are statistical "apples and oranges."

On the other hand, substantive theory argues for 28-day months. A large, consistent body of research on trauma deaths shows that the incidence rate rises sharply on Fridays, Saturdays, and Sundays, with Saturday usually being the single highest day of the week (Dobrin et al., 1996; Kposowa and Breault, 1998; Lester, 1979; Wolfgang, 1958). Researchers often attribute the weekend peak to increased leisure time and to the informal socializing and alcohol consumption that comes with it. Whatever its source, weekend peaks should be distributed equally and evenly across observations. Whereas each 28-day month has the same number of weekends, calendar months do not.

Table 8.4. Estimation and Diagnosis for Two Trauma Patient Time Series

$$\nabla^{12} Calendar_t = \theta_0 + (1 - \theta_2 B_2 - \theta_{11} B^{11} - \theta_{12} B^{12}) a_t$$

		Estimate	SE	t	Diagnosis
N = 156	$\hat{\theta}_0$	.0903	.5729	.16	RSE = 9.0452
Mean = 45.14	$\hat{\theta}_2$	−.1269	.0691	−1.84	Q_{24} = 23.0
Variance = 108.01	$\hat{\theta}_{11}$	−.1716	.0704	−2.44	Z_{KS} = 0.522
Z_{KS} = 0.84	$\hat{\theta}_{12}$	.6105	.0714	8.55	

$$\nabla^{13} Lunar_t = \theta_0 + (1 - \theta_2 B_2 - \theta_6 B^6 - \theta_{12} B^{12} - \theta_{13} B^{13}) a_t$$

		Estimate	SE	t	Diagnosis
N = 169	$\hat{\theta}_0$	.0500	.5849	.09	RSE = 8.7598
Mean = 41.59	$\hat{\theta}_2$	−.1363	.0608	−2.24	Q_{26} = 15.4
Variance = 90.90	$\hat{\theta}_6$	−.1312	.0609	−2.15	Z_{KS} = 0.405
Z_{KS} = 0.81	$\hat{\theta}_{12}$	−.1613	.0623	−2.59	
	$\hat{\theta}_{13}$	.6645	.0606	10.96	

So what? The reader is now directed back to Figure 8.2. In July 2003, a potential regime change is apparent in the calendar month time series. In fact, *nothing* changed in the underlying process—nothing that we or other knowledgeable people can think of, at least. The *appearance* of a regime change in the calendar month time series is a visual artifact of calendar month aggregation. Pounding "square" data into a "round" construct often accentuates minor anomalies in a time series. The potential regime change that is so apparent in the calendar month time series fades into the background noise of the 28-day monthly time series.

The widespread preference for calendar months is difficult to explain, given the strong *theoretical* basis for 28-day months in many social processes. In our experience, the preference for calendar months is based on superstition, bureaucratic demands, and misconceptions. Whereas calendar months are simply called "months," for example, 28-day months are often called "lunar" months. To avoid the image problem created by this unfortunate name, we propose the alternative name of "retail" months. Analysts working for agencies have told us that they avoid 28-day months because their agencies report calendar month statistics. Statistics from analyses of 28-day month time series are easily converted to calendar month statistics, of course. Finally, some analysts point to the fact that the quotient of 28 and 365 has a remainder that runs into the new year. To those analysts, we point out that the quotient of 12 and 365 also has a remainder. The calendar month remainder stays out of sight, however, and out of mind.

8.1.3 Worldview

In Chapter 6.4.5, discussing the threats to statistical conclusion validity associated with missing data, we offered the example of an annual time series of physician expenditures reported by two U.S. government agencies. Although sociologically naïve analysts might expect the numbers reported by the Health Care Financing Administration (1965–76) and the Social Security Administration (1949–73) to agree, they do not. To the extent that discrepancies between the two time series lead to biased estimates of model parameters, they are most appropriately analyzed as uncontrolled threats to statistical conclusion validity. Questions about the nature of the discrepancy, on other other hand, are most appropriately analyzed as uncontrolled threats to construct validity.

In Chapter 7.5.2, we discussed the somewhat larger discrepancy in annual motor vehicle fatality time series reported by the National Highway Traffic Safety Administration (NHTSA) and the National Center for Health Statistics (NCHS). In that example, the discrepancy was attributed to differences in the worldviews of the medical examiners and traffic engineers who administer those two agencies. Whereas medical examiners collect data for the purpose of filing accurate death certificates, traffic engineers collect data for the purpose of determining the causes of the vehicle crashes that lead to the fatalities. Discrepancies between the two fatality counts can be explained almost entirely by the different motives of the two professions.

Although the different worldviews of bureaucrats are often explained by the different mandates of their bureaucracies, darker motives cannot be discounted. Morgenstern (1963) attributes discrepancies in national accounts and transfers to the national interests and motives.[4] Campbell's Law of data corruption, which we will discuss more fully in Chapter 9.1, explains discrepancies in terms of the selfish competing motives of stakeholders. On an optimistic note, Campbell's Law allows for the possibility that data are sometimes relegated to archives and never used. These data are free of corruption.

What can be done about corrupt data? First, many forms of data corruption are inconsequential to the results. If traffic fatalities are consistently under- or over-reported, for example, the pre- and post-intervention levels are likely to be affected equally. For purposes of inferential validity, then, the corrupted, biased fatality counts can be ignored. Otherwise, the best that can be done is to become aware of potential corrupting influences. We will have more to say about this in Chapter 9, when we discuss external validity.

---

4. Morgenstern begins with the tantalizing Latin aphorism, *Qui numerare incipit errare incipit.* In English, this roughly translates to "Whoever begins to count begins to make mistakes."

8.2 THREATS ON THE RIGHT-HAND SIDE

The right-hand-side threats to construct validity arise from misspecifications of the theoretical relationship between I_t and Y_t. The transfer function, $X(I_t)$, describes the *response* of Y_t to *change* in I_t. Although the response can be informed by facts, proper specification relies on a theory of the phenomenon within the rules of hypothesis testing. The theory must be testable, after all. With that said, in our experience the two most common threats to construct validity involve "fuzzy" onsets and responses. Though less common, a third threat involves a misguided attempt to equate *detection* of an intervention with theoretically informed *modeling* of the intervention.

8.2.1 "Fuzzy" Onsets

The onset of an intervention is assumed to occur homogeneously across all subunits. If the unit of analysis is a classroom, for example, I_t is assumed to turn on or off at the same time for each student. If the unit of analysis is a community, I_t is assumed to turn on or off at the same time for each household. Violations of the homogeneity assumption lead to biased estimates of $X(I_t)$. An example illustrates both the nature of this bias and the ideal method for controlling the "fuzzy" intervention threat to statistical conclusion validity.

To estimate the impact of a housing program on mortgage loan activity, Mushkatel and Wilson (1982) analyze housing loan time series for the Denver metropolitan area before and after the onset of the program. Finding no impact, they discover that the program was implemented in high- and low-income neighborhoods at different times. Disaggregating the metropolitan area time series into lower-level time series, they find that the program had large, significant impacts on mortgage loan activity across the Denver metropolitan area.

The experience of Mushkatel and Wilson (1982) is typical in one respect. The biased estimate of $X(I_t)$ is almost always in the direction of a null finding. It might be tempting to treat the "fuzzy" intervention as a threat to statistical conclusion validity, especially given that the biased estimate of $X(I_t)$ favors the H_0. Given the ideal method of controlling this threat, however, it clearly belongs to the construct validity category.

The ideal method of controlling the threat consists of re-specifying I_t so that it conforms more closely to theory. Mushkatel and Wilson (1982) controlled the "fuzzy" intervention threat by disaggregating their higher-level time series into several lower-level component time series, each with its own I_t. This ideal method of control is not always feasible, of course. If the higher-level time series was selected because the lower-level component time series have undesirable

statistical properties, the threat to statistical conclusion validity is more appropriately controlled by statistical means such as a transformation. It happens more
often that the use of a high-level time series is dictated by data availability. This
is particularly true of time series constructed from data stored in government
archives.

8.2.2 "Fuzzy" Responses

Judging from the literature, the four impact models presented in Figure 5.1
adequately describe most of the impacts enountered by social and behavioral
scientists. Hybrid models composed of two or more of the four models extend
the range of the four component models. Although the estimated parameters of
the first-order transfer function might provide evidence for or against a particular
impact pattern, construct validity demands a theoretical specification of the
impact model prior to estimation. Practical considerations sometimes make it
difficult or impossible to realize this ideal. Reliable estimates of the transfer
function's parameters assume a long post-intervention time series segment. Even
when N_{post} is large, however, a "fuzzy" response to the intervention may pose a
serious threat to construct validity.

The annual neonatal tetanus death rate time series plotted in Figure 8.4
illustrates what surely must be a worst-case scenario for this threat to construct
validity. Veney (1993) used this time series to evaluate the effectiveness of a 1974
Sri Lankan prenatal tetanus immunization program. Given that the time series

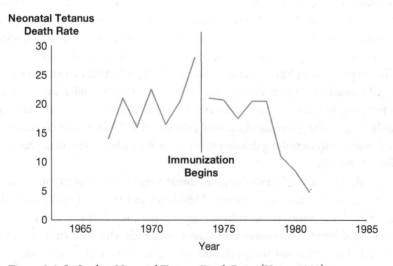

Figure 8.4 Sri Lankan Neonatal Tetanus Death Rates (Veney, 1993)

has only $N=15$ observations, *ARIMA* modeling is difficult at best. Still, assuming an abrupt, permanent impact, the "best" *ARIMA* model is

$$Tetanus_t = \nabla^{-1}(\theta_0 + \omega_0 I_t + a_t)$$

Parameter estimates for this "best" *ARIMA* model are reported as Model 1 in Table 8.5. Since the estimate of $\hat{\omega}_0 = -6.83$ is too small to reject H_0, one might infer that prenatal immunization has no impact on neonatal tetanus deaths. But that inference would be unwarranted not only on grounds of statistical conclusion validity—a time series of $N = 15$ observations is too short to reject a reasonable H_0—but also on construct validity grounds. Population theory (*e.g.*, Anderson and May, 1992, pp. 149–152) predicts a *dynamic* response to an immunization program, *not* the static response implied by the zero-order transfer function in Model 1.

Unfortunately, the tetanus time series is too short to support a reliable estimate of a first-order transfer function. In addition to the insufficient number of observations, the program was implemented in fits and starts, producing a "fuzzy" response to the intervention. To control the implied threat to construct validity, Veney redefined I_t to be equal to zero from 1967 through 1973 and from 1974 through 1981, equal to the proportion of the at-risk population that was inoculated. The "best" *ARIMA* model for this time series is

$$Tetanus_t = \theta_0 + \omega_0 I_t + a_t$$

Parameter estimates are reported as Model 2 in Table 8.5. Redefining I_t produces a better-fitting model—*RSE*=4.35 versus *RSE*=5.02—but more important a model that provides a more accurate test of the underlying theory. Since the estimate of $\hat{\omega}_0 = -21.67$ is large enough to reject H_0, moreover, we infer correctly

Table 8.5. ESTIMATION AND DIAGNOSIS, *Tetanus_t*

		Estimate	SE	t	Diagnosis
Model 1	$\hat{\theta}_0$	−.1692	1.3940	−0.12	$RSE = 5.0259$
	$\hat{\omega}_0$	−6.8308	5.2157	−1.31	$Q_5 = 3.9$
					$Z_{KS} = 0.49$
Model 2	$\hat{\theta}_0$	20.7115	1.4692	14.10	$RSE = 4.3502$
	$\hat{\omega}_0$	−21.6691	6.4568	−3.36	$Q_5 = 1.5$
					$Z_{KS} = 0.51$
Model 3	$\hat{\theta}_0$	13.857	3.070	4.51	$RSE = 0.8605$
	$\hat{\omega}_0$	28.251	7.524	3.90	$Q_5 = 6.2$
	$\hat{\omega}_1$	1.482	0.686	2.16	$Z_{KS} = 0.947$
	$\hat{\omega}_2$	−3.790	0.886	−4.28	

that prenatal immunization has a large, statistically significant impact on neonatal tetanus deaths.

Parameter estimates for a three-segment model of the tetanus time series are reported as Model 3 in Table 8.5. These estimates are even more difficult to interpret. Taken jointly, $\hat{\omega}_0$, $\hat{\omega}_1$, and $\hat{\omega}_2$ are large enough to reject H_0, so one might want to infer that the immunization program had an impact. The *nature* of the impact is not obvious, however. From one perspective, the vaccination program has a positive impact. From another perspective, the impact is arguably negative. Can these contrary — or at least *inconsistent*—effects be reconciled? Unfortunately, the multiple analyses reported in Table 8.5 suggests post facto rationalization. No one seriously doubts the effectiveness of national tetanus vaccination programs, but this particular time series experiment cannot provide valid, sufficient evidence for that inference.

8.2.3 Detection Modeling

A visual inspection of the tetanus time series reveals another shortcoming of this particular experiment. The level of the time series rises at a roughly linear rate prior to 1974, then falls at a roughly linear rate. Whatever impact the vaccination had, the tetanus death rate *appears* to have been realized in the pre- and post-intervention secular trends. In light of this visual evidence, analysts might be tempted to build a model that compares secular trends before and after the intervention. We urge readers to resist the temptation to build such a model, however, and indeed to avoid thinking in terms of secular trends.

A review of the applied literature reveals two competing impact theories for time series experiments. The first theory, associated with Box and Jenkins (1970; Box and Tiao, 1975) and described in Chapter 5, relies on a first-order dynamic transfer function to map I_t into Y_t. We write this dynamic transfer function as

$$X(I_t) = \frac{\omega_0}{1 - \delta_1 B} \nabla^j I_t \qquad \text{where } j = 0 \text{ or } 1$$

Depending on whether $j=0$ or 1, the impact can be either permanent or temporary in duration. And depending on the value of δ_1, the impact can be either abrupt or gradual in onset. Distinct transfer functions can be coupled to form a hybrid impact model. The impact theory implied by this $X(I_t)$ is flexible and realistic in our experience.

The second impact theory is less flexible in our experience and not at all realistic. Developed by Kepka (1972) and popularized by Bower et al. (1974),

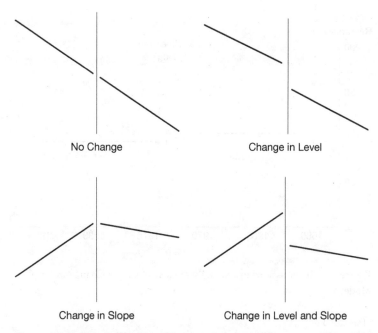

No Change   Change in Level

Change in Slope   Change in Level and Slope

Figure 8.5 Impact Defined by Changes in Levels and Slopes

this theory relies on a static transfer function model:

$$X(I_t) = \omega_0 I_t + \omega_1 t + \omega_2 (I_t \times t) \qquad \text{where } t = 1, 2, \ldots, N$$

This static transfer function yields the four models shown in Figure 8.5. Under this system, an impact can be realized as a *change in level*, a *change in slope*, a *change in both level and slope*, or *no-in change*.

The time series plotted in Figures 8.6 and 8.7 illustrate the salient shortcomings of the static transfer function model. These data are annual readmission rates for the Vermont state psychiatric hospital before and after implementation of a diversion program. A similar Massachusetts program had been evaluated with a simple change in level model. Where $I_t = 0$ before and $I_t = 1$ after implementation of the diversion program, the change-in-level model is

$$Readmit_t = \omega_0 I_t$$

Since this is the special case of the static transfer function model where $\omega_1 = \omega_2 = 0$, the change-in-level model is nested within the static transfer function model. We will not go to the trouble of calculating likelihood ratios, however, because these data do not satisfy the basic likelihood assumptions.

Judged in terms of a simple change-in-level, the Massachusetts program had no significant impact on readmissions. Noting that the Massachusetts time series

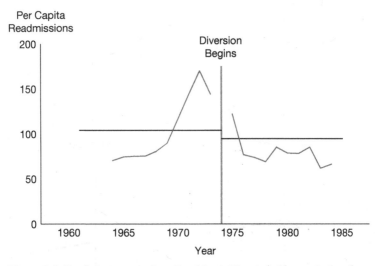

Figure 8.6 Readmissions to a State Psychiatric Hospital: Change-in-Level Model

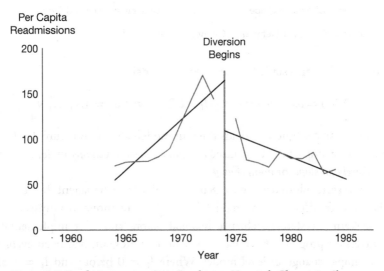

Figure 8.7 Readmissions to a State Psychiatric Hospital: Change-in-Slope Model

followed strong secular trends, Pandiani and Girardi (1993) argue that this null finding is a spurious artifact of the model. To demonstrate this point, they estimate both the change-in-level model and the more general change-in-slope model for the Vermont diversion program. Parameter estimates for the models are reported as Model 1 and Model 2 in Table 8.6.

Consistent with the visual evidence in Figure 8.6, the impact estimate from the change-in-level model is not statistically significant. We agree with Pandiani

Table 8.6. Parameter Estimates for Pandiani and Girardi (1993)

		Estimate	SE	t	
Model 1	$\hat{\theta}_0$	104.18	9.53	10.93	$RSE = 30.13$
	$\hat{\omega}_0$	−19.46	13.16	−1.48	$F_{1,19} = 2.19$
Model 2	$\hat{\theta}_0$	43.90	11.44	3.84	$RSE = 16.74$
	$\hat{\omega}_0$	118.14	28.44	4.16	$F_{3,17} = 17.2$
	$\hat{\omega}_1$	10.96	1.84	5.95	
	$\hat{\omega}_2$	−15.79	2.44	−4.34	

and Girardi, of course, and dismiss this estimate as a spurious artifact. The impact estimate from the change-in-slope model, on the other hand, is *highly* significant. We disagree with Pandiani and Girardi on the proper interpretation of this estimate, however. Although the change-in-slope model does indeed provide a "better" fit to the time series, the visual evidence in Figure 8.7 raises many questions. The fact that the impact on readmissions is visually apparent two years before the diversion program is implemented casts doubt on the nominal interpretation of the parameter estimates.

8.3 CONCLUSION

In Chapter 7, we alluded to discrepancies in the motor vehicle fatality counts reported by the NHTSA and the NCHS. Disrepancies between the data reported by these two agencies are small enough to be ignored for many purposes. We attributed the discrepancies to differences in the worldviews of the traffic engineers and medical examiners who collect, code, and analyze these data. The principle that different motives and interests can lead to different facts was offered as a threat to construct valiidity. Others might see this principle as a threat to external validity, of course, and that disagreement hints at the demarcation problem that we solved with this arbitrary rule: Construct validity is limited to questions of whether an observed effect can be generalized to alternative cause-and-effect measures. All other questions of generalizability—to other people, other places, and other times—are in the external validity domain.

Accepting this arbitrary definition, it was useful to divide the plausible threats to construct validity into those that arise from the left-hand-side time series, Y_t, and those that arise from the intervention model, $X(I_t)$. The "talking out" time series (Figure 5.13) and the self-injurious behavior time series (Figure 5.18) are examples of *primary* data. Primary data are collected by researchers from direct observation to test specific hypotheses deduced from their theories. In this ideal situation, we demonstrated the alternative ways in which Y_t could be constructed to facilitate an optimal test of the null hypothesis.

Primary data are a luxury in many instances. Researchers often have no choice but to use *secondary* data that were collected by third parties for purposes unrelated to any hypothesis test. These data languish in an archive until discovered by an imaginative researcher who realizes that the data are relevant to some phenomenon and, perhaps, suited to testing some hypothesis. Even in those less-than-ideal instances, however, an optimal time series can be constructed by limiting the timeframe and otherwise paying attention to regime changes.

Threats to construct validity that arise from the right-hand-side intervention model, $X(I_t)$, are controlled by paying close attention to the underlying theory. Even a minimal theory should specify the onset and duration of an impact. The flexible set of transfer function models developed in Chapter 5 can accommodate most of the theoretical specifications found in the social and behavioral sciences. An alternative set of models developed by Kepka (1972) and popularized by Bower et al. (1974) is less flexible in our experience and should be avoided.

9

External Validity

The second criterion is that of external validity, representativeness, or generalizability: to what populations, settings, and variables can this effect be generalized?

—CAMPBELL (1957, P. 297)

External validity asks the question of generalizability: to what populations, settings, and variables can this effect be generalized?

—CAMPBELL AND STANLEY (1966, P. 5)

We shall use the term external validity to refer to the approximate validity with which conclusions are drawn about the generalizability of a causal relationship to and across populations of persons, settings, and times.

—COOK AND CAMPBELL (1979, P. 39)

External validity concerns inferences about the extent to which a causal relationship holds over variations in persons, settings, treatments, and outcomes.

—SHADISH ET AL. (2002, P. 83)

Although many aspects of external validity are challenged and debated, the *meaning* of this last validity has not changed in the more than 60 years since it was coined. External validity is an indicator or measure of the *generalizability* of an observed finding. Threats to external validity, simply stated, are factors other than a causal variable that limit the generality of a finding. We have narrowed the domain of external validity by excluding generalizations across alternative measures or constructs. Those questions belong to the construct validity domain. Otherwise, in the social and behavioral sciences, threats to external

Table 9.1. THREATS TO EXTERNAL VALIDITY (SHADISH ET AL., 2002)

Interaction of the causal relationship with units
Interaction of the causal relationship over treatment variations
Interaction of the causal relationship with outcomes
Interaction of the causal relationship with settings
Context-dependent mediation

validity almost always imply a contrived, artificial milieu. Impacts observed in a laboratory are less general than impacts observed in the field, for example, and threats to external validity become less plausible with distance from the controlled environment.

Students often have a difficult time distinguishing external validity from construct validity, and this is understandable. We can now confess that our half-hearted attempt to draw a sharp demarcation line between the two validities in Chapter 8 was little more than a useful literary device. Applied to the common threats to external validity, its usefulness vanishes quickly. Unlike the threats to the other validities, which are tied to features of design or construction, the threats to external validity reduce to this single control: replicate, replicate, replicate.

Campbell (1957; Campbell and Stanley, 1966) originally listed four threats to external validity. Cook and Campbell (1979) narrowed the list to three. Shadish et al. (2002) expanded the number to the five threats listed in Table 9.1. In principle, any of these five threats might be plausible in a time series experiment, but it is unlikely that all five would be plausible in any single time series experiment. This is because some of the five threats apply to primary data only. At least one threat arises when either primary or secondary data change over time. Finally, although the five threats pertain narrowly to specific contingencies, it will be useful to divide them into two categories: threats that arise from variation in subjects and situations and threats that arise from variation in timeframes.

9.1 SUBJECTS AND SITUATIONS

Campbell's original interest in external validity focused on the relative *reactivity*—or *non*reactivity— of a measurement. In simple terms, a reactive measurement is one that *changes* the phenomenon under observation so as to bias the empirical result:

> Whenever the measurement process is not a part of the normal environment it is probably reactive ... Measurement of a person's height is relatively nonreactive. However, measurement of weight ... would ... be reactive

in that the process of measuring would stimulate weight reduction. A photograph of a crowd taken in secret from a second story window would be nonreactive, but a news photograph of the same scene might very well be reactive, in that the presence of the photographer would modify the behavior of people seeing themselves being photographed.—Campbell (1957, p. 299)

"Reactivity" relied on the commonsense notion that people would change their behaviors if they suspected that they were being watched. Blinding or masking with a placebo was a fairly obvious way to control this threat in an experimental trial. To test the effectiveness of a common cold vaccine, for example, Diehl et al. (1938) used a placebo control design diagrammed as

$$\text{Vaccine} \quad \ldots \quad O \quad X \quad O \quad \ldots$$
$$\text{Placebo} \quad \ldots \quad O \quad . \quad O \quad \ldots$$

Vaccinated subjects reported a 73 percent reduction in cold symptoms, suggesting that the vaccine was spectacularly effective. Control subjects who were injected with a saline placebo reported a 63 percent reduction in symptoms, however, suggesting that the vaccine had a larger effect on subjects' imaginations than on their immune systems.

In both laboratory trials and "real-world" immunization programs, the intervention is expected to impact immune systems. Whether it achieves this goal or not, however, the intervention is likely to impact expectations, hopes, dreams, and fears. The practical problem of controlling the implied threat to external validity amounts to untangling these two impacts and, in experimental trials, that is done with a placebo control group.

Controlling the analogous threat to external validity in a nonexperimental trial requires ingenuity and imagination. One approach to controlling the threat involves using *secondary* data to test hypotheses that might ordinarily be tested with *primary* data. To study cohesion and disintegration of Wehrmacht units in World War II, for example, Shils and Janowitz (1948) analyzed letters written by German prisoners to their families. On the one hand, these data were undoubtedly less "reactive" than the alternative primary data—face-to-face interviews. But on the other hand, it is likely that the data dictated the hypothesis to be tested, not vice versa. Abandoning one's hypothesis of interest is not a reasonable method of controlling threats to external validity.

Had the German prisoners known that their letters were being analyzed, of course, the threats to external validity might have persisted in a different form. Abel's (1938) analyses of essays written by Nazi Party members illustrate how deception can be used to secure a stronger degree of control over threats to external validity. To collect the opinions of young Nazi Party members, Abel offered a cash prize for the "best" biographical essay of a Nazi movement leader. It is unlikely that the 600-plus respondents suspected what the ultimate use of their essays would be. To the extent that the essayists would want to exhibit their enthusiam for the Nazi cause, however, the sham contest might have generated another variation of the threat to external validity.

Webb et al. (1966) offer a systematic development of the approach. The title of this book—*Unobtrusive Measures: Non-Reactive Research in the Social Sciences*—says much. Webb *et al.* (1966) saw the use of secondary data as a method to control threats to external validity, particularly "reactive arrangements." Secondary data have a compensating advantage nevertheless in that the people who created the data presumably had no interest in the hypothesis that the data were used to test. Analyses of household and bank accounts of antebellum plantations by Fogel and Engerman (1974) illustrate this principle.

Mundane household accounts and records collected and archived by governments are another matter. Since these data were generated *sine ira et studio*, the plausible threats to external validity associated with letters and essays— and with primary data for that matter—are a minor concern at worst. But this advantage need not inhere to all archival data. Comparing census and election records in Chicago, Campbell (1976, pp. 49–50) argued that whereas Census workers had no incentive to "fix" their data, precinct bosses in the dominant political party were rewarded for producing high vote totals:

> Surrounding the voting process, there are elaborate precautionary devices designed to ensure its honesty; surrounding the census-taking process, there are few, and these could be easily evaded. Yet, in our region, the voting statistics are regarded with suspicion while the census statistics are widely trusted (despite under-enumeration of young adult, black males). I believe this order of relative trust to be justified. The best explanation for it is that votes have continually been used – have had real implications as far as jobs, money, and power are concerned – and have therefore been under great pressure from efforts to corrupt. On the other hand, until recently our census data were unused for political decision-making. (Even the constitutional requirement that electoral districts be changed to match population distribution after every census was neglected for decades.)

In light of this general phenomenon, Campbell (1976, p. 49) proposed what some call "Campbell's Law of data corruption." When data are used to evaluate the work of the people who generate or collect the data, Campbell's Law holds that the data are subject to corruption. When crime rates are used to evaluate the effectiveness of police, for example, crime rates drop (Seidman and

Couzens, 1974; Meehan, 2000). When achievement tests are used to evaluate the effectiveness of teachers, test scores rise (Koretz, 1992, 2002).[1]

The threats implied by Campbell's Law are not necessarily threats to external validity. An abrupt change in the crime rate might reflect a coincident change in the way that crime incidents are recorded, for example—instrumentation as a threat to internal validity, in other words. Or if bureaucratic recordkeeping processes vary by subpopulation or jurisdiction, the confound might pose a threat to construct validity. This is surely the case when the indicator loses its nominal meaning.

In light of the interpretive ambiguities associated with archival data, Webb et al. (1966) describe how measures of accretion and decay can be used as secondary data. The relative significance of encyclopedia articles could be measured by the accretion of fingerprint smudges on their pages, for example; the relative popularity of museum exhibits could be measured by the wear and tear on floor tiles in front of the exhibits.

Accretion and decay seem to have straightforward interpretations, at least compared to written records. But accretion and decay are subject to the same threats to construct validity. Finding what appeared to be inscriptions on bones in a French cave, for example, François Bordes interpreted the bone markings as the work of a cave artist. This interpretation proved incorrect. Binford (1981) found identically marked bones in an area that had no caves. The markings that Bordes had interpreted as abstract art were created by an acid secreted from the roots of grasses that grew over the shallowly buried bones.

In principle, we can infer much about a neighborhood from its graffiti. Likewise, we can read prisoners' tattoos to draw inferences about their criminal careers. Inferences drawn from measures like these require interpretation, and therein lies the potential threat to construct validity. Measures of accretion and decay are no different in that respect than facial expressions, gaits and postures, or polygraph records.

9.2 TIMEFRAMES

From a methodological perspective, the two most important time series in this book are Kroeber's skirt widths (Figure 1.1) and Directory Assistance

---

1. Enemy fatality counts are another example, albeit a grisly one. Near the end of the Vietnam War, Campbell (1976, p. 53) said, "Pressure to score well in this regard was passed down from higher officers to field commanders. The realities of guerrilla warfare participation by persons of a wide variety of sexes and ages added a permissive ambiguity to the situation. Thus poor Lt. Calley was merely engaged in getting bodies to count for the weekly effectiveness report when he participated in the tragedy at My Lai. His goals had been corrupted by the worship of a quantitative indicator, leading both to a reduction in the validity of that indicator for its original military purposes, and a corruption of the social processes it was designed to reflect."

calls to Cincinnati Bell (Figure 1.5). Whereas Kroeber thought that the broad up-and-down movement in his time series was *un*natural, in fact these movements are typical of time series generated by integrated processes. Abrupt changes in level, on the other hand, such as those that we see in the Directory Assistance time series, are not generated by natural processes. Having observed a change of this sort, it is reasonable to suspect *un*natural, exogenous causes.

Controlling the common threats to internal and statistical conclusion validities amounts to recognizing the differences between these two time series. Other natural patterns of change can pose threats to external validity, however. One wholly natural pattern of change that we call "temporal drift" poses a threat to construct or external validity. The best-known examples of this threat occur in long historical time series of economic wealth:

> The difficulties in measuring economic growth, supply of empirical data apart, lie precisely in this point: modern economic growth implies major structural changes and correspondingly large modifications in social and institutional conditions under which the greatly increased product *per capita* is attained. Yet for purposes of measurement, the changing components of the structure must be reduced to a common denominator; otherwise it would be impossible to compare the product of the economy of the United States with that of China, or the product of an advanced country today with its output a century ago when many of the goods and industries that loom so large today were unknown. (Kuznets, 1959, p. 15)

Tiny changes in the nature of wealth can be ignored over short timeframes. Over longer timeframes, the sequence of tiny changes may accumulate, rendering time series segments noncomparable. A drift hypothesis might explain the evolving, changing variance in Beveridge's wheat price time series (Figure 3.12), for example. Semantic drift suggests other examples. The meanings of words, phrases, and concepts change constantly. The rate of change is ordinarily so gradual that changes in meaning pass unnoticed over short timeframes. Over a long enough timeframe, however, older and newer meanings are likely to differ radically. Kroeber's skirt-width time series (Figure 1.1) might also be explained as drift or, more to the point, as the integration of tiny annual changes in fashion.

The tendency to overlook temporal drift reflects our natural science heritage. When neutrino physicists assume that the behavior of these tiny particles is constant across even the longest timeframes, their assumption is at least approximately warranted. When social and behavioral scientists use an analogous assumption, however, it is almost never warranted. Over a long enough timeframe, the meanings of virtually all social and behavioral phenomena drift. The complicating effects of drift can sometimes be ignored or modeled. But on other occasions, drift can pose a serious threat to external validity.

On the other hand, replication per se can provide a degree of control for threats to external validity that arise from a specific timeframe. To illustrate, consider the hypothetical case of a psychologist who wants to evaluate the impact of a pedagogic technique on achievement scores. Concerned for internal validity, the investigation begins in a laboratory where experimental control is nearly absolute. But then, to control external validity, the prudent psychologist replicates the intervention in a classroom, in a school, and finally in a school system. We are tempted to diagram this design as

Laboratory	...	O O O O X O O O O ...
Classroom	...	O O O O X O O O O ...
School	...	O O O O X O O O O ...
School District	...	O O O O X O O O O ...

But to the extent that comparisons across the levels of aggregation provide the same sort of control provided by the placebo control group vaccine trial, this diagram is deceptive. Although it appears that the laboratory, classroom, school, and school system time series experiments occurred simultaneously, the four experiments would more likely occur over a period of years and in sequence. After all, the four studies are replications designed to control threats to external validity posed by subjects and situations. At the same time, however, the replications control threats posed by narrow, short timeframes.

Threats to external validity can also arise from short-run temporal variations. The impact of an intervention may vary by time of day or day of the week, for example. The two British Breathalyzer time series (Figure 7.7) illustrate the general principle. Day-of-the-week variation was discussed in Chapter 8.1. Unmodeled weekday cycles that reflect the natural ebb and flow of social life can pose a threat to construct validity. When the impact of an intervention varies by weekday, however, threats to external validity are plausible. The same principle applies to variation by month or even by historical era. Re-analyses of the Hovland-Sears time series (Figure 1.3), for example, find that, contrary to the frustration-aggression hypothesis, the weak negative correlation between lynchings and cotton prices was limited to the World War I years.

The threat to external validity in each of these examples limits an observed effect to a specific era, a recurring season, or a weekday. Unfortunately, we know of no simple methods for controlling these external validity threats. Temporal limitations can sometimes be discovered through experimentation, and that is often the best that can be done. When a temporal limitation is discovered, of course, the limitation can be incorporated into the larger theory that motivated the time series experiment in the first place.

9.3 THE ROLE OF DESIGN

To highlight the analogy to internal validity, Campbell (1957; Campbell and Stanley, 1966) offered a list of four *threats* to external validity and two external design structures that had been used to control the threats. This aspect of the analogy was weak at best. While the two validities serve a common function in a larger, broader sense of the word, the common use of *experimental* "design" structures to control threats to internal and external validity is a coincidental accident at most. The impact of the coincidental accident is small and, moreover, disproportionately distributed across the four threats. Although a generation of social scientists was led to believe that the *Solomon Four-Group* design was important enough to commit to memory, for example, its use was limited to a small subgenre of applied marketing research. Very few social scientists will ever encounter a situation warranting the expense of a Solomon Four-Group design.

Based on its prevalence in the behavioral, biomedical, and social science applications, the most important threat to external validity—indeed, the *only* important threat to external validity— is the threat called "reactive arrangements" or "reactivity." As Campbell analyzed this threat, it was commonly encountered in testing the effects of experimental interventions on human subjects. For example,

> Half of my own students fail to answer the following question correctly: When one adds a placebo control group in a pharmaceutical experiment, is this done to improve internal or external validity? As I read Campbell (1957) and Campbell and Stanley (1966), the correct answer is external validity.—Campbell (1986, p. 67)

A placebo control group can be used to control this threat to external validity whenever a reaction to an intervention is expected *and* a sham treatment is ethically permitted. Where placebo-like reactions arise from variations in populations and situations, on the other hand, the implied threats to external validity can only be controlled by means of replication across populations and situations. Controlling threats to external validity by replication is time-consuming, to say the least, and that is why experimenters prefer control by design. Threats to external validity can be controlled by design only in rare instances, unfortunately.

The time series in Figures 9.1 and 9.2 are an exception. Prior to March 2008, prophylactic antibiotics were prescribed for virtually all U.K. patients who were scheduled for major oral surgeries. In March 2008, the National Institute for Health and Clinical Excellence (NICE) announced a new set of guidelines that restricted antibiotic prophylaxis to patients at moderate to high risk for infectious endocarditis. The time series in Figure 9.1 show the number of antibiotic prescriptions written by dental surgeons and general-practice physicians. The time series in Figure 9.2 show the number of prescriptions broken down by

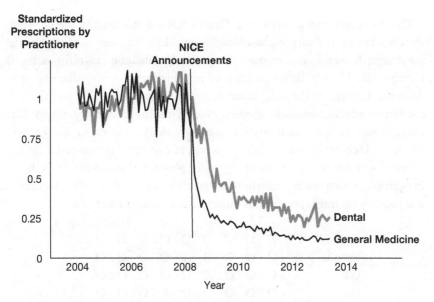

Figure 9.1 U.K. Standardized Prescriptions by Practitioner

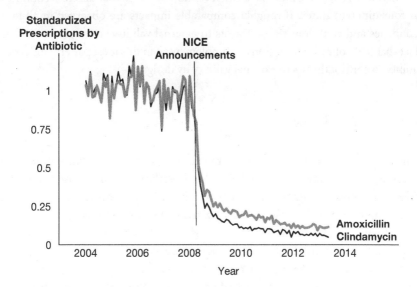

Figure 9.2 U.K. Standardized Prescriptions by Antibiotic

amoxicillin and clindamycin, two antibiotics. To facilitate comparison across practitioners and antibiotics, all of the time series were divided by their respective pre-intervention means. The March 2008 announcement has a large, gradually accruing impact on all of the time series. Dayer et al. (2015) report no significant differences in the impact across practitioners and antibiotics. We agree.

The consensus impact shown in Figures 9.1 and 9.2 renders the common threats to external validity implausible *by design*. Most situations lack the potential for design, however, and even in this particular situation, an obvious threat remains: Would a similar announcement of guidelines have a similar impact in Australia, Canada, or the U.S.? Since Australia, Canada, the U.K., and the U.S. are developed economies with modern, rational health care delivery systems, one might expect guideline announcements to have similar impacts in each of these countries. Despite their similarities, however, idiosyncratic nation-to-nation differences in health care systems will always be a plausible threat to external validity. In principle, a comparative case study design of the sort used by political scientists and sociologists might control this threat. In this particular instance:

```
Australia  ...  O  O  O  O  O  O  X  O  O  ...
Canada     ...  O  O  O  O  X  O  O  O  O  ...
U.K.       ...  O  O  O  X  O  O  O  O  O  ...
U.S.       ...  O  O  O  O  X  O  O  O  ...
```

This ideal design assumes that an intervention occurs in four different countries at four different times. If roughly comparable impacts are observed in all four countries and at all four times, threats to external validity are implausible. The fact that few policy interventions are implemented in this ideal pattern limits our ability to control threats to external validity by design.

9.4 CONCLUSION

There is virtually no disagreement on the meaning of external validity. A *threat* to external validity is any factor that limits the generalizability of an observed result. Removing those threats that limit generalizability across measures or constructs, the common threats to external validity accrue from variations across subjects and situations and to variations across timeframes. Unlike all threats to statistical conclusion and internal validities and some threats to construct validity, threats to external validity cannot ordinarily be controlled by design. Threats associated with variations in persons and situations can be mitigated to some extent by using unobtrusive secondary data instead of relatively obtrusive primary data. Secondary data are not likely to mitigate threats associated with timeframes, however.

Nor is there any disagreement on how threats to external validity are to be controlled. In rare instances, natural features of the environment can be harnessed to control threats. In most instances, however, regardless of the source or nature of the threat, it can only be controlled by *replication*—across subjects, situations, and timeframes. This seldom happens, unfortunately, because the academic incentive structure discourages replication. Journals eschew replications. Worse, once an effect (or lack of an effect) has been demonstrated, it is accepted without question. Replications that fail to find the established effect are assumed to be flawed and are relegated to the file drawer.

It appears now that many of the established effects may be incorrect. Social scientists organized as the *Open Science Collaboration* recently attempted to replicate 100 experimental and correlational studies published in three mainstream psychology journals. Sixty percent of the replications failed to reproduce the published effect, leading to a "reproducibility crisis":

> Reproducibility is a defining feature of science, but the extent to which it characterizes current research is unknown. Scientific claims should not gain credence because of the status or authority of their originator but by the replicability of their supporting evidence. Even research of exemplary quality may have irreproducible empirical findings because of random or systematic error. (Open Science Collaboration, 2015, p. 943)

Although many explanations for the crisis have been proposed, from our perspective, the reproducibility crisis is the obvious consequence of ignoring threats to external validity that stem from uncontrolled variations in persons, situations, and timeframes.

Van Bavel et al. (2015) reinforce our interpretation of the reproducibility crisis. Re-analyzing the Open Science Collaboration (2015) report, Van Bavel et al. (2015. p. 5) found that

> the contextual sensitivity of research topics in psychology was associated with replication success, even after statistically adjusting for several methodological characteristics. This analysis focused on broad, macrolevel contextual influences—time, culture, location, and population—and, ultimately, collapsed across these very different sources of variability. Future work should test these (and other) factors separately and begin to develop a more nuanced model of the influence of context on reproducibility. Moreover, the breadth of contextual sensitivity surveyed in our analysis might represent an underestimation of a host of local influences that may determine whether an effect is replicated. These additional influences range from obvious but sometimes overlooked factors, such as the race or gender of an experimenter, temperature, and time of day, to the more amorphous (*e.g.*, how the demeanor of an experimenter conducting a first-time test of a hypothesis she believes is credible may differ from that of an experimenter assessing whether a study will replicate). Although it is difficult for any single researcher to anticipate and specify every potential moderator, that is the

central enterprise of future research. The lesson here is not that context is too hard to study but rather that context is too important to ignore.

Since the original studies and their replications differed by time, culture, location, and population, we infer that the original findings were spurious causal artifacts of these variables, at least in part. Failing to control the effects of the experimenter's personal characteristics, including race, sex, attractiveness, and so forth; the effects of local ambience; and the effects of a host of other contextual variables, the original finding may not be reproducible.

The pessimistic implication of the reproducibility crisis is that "most published research findings are false" (Ioannidis, 2005). While we do not reject the kernel of this claim, the implied pessimism is unwarranted in our opinion. When we successfully control threats to internal or statistical conclusion validity, we learn nothing new. When we fail to control threats to external validity, on the other hand, we learn something about the conditions under which an intervention has no effect. By exploring the surface of possible contextural variations, we can place bounds on when, where, and how the intervention works to produce the effect. No feature of experimental design can replace the tedious, time-consuming effort to replicate the original result. In that sense, external validity is the engine of knowledge.

REFERENCES

Aaronson, D.E., C.T. Dienes and M.C. Musheno (1978) Changing the public drunkenness laws: The impact of decriminalization. *Law and Society Review*, 12, 405–436.

Abadie, A., A. Diamond and J. Hainmueller (2010) Synthetic control methods for comparative case studies: Estimating the effect of California's tobacco control program. *Journal of the American Statistical Association*, 105, 493–505.

Abadie, A., A. Diamond and J. Hainmueller (2011) Synth: An R package for synthetic control methods in comparative case studies. *Journal of Statistical Software*, 42, 1–17.

Abadie, A. and J. Gardeazabal (2003) The economic cost of conflict: A case study of the Basque country. *American Economic Review*, 93, 113–132.

Abel, T.F. (1938) *Why Hitler Came into Power*. New York: Prentice-Hall.

Abraham, B. (1981) Missing observations in time series. *Communications in Statistics Theory, A*, 10, 1643–1653.

Agresti, A. and B. Finlay (1997) *Statistical Methods for the Social Sciences*, 3rd Edition. Upper Saddle River, NJ: Prentice-Hall.

Akaike, H. (1974) A new look at the statistical model identification. *IEEE Transactions on Automatic Control*, 19, 716–723.

Anderson, D.M., B. Hansen and D.I. Rees (2013) Medical marijuana laws, traffic fatalities, and alcohol consumption. *Journal of Law and Economics*, 56, 333–363.

Anderson, R.M. and R.M. May (1992) *Infectious Diseases of Humans: Dynamics and Control*. Oxford: Oxford University Press.

Andrews, D.W.K. (1993) Tests for parameter instability and structural change with unknown change point. *Econometrica*, 61, 821–856.

Aristotle (1984) *Posterior Analytics*. Pp. 114–166 in J. Barnes (ed.) *Complete Works of Aristotle: The Revised Oxford Translation*. Princeton, NJ: Princeton University Press.

Bacon, F. (2000) *The New Organon*, in L. Jardine and M. Silverthorne (eds.). New York: Cambridge University Press.

Barron, D.N. (1992) The analysis of count data: Overdispersion and autocorrelation. *Sociological Methodology*, 22, 179–220.

Bechtold, H.T. (1959) Construct validity: A critique. *American Psychologist*, 14, 619–629.

Beck, L.W. (1950) Constructions and inferred entities. *Philosophy of Science*, 17, 74–86.

Becker, H.S. (1953) Becoming a marijuana user. *American Journal of Sociology*, 59, 235–243.

Berger, J.O. (2003) Could Fisher, Jeffreys and Neyman have agreed on testing? *Statistical Science*, 18, 1–32.

Berger, J.O. and M. Delampady (1987) Testing precise hypotheses. *Statistical Science*, 2, 317–352.

Beveridge, W.H. (1922) Wheat prices and rainfall in western Europe. *Journal of the Royal Statistical Society*, 85, 412–475.

Bhattacharyya, M.N. and A.P. Layton (1979) Effectiveness of seat belt legislation on the Queensland road toll: An Australian case study in intervention analysis. *Journal of the American Statistical Association*, 74, 596–603.

Binford, L.R. (1981) *Bones: Ancient Men and Modern Myths*. New York: Academic Press.

Bower, C.R., W.L. Padia and G.V. Glass (1974) *TMS: Two FORTRAN IV Programs for Analysis of Time-series Experiments*. Laboratory of Educational Research, University of Colorado, Boulder.

Box, G.E.P. (1979) Robustness in the strategy of scientific model building. *Robustness in statistics*, 1, 201–236.

Box, G.E.P. and D.R. Cox (1964) An analysis of transformations. *Journal of the Royal Statistical Society. Series B (Methodological)*, 211–252.

Box, G.E.P. and G.M. Jenkins (1970) *Time Series Analysis: Forecasting and Control*. San Francisco: Holden-Day.

Box, G.E.P. and D.A. Pierce (1970) Distribution of residual autocorrelations in autoregressive-integrated moving average time series models. *Journal of the American Statistical Association*, 65, 1509–1526.

Box, G.E.P. and G.C. Tiao (1975) Intervention analysis with applications to economic and environmental problems. *Journal of the American Statistical Association*, 70, 70–79.

Box, G.E.P. and G.C. Tiao (1976) Comparison of forecast and actuality. *Journal of the Royal Statistical Society, C*, 25, 195–200.

Box-Steffensmeier, J.M., J.R. Freeman, M.P. Hitt and J.C.W. Pevehouse (2015) *Time Series Analysis for the Social Sciences*. New York: Cambridge University Press.

Brandt, P.T. and J.T. Williams (2001) A linear Poisson autoregressive model: The Poisson AR(p) model. *Political Analysis*, 9, 164–184.

Bunge, M. (1959) *Causality and Modern Science*, 3rd Edition. New York: Dover.

Burnham, K.P. and D.R. Anderson (2002) *Model Selection and Inference: A Practical Information-Theoretical Approach*, 2nd Edition. New York: Springer-Verlag.

Burnham, K.P. and Anderson, D.R. (2004) Multimodel inference: Understanding AIC and BIC in model selection. *Sociological Methods and Research*, 33, 261–304.

Burns, D.M., C. Berry, B. Rosbrook, J. Goodman, E. Gilpin, D. Winn and D. Bal (1991) Reducing tobacco consumption in California: Proposition 99 seems to work. *Journal of the American Medical Association*, 265, 1257–1257.

Cameron, A.C. and P.K. Trivedi (1998) *Regression Analysis of Count Data*. New York: Cambridge University Press.

Campbell, D.T. (1957) Factors relevant to the validity of experiments in social settings. *Psychological Bulletin*, 54, 297–312.

Campbell, D.T. (1960) Recommendations for APA test stanadards regarding construct, trait, or discriminant validity. *American Psychologist*, 15, 546–553.

Campbell, D.T. (1963) From description to experimentation: Interpreting trends as quasi-experiments. Pp. 212–243 in C.W. Harris (ed.) *Problems in Measuring Change.* Madison: University of Wisconsin Press.

Campbell, D.T. (1969) Reforms as experiments. *American Psychologist,* 24, 409–429.

Campbell, D.T. (1971) Methods for the Experimenting Society. Address to the American Psychological Association, September 5, 1971, Washington D.C.

Campbell, D.T. (1974) Evolutionary epistemology. Pp. 413–463 in P.A. Schilpp (ed.) *The Philosophy of Karl Popper.* LaSalle, IL: Open Court.

Campbell, D.T. (1975) III. "Degrees of freedom"and the case study. *Comparative Political Studies,* 8, 178–193.

Campbell, D.T. (1976) Assessing the impact of planned social change. No. 8 in the Occasional Paper Series, Public Affairs Center, Dartmouth College.

Campbell, D.T. (1986) Relabeling internal and external validity for applied social scientists. Pp. 67–77 in W.M.K. Trochim (ed.) *Advancements in Quasi-Experimental Design and Analysis, New Directions for Program Evaluation, No. 31.* San Francisco: Jossey-Bass.

Campbell, D.T. (1991[1971]) Methods for the experimenting society. *American Journal of Evaluation,* 12, 223–260.

Campbell, D.T. and A.E. Erlebacher (1970) How regression artifacts in quasi-experimental evaluations can mistakenly make compensatory education look harmful. In J. Helmuth (ed.) *The Disadvantaged Child, Volume III, Compensatory Education: A National Debate.* New York: Brunner-Mazel.

Campbell, D.T. and D.A. Kenny (1999) *A Primer on Regression Artifacts.* New York: Guilford Press.

Campbell, D.T. and H.L. Ross (1968) The Connecticut crackdown on speeding. *Law and Society Review,* 3, 33–53.

Campbell, D.T. and J.C. Stanley (1966) *Experimental and Quasi-experimental Designs for Research.* Skokie, IL: Rand McNally.

Chen, C. and L-M. Liu (1993) Forecasting time series with outliers. *Journal of Forecasting,* 12, 13–35.

Chree, C. (1913) Some phenomena of sunspots and of terrestrial magnetism at Kew Observatory. *Philosophical Transactions of the Royal Society of London, A,* 212, 75–116.

Cobb, L. and S. Zacks (1985) Applications of catastrophe theory for statistical modeling in the biosciences. *Journal of the American Statistical Association,* 80, 793–802.

Cohen, J. (1988) *Statistical Power Analysis for the Behavioral Sciences,* 2nd Edition. Englewood Cliffs, NJ: L.E. Erlbaum Associates.

Cohen, J. (1992) A power primer. *Psychological Bulletin,* 112, 155–159.

Cohen, J. (1994) The earth is round ($p < .05$). *American Psychologist,* 49, 997–1003.

Coleman, B.J. and C.D. Wiggins (1996) Using interrupted time series analysis to assess an allegedly damaging event. *Litigation Economics Digest* 1, 3–18.

Coleman, J.S. (1964) *Introduction to Mathematical Sociology.* Glencoe, IL: The Free Press.

Cook, T.D. and D.T. Campbell (1976) The design and conduct of quasi-experiments and true experiments in field settings. Pp. 223–336 in M.D. Dunnette (ed.) *Handbook of Industrial and Organizational Psychology.* Chicago: Rand McNally.

Cook, T.D. and D.T. Campbell (1979) *Quasi-experimentation: Design and Analysis Issues for Field Settings.* Boston: Houghton-Mifflin.

Cronbach, L.J. (1982) *Designing Evaluations of Educational and Social Programs*. San Francisco: Jossey-Bass.

Cronbach, L.J. and P.E. Meehl (1955) Construct validity in psychological tests. *Psychological Bulletin*, 52, 281–302.

Crosbie, J. (1993) Interrupted time-series analysis with brief single-subject data. *Journal of Consulting and Clinical Psychology*, 61, 966–974.

Dayer, M.J., S. Jones, B. Prendergast, L.M. Baddour, P.B. Lockhart and M.H. Thornhill (2015) Incidence of infective endocarditis in England, 2000–2013: A secular trend, interrupted time-series analysis. *Lancet*, 385, 1219–1228.

Deutsch, S.J. and F.B. Alt (1977) The effect of Massachusetts' gun control law on gun-related crimes in the City of Boston. *Evaluation Quarterly*, 1, 543–568.

Dickey, D.A., W.R. Bell and R.B. Miller (1986) Unit roots in time series models: Tests and implications. *American Statistician*, 40, 12–26.

Dickey, D.A. and W.A. Fuller (1979) Distribution of the estimators for autoregressive time series with a unit root. *Journal of the American Statistical Association*, 74, 427–431.

Diehl, H.S., A.B. Baker and D.W. Cowan (1938) Cold vaccines: An evaluation based on a controlled study. *Journal of the American Medical Association*, 2, 1168–1173.

Dienes, Z. (2011) Bayesian versus orthodox statistics: Which side are you on? *Perspectives on Psychological Science*, 6, 274–290.

Dobrin, A., B. Wiersema, C. Loftin and D. McDowall (1996) *Statistical Handbook of Violence in America*. Phoenix: Oryx.

Dollard, J., L.W. Doob, N.E. Miller, O.H. Mowrer and R.R. Sears (1939) *Frustration and Aggression*. New Haven: Yale University Press.

Edgington, E.S. (1996) Randomized single-subject experimental designs. *Behavioral Research and Therapy*, 34, 567–574.

Edwards, A.W.F. (1972) *Likelihood. An Account of the Statistical Concept of Likelihood and its Application to Scientific Inference*. Cambridge: Cambridge University Press.

Edwards, W., H. Lindman and L.J. Savage (1963) Bayesian statistical inference for psychological research. *Psychological Review*, 70, 193–242.

Efron, B. (1976) Discussion. *Annals of Statistics*, 4, 483–484.

Elliott, G., T.J. Rothenberg and J.H. Stock (1996) Efficient tests for an autoregressive unit root. *Econometrica*, 64, 813–836.

Elton, C.S. (1924) Fluctuations in the numbers of animals: Their causes and effects. *British Journal of Experimental Biology*, 2, 119–163.

Elton, C.S. and M. Nicholson (1942) The ten-year cycle in numbers of the lynx in Canada. *Journal of Animal Ecology*, 11, 215–244.

Enders, W. (2010) *Applied Econometric Time Series*, 3rd Edition. New York: Wiley.

Engle, R.F. and C.W.J. Granger (1987) Co-integration and error correction: Representation, estimation, and testing. *Econometrica*, 55, 251–276.

Evans, R. (1997) Soothsaying or science? Falsification, uncertainty and social change in macroeconomic modelling. *Social Studies of Science*, 27, 395–438.

Ewald, P.W. (1994) *Evolution of Infectious Disease*. New York: Oxford University Press.

Falcon, A. (2014) Aristotle on Causality. In E.N. Zalta (ed.) *The Stanford Encyclopedia of Philosophy*, http://plato.stanford.edu/.

Fisher, R.A. (1921) Studies in crop variation: An examination of the yield of dressed grain from Broadbalk. *Journal of Agricultural Science*, 11, 107–135.

Fisher, R.A. (1922a) On the interpretation of χ^2 from contingency tables, and the calculation of P. *Journal of the Royal Statistical Society*, 85, 87–94.

Fisher, R.A. (1922b) IX. On the mathematical foundations of theoretical statistics. *Philosophical Transactions of the Royal Society of London, A*, 222, 309–368.

Fisher, R.A. (1925) *Statistical Methods for Research Workers*. London: Oliver and Boyd.

Fisher, R.A. (1929) The statistical method in psychical research. *Proceedings of the Society for Psychical Research*, 39, 189–192.

Fisher, R.A. (1935) *Design of Experiments*. London: Oliver and Boyd.

Fisher, R.A. (1935) The fiducial argument in statistical inference. *Annals of Eugenics*, 6, 391–398.

Fisher, R.A. (1955) Statistical methods and scientific induction. *Journal of the Royal Statistical Society, B*, 17, 69–78.

Fisher, R.A. (1970) *Statistical Methods and Scientific Inference*, 3rd Edition. New York: Hafner Press.

Florence, P.S. (1923) Recent researches in industrial fatigue. *Economic Journal*, 33, 185–197.

Fogel, R.W. and S.L. Engerman (1974) *Time on the Cross: The Economics of American Negro Slavery*. Boston: Little, Brown.

Fox, K.K., W.L. Whittington, W.C. Levine, J.S. Moran, A. Zaidi and A.K. Nakashima (1998) Gonorrhea in the United States, 1981–1996: Demographic and geographic trends. *Sexually Transmitted Diseases*, 25, 386–393.

Franke, R.H. (1980) Worker productivity at Hawthorne. *American Sociological Review*, 45, 1006–1027.

Franke, R.H. and J.D. Kaul (1978) The Hawthorne experiments: First statistical interpretation. *American Sociological Review*, 43, 623–643.

Frick, R.W. (1996) The appropriate use of null hypothesis testing. *Psychological Methods*, 1, 379–390.

Friedman, M. (1948) A monetary and fiscal framework for economic stability. *American Economic Review*, 38, 245–264.

Friesema, H.P., J.A. Caporaso, G. Goldstein, R.L. Lineberry and R. McCleary (1978) *Aftermath: Communities After Natural Disaster*. Beverly Hills: Sage.

Friman, P.C., K.E. Hoff, C. Schnoes, K.A. Freeman, D.W. Woods and N. Blum (1999) The bedtime pass: An approach to bedtime crying and leaving the room. *Archives of Pediatric and Adolescent Medicine*, 153, 1027–1029.

Fruhwirth-Schnatter, S. (1995) Bayesian model discrimination and Bayes factors for linear Gaussian state space models. *Journal of the Royal Statistical Society, B*, 57, 237–246.

Fuller, W. A. (1996) *Introduction to Statistical Time Series*. New York: Wiley.

Garey, K.W., D. Lai, T.K. Dao-Tran, L.O. Gentry, L.Y. Hwang and B.R. Davis (2008) Interrupted time series analysis of vancomycin compared to cefuroxime for surgical prophylaxis in patients undergoing cardiac surgery. *Antimicrobial Agents and Chemotherapy*, 52, 446–451.

Gautier, P.A., A. Siegmann and A. Van Vuuren (2009) Terrorism and attitudes towards minorities: The effect of the Theo van Gogh murder on house prices in Amsterdam. *Journal of Urban Economics*, 65, 113–126.

Geweke, J. and C. Whiteman (2006) Bayesian forecasting. Pp. 1–80 in G. Elliott, C.W.J. Granger and A. Timmermann (eds.), *Handbook of Economic Forecasting, Volume 1*. Amsterdam: Elsevier.

Ghosh, J.K., M. Delampady and T. Samanta (2006) *An Introduction to Bayesian Analysis: Theory and Methods*. New York: Springer.

Gigerenzer, G., Z. Swijtink, T. Porter, L. Daston, J. Beatty and L. Kruger (1989) *The Empire of Chance: How Probability Changed Science and Everyday Life*. Cambridge: Cambridge University Press.

Gill, J. (1999) The insignificance of null hypothesis significance testing. *Political Research Quarterly*, 52, 647–674.

Glantz, S.A. (1993) Changes in cigarette consumption, prices, and tobacco industry revenues associated with California's Proposition 99. *Tobacco Control*, 2, 311–314.

Glantz, S.A. and E.D. Balbach (2004) *Tobacco War: Inside the California Battles*. Berkeley: University of California Press.

Glass, G.V. (1968) Analysis of data on the Connecticut speeding crackdown as a time-series quasi-experiment. *Law and Society Review*, 3, 55–76.

Glass, G.V., V.L. Willson and J.M. Gottman (1975) *Design and Analysis of Time Series Experiments*. Boulder: Colorado Associated University Press.

Glymour, C. (1986) Comment: Statistics and metaphysics. *Journal of the American Statistical Association*, 81, 964–966.

Goodman, S.N. (1999) Toward evidence-based medical statistics. 1: The P value fallacy. *Annals of Internal Medicine*, 130, 995–1004.

Goodman, S.N. (2008) A dirty dozen: Twelve P-value misconceptions. *Seminars in Hematology*, 45, 135–140.

Goodman, S.N. and J.A. Berlin (1994) The use of predicted confidence intervals when planning experiments and the misuse of power when interpreting results. *Annals of Internal Medicine*, 121, 200–206.

Granger, C.W.J. (1969) Investigating causal relationships by econometric models and cross-spectral methods. *Econometrica*, 37, 424–438.

Granger, C.W.J. (1981) Some properties of time series data and their use in econometric model specification. *Journal of Econometrics*, 16, 121–130.

Granger, C. W.J. (1991) Developments in the nonlinear analysis of economic series. *The Scandinavian Journal of Economics*, 263–276.

Granger, C.W.J. (1992) Forecasting stock market prices: Lessons for forecasters. *International Journal of Forecasting*, 8, 3–13.

Granger, C.W.J. and P. Newbold (1977) *Forecasting Economic Time Series*. New York: Academic Press.

Gregory, A.W. and B.E. Hansen (1996) Tests for cointegration in models with regime and trend shifts. *Oxford Bulletin of Economics and Statistics*, 58, 555–560.

Gregory, A.W., J. Nason and D.G. Watt (1996) Testing for structural breaks in cointegrated relationships. *Journal of Econometrics*, 71, 321–342.

Hacking, I. (2001) *An Introduction to Probability and Inductive Logic*. New York: Cambridge University Press.

Hájek, A. (2012) Interpretations of probability. In E.N. Zalta (ed.), *The Stanford Encyclopedia of Philosophy*, http://plato.stanford.edu.

Hall, R.V., R. Fox, D. Willard, L. Goldsmith, M. Emerson, M. Owen, F Davis and E. Porcia (1971) The teacher as observer and experimenter in the modification of disputing and talking-out behaviors. *Journal of Applied Behavior Analysis*, 4, 141–149.

Hamilton, J.D. (1994) *Time Series Analysis*. Princeton, NJ: Princeton University Press.

Hansen, B.E. (2001) The new econometrics of structural change: Dating breaks in U.S. labor productivity. *Journal of Economic Perspectives*, 15, 117–128.

Harvey, A.C. (1989) *Forecasting, Structural Time Series Models and the Kalman Filter*. New York: Cambridge University Press.

Harvey, A.C. and C. Fernandes (1989) Time series models for count or qualitative observations. *Journal of Business and Economic Statistics*, 7, 407–417.

Hawton, K., H. Bergen, S. Simkin, A. Brock, C. Griffiths, E. Romeri, K.L. Smith, N. Kapur and D. Gunnell (2009) Effect of withdrawal of co-proxamol on prescribing and deaths from drug poisoning in England and Wales: Time series analysis. *BMJ*, 338, b2270.

Hay, R.A., Jr. and R. McCleary (1979) Box-Tiao time series models for impact assessment. *Evaluation Review*, 3, 245–292.

Hennigan, K.M., M.L. Del Rosario, L. Heath, T.D. Cook, J.D. Wharton and B. Calder (1982) Impact of the introduction of television on crime in the United States: Empirical findings and theoretical implications. *Journal of Personality and Social Psychology*, 42, 461–477.

Hepworth, J.T. and S.G. West (1989) Lynchings and the economy: A time-series reanalysis of Hovland and Sears. *Journal of Personality and Social and Psychology*, 55, 239–247.

Holland, P.W. (1986) Statistics and causal inference. *Journal of the American Statistical Association*, 81, 945–960.

Homel, R. (1988) *Policing and Punishing the Drinking Driver: A Study of General and Specific Deterrence*. New York: Springer-Verlag.

Hovland, C.I. and R.R. Sears (1940) Minor studies of aggression IV. Correlation of lynchings with economic indices. *Journal of Psychology*, 9, 30–310.

Howson, C. and P. Urbach (2006) *Scientific Reasoning: The Bayesian Approach*, 3rd Edition. Chicago: Open Court Publishing.

Hróbjartsson, A. and P.C. Gotzsche (2001) Is the placebo powerless? An analysis of clinical trials comparing placebo with no treatment. *New England Journal of Medicine*, 344, 1594–1603.

Hu, T., H. Sung and T.E. Keeler (1995) Reducing cigarette consumption in California: Tobacco taxes vs. an anti-smoking media campaign. *American Journal of Public Health*, 85, 1218–1222.

Huitema, B.E. (2004) Analysis of interrupted time-series experiments using ITSE: A critique. *Understanding Statistics*, 3(1), 27–46.

Ioannidis, J.P.A. (2005) Why most published research findings are false. *PLoS Medicine*, 2, e124.

Izenman, A.J., J.R. Wolf and H.A. Wolfer (1983) An historical note on the Zurich sunspot relative numbers. *Journal of the Royal Statistical Society, A*, 146, 311–318.

Jeffreys, H. (1935) Some tests of significance, treated by the theory of probability. *Proceedings of the Cambridge Philosophy Society*, 31, 203–222.

Jeffreys, H. (1961) *Theory of Probability*, 3rd Edition. Oxford: Oxford University Press.

Johansen, S., R. Mosconi and B. Nielsen (2000) Cointegration analysis in the presence of structural breaks in the deterministic trend. *Econometrics Journal*, 34, 216–249.

Kadane, J. (2011) *Principles of Uncertainty*. Boca Rato: CRC Press.

Keeling, C.D., R.B. Bacastow, A.F. Carter, S.C. Piper, T.P. Whorf, M. Heimann, W.G. Mook and H. Roeloffzen (1989) A Three-Dimensional Model of Atmospheric CO_2 Transport Based on Observed Winds. I. Analysis of Observational Data. *Geophysical Monograph 55*. Washington D.C.: American Geophysical Union.

Kendall, M.G. (1963) Ronald Aylmer Fisher, 1890–1962. *Biometrika*, 50, 1–15.

Kendall, M.G. and A. Stuart (1979) *The Advanced Theory of Statistics*, Volume 2, 4th Edition. London: Charles Griffin.

Kepka, E.J. (1972) Model Representation and the Threat of Instability in the Interrupted Time Series Quasi-experiment. Unpublished Ph.D. Dissertation, Northwestern University.

Kmenta, J. (1986) *Elements of Econometrics*, 2nd Edition. New York: MacMillan.

King, D.R. (1978) The brutalization effect: Execution publicity and the incidence of homicide in South Carolina. *Social Forces*, 57, 683–687.

Kirby, K.C., M.E. Kerwin, C.M. Carpendo, B.J. Rosenwasser and R.S. Gardener (2008) Interdependent group contingency management for cocaine-dependent methadone maintenance patients. *Journal of Applied Behavior Analysis*, 41, 579–595.

Koretz, D.M. (1992) What happened to test scores and why? *Educational Measurement, Issues and Practices*, 11, 7–11.

Koretz, D.M. (2002) Limitations in the use of achievement tests as measures of educators' productivity. *Journal of Human Resources*, 37, 752–777.

Kposowa, A.J. and K.D. Breault (1998) Temporal factors and homicide in the United States. *Journal of Interpersonal Violence*, 13, 590–604.

Kroeber, A.L. (1919) On the principle of order in civilization as exemplified by changes of fashion. *American Anthropologist*, 21, 235–263.

Kroeber, A.L. (1969) *Configurations of Cultural Growth*. Berkeley: University of California Press.

Krueger, J. (2001) Null hypothesis significance testing: On the survival of a flawed method. *American Psychologist*, 56, 16–26.

Kruschke, J.K. (2011) Bayesian assessment of null values via parameter estimation and model comparison. *Perspectives on Psychological Science*, 6, 299–312.

Kruschke, J.K. (2013) *Doing Bayesian Data Analysis: A Tutorial with R and BUGS*. Amsterdam: Academic Press.

Kruschke, J.K., H. Aguinis and H. Joo (2012) The time has come: Bayesian methods for data analysis in the organizational sciences. *Organizational Research Methods*, 15, 722–752.

Kuhn, L., L.L. Davidson and M.S. Durkin (1994) Use of Poisson regression and time series analysis for detecting changes over time in rates of child injury following a prevention program. *American Journal of Epidemiology*, 140, 943–955.

Kuhn, T.S. (1996) *The Structure of Scientific Revolutions*, 3rd Edition. Chicago: University of Chicago Press.

Kuhn, T.S. (2000) What are scientific revolutions? Pp. 13–32 in J. Conant and J. Haugeland (eds.) *The Road Since Structure*. Chicago: University of Chicago Press.

Lai, A. (2011) London cholera and the blind-spot of an epidemiology theory. *Significance*, 8, 82–85.

Leek, J.T. and R.D. Peng (2015) Statistics: P-values are just the tip of the iceberg. *Nature*, 520, 612.

Legge, J.S. (1983) The unintended consequences of policy change: The effect of a restrictive abortion policy. *Administration and Society*, 15, 243–256.

Lenhard, J. (2006) Models and statistical inference: The controversy between Fisher and Neyman-Pearson. *British Journal of Philosophical Science*, 57, 69–91.

Lester, D. (1979) Temporal variation in suicide and homicide. *American Journal of Epidemiology*, 109, 517–520.

Lieberson, S. (1991) Small N's and big conclusions: An examination of the reasoning in comparative studies based on a small number of cases. *Social Forces*, 70, 307–320.

Lin, B., D.L. MacKenzie and T.R. Gulledge, Jr. (1986) Using *ARIMA* models to predict prison populations. *Journal of Quantitative Criminology*, 2, 251–264.

Lipsey, M. (1990) *Design Sensitivity: Statistical Power for Experimental Research*. Sherman Oaks, CA: Sage.

Liu, L.-M. (1999) *Forecasting and Time Series Analysis Using the SCA Statistical System*. Villa Park, IL: Scientific Computing Associates.

Ljung, G.M. and G.E.P. Box (1978) On a measure of lack of fit in time series models. *Biometrika*, 65, 297–303.

MacCorquodale, K. and P.E. Meehl (1948) On a distinction between hypothetical constructs and intervening variables. *Psychological Review*, 55, 95–107.

MacKinnon, J.G. (1994) Approximate asymptotic distribution functions for unit-root and cointegration tests. *Journal of Business and Economic Statistics*, 12, 167–176.

Maddala, G.S. and I-M. Kim (1998) *Unit Roots, Cointegration, and Structural Change*. New York: Cambridge University Press.

Manski, C.F. (2013) Identification of treatment response with social interactions. *Econometrics Journal*, 16, 1–23.

Masson, M.E.J. (2011) A tutorial on a practical Bayesian alternative to null-hypothesis significance testing. *Behavior Research Methods*, 43, 679–690.

Mausner, J.S. and S. Kramer (1985) *Epidemiology: An Introductory Text*, 2nd Edition. Philadelphia: W.B. Saunders.

Mayr, E. (1997) *This Is Biology: The Science of the Living World*. Cambridge, MA: Harvard University Press.

McCain, L.J. and R. McCleary (1979) The statistical analysis of the simple interrupted time-series quasi-experiment. Pp. 233–293 in T.D. Cook and D.T. Campbell (eds.), *Quasi-Experimentation: Design and Analysis Issues for Field Settings*. Chicago: Rand-McNally.

McCleary, R. (2000) Evolution of the time series experiment. Pp. 215–234 in L. Bickman (ed.) *Research Design: Donald Campbell's Legacy*. Thousand Oaks, CA: Sage.

McCleary, R., R.A. Hay, Jr., D. McDowall and E.E. Meidinger (1980) *Applied Time Series Analysis for the Social Sciences*. Beverly Hills: Sage.

McCleary, R. and D. McDowall (1984) A time series approach to causal modeling: Swedish population growth, 1750–1849. *Political Methodology*, 10, 357–375.

McCleary, R. and M.C. Musheno (1980) Floor effects in the time series quasi-experiment. *Political Methodology*, 7, 351–362.

McCleary, R., B.C. Nienstedt and J.M. Erven (1982) Uniform Crime Reports as organizational outcomes: Three time series experiments. *Social Problems*, 29, 361–372.

McCleary, R. and J.E. Riggs (1982) The impact of Australia's 1975 Family Law Act on divorce rates: A general model for evaluating legal impacts. Pp. 7–18 in G.H. Forehand (ed.) *New Directions in Program Evaluation: Applications of Time Series Analysis in Evaluation*. San Francisco: Jossey-Bass.

McCleary, R., P. Touchette, D.V. Taylor and J.L. Barron (1999) Contagious models for self-injurious behavior. Poster presentation, 32nd Annual Gatlinburg Conference on Research and Theory in Mental Retardation.

McDowall, D. and K. Curtis (2015) Seasonal variation in homicide and assault across large U.S. cities. *Homicide Studies*, 19, 303–325.

McDowall, D., R. McCleary, E.E. Medinger and R.A. Hay, Jr. (1980) *Interrupted Time Series Analysis. Volume 21, University Papers Series: Quantitative Applications in the Social Sciences*. Beverly Hills: Sage.

McLeod, A.I. and E.R. Vingilis (2005) Power computations for intervention analysis. *Technometrics*, 47, 174–181.

McSweeney, A.J. (1978) The effects of response cost on the behavior of a million persons: Charging for directory assistance in Cincinnati. *Journal of Applied Behavioral Analysis*, 11, 47–51.

Meehan, A.J. (2000) The organizational career of gang statistics: The politics of policing gangs. *Sociological Quarterly*, 41, 337–370.

Meltzer, A., C. Goodman, K. Langwell, J. Cosler, C. Baghelai and J. Bobula (1980) *Develop Physician and Physician Extender Data Bases. G-155, Final Report*. Applied Management Sciences, Inc., Silver Spring, MD.

Mill, J.S. (2009[1843]) *A System of Logic: Ratiocinative and Inductive*. Project Gutenberg EBook 27942.

Mills, T.C. (1991) *Time Series Techniques for Economists*. New York: Cambridge University Press.

Winship, C. and S.L. Morgan (2007) *Counterfactuals and Causal Inference*. New York: Cambridge University Press.

Morgenstern, O. (1963) *On the Accuracy of Economic Observations*. Princeton, NJ: Princeton University Press.

Mulaik, S.A., N.S. Raju and R.A. Harshman (1997) There is a time and a place for significance testing. Pp. 65–115 in L.L. Harlow, S.A. Mulaik and J.H. Steiger (eds.) *What If There Were No Significance Tests?* New York: Psychology Press.

Murray, M.P. (1994) A drunk and her dog: An illustration of cointegration and error correction. *American Statistician*, 48, 37–39.

Mushkatel, A.J. and L.A. Wilson II (1982) The effects of geographic targeting and programmatic change: The Denver Community Development Agency. *New Directions for Program Evaluation*, 16, 49–63.

Nerlove, M. (1964) Spectral analysis of seasonal adjustment procedures. *Econometrica*, 32, 241–285.

Neter, J., W. Wasserman and G.A. Whitmore (1993) *Applied Statistics*, 4th Edition. Boston: Allyn and Bacon.

Neyman, J. (1934) On the two different aspects of the representative method: The method of stratified sampling and the method of purposive selection. *Journal of the Royal Statistical Society*, 97, 558–625.

Neyman, J. (1956) Note on an article by Sir Ronald Fisher. *Journal of the Royal Statistical Society, B*, 18(2), 288–294.

Neyman, J. (1990[1923]) On the application of probability theory to agriculture experiments: Essay on principles (Section 9). *Statistical Science*, 5, 465–480.

Neyman, J. and E.S. Pearson. (1928a) On the use and interpretation of certain test criteria for purposes of statistical inference: Part I. *Biometrika*, 20A, 175–240.

Neyman, J. and E.S. Pearson (1928b) On the use and interpretation of certain test criteria for purposes of statistical inference: Part II. *Biometrika*, 20A, 263–294.

Ng, S., and P. Perron (1995) Unit root tests in ARMA models with data-dependent methods for the selection of the truncation lag. *Journal of the American Statistical Association*, 90, 268–281.

Nickerson, R.S. (2000) Null hypothesis significance testing: A review of an old and continuing controversy. *Psychological Methods*, 5, 241–301.

Norpoth, H. (1984) Economics, politics, and the cycle of presidential popularity. *Political Behavior*, 6, 253–273.

Norpoth, H. (1986) Transfer function analysis. Chapter 10, pp. 241–273 in W. D. Berry and M. S. Lewis-Beck (eds.) *New Tools for Social Scientists*. Beverly Hills: Sage.

Norpoth, H. (1987a) Guns and butter and government popularity in Britain. *American Political Science Review*, 81, 949–959.

Norpoth, H. (1987b) The Falklands war and government popularity in Britain: Rally without consequence of surge without decline? *Electoral Studies*, 6, 3–16.

Norpoth, H. and T. Yantek (1983) Macroeconomic conditions and fluctuations of presidential popularity: The question of lagged effects. *American Journal of Political Science*, 27, 785–807.

Norton, D.F. and M.J. Norton (2000) *David Hume: A Treatise of Human Nature*. Oxford: Oxford University Press.

O'Grady, K.E. (1988) MMPI and Rorschach: Three decades of research: A time series re-analysis. *Professional Psychology: Research and Practice*, 19, 132–133.

Open Science Collaboration (2015) Estimating the reproducibility of psychological science. *Science*, 349, 943–952.

Ozdowski, S.A. and J. Hattie (1981) The impact of divorce laws on divorce rate in Australia: A time series analysis. *Australian Journal of Social Issues*, 16, 3–17.

Pandiani, J.A. and L.M. Girardi (1993) Diversion of admissions from state hospitals: A re-examination. *Hospital and Community Psychiatry*, 44, 579–580.

Parsonson, B.S. and D.M. Baer (1986) The graphic analysis of data. Pp. 157–186 in A. Poling and R.W. Fuqua (eds.) *Research Methods in Applied Behavior Analysis: Issues and Advances*. New York: Plenum Press.

Patterson, K. (2011) *Unit Root Tests in Time Series, Volume 1: Key Concepts and Problems*. New York: Palgrave Macmillan.

Pawitan, Y. (2013) *In All Likelihood: Statistical Modelling and Inference Using Likelihood*. New York: Oxford University Press.

Pearson, K. (1900) On the criterion that a given system of deviations from the probable in the case of a correlated system of variables is such that it can be reasonably supposed to have arisen from random sampling. *Philosophy Magazine*, Series 5, 50, 157–172.

Phillips, P.C.B. and P. Perron (1988) Testing for a unit root in time series regression. *Biometrika*, 75, 335–346.

Pitcher, B.L. (1981) The Hawthorne experiments: Statistical evidence for a learning hypothesis. *Social Forces*, 60, 133–149.

Polyson, P., R. Peterson and C. Marshall (1986) MMPI and Rorschach: Three decades of research. *Professional Psychology: Research and Practice*, 17, 476–478.

Price, D.D., D.G. Finniss and F. Benedetti (2008) A comprehensive review of the placebo effect: Recent advances and current thought. *Annual Review of Psychology*, 59, 565–590.

Quandt, R. (1960) Tests of a hypothesis that a linear regression obeys two separate regimes. *Journal of the American Statistical Association*, 55, 324–330.

Raftery, A.E. (1995) Bayesian model selection in social research. Pp. 111–195 in P.V. Marsden (ed.) *Sociological Methodology 1995*. Cambridge, MA: Blackwell.

Reed, D. (1978) *Whistlestop: A Community Alternative for Crime Prevention*. Unpublished Ph.D. Dissertation, Northwestern University.

Reichardt, C.S. (2011) Criticisms of and an alternative to the Shadish, Cook, and Campbell validity typology. Pp. 43–53 in H.T. Chen, S.I. Donaldson and M.M. Mark (eds.), *Advancing Validity in Outcome Evaluation: Theory and Practice. New Directions for Evaluation, Number 130*(Vol. 101). San Francisco: Wiley/Jossey-Bass.

Richardson, J. and A.L. Krober (1940) Three centuries of women's dress fashions: A quantitative analysis. *Anthropological Records*, 5, 111–153.

Rindskopf, D.M. (1997) Testing "small," not null, hypotheses: Classical and Bayesian approaches. Pp. 319–332 in L.L. Harlow, S.A. Mulaik and J.H. Steiger (eds.) *What If There Were No Significance Tests?* Mahway, NJ: L.E. Erlbaum and Associates.

Rivara, F.P. and A.L. Kellermann (2007) Reducing the misuse of firearms. Chapter 17, pp. 311–331 in L.S. Doll, S.E. Bonzo, D.A. Sleet and J.A. Mercy (eds.) *Handbook of Injury and Violence Prevention*. New York: Springer.

Roethlisberger, F. and W.J. Dickson (1939) *Management and the Worker*. Cambridge: MA: Harvard University Press.

Ross, H.L., D.T. Campbell and G.V. Glass (1970) Determining the social effects of a legal reform: The British "breathalyzer" crackdown of 1967. *American Behavioral Scientist*, 13, 493–509.

Ross, H.L. and R. McCleary (1983) Methods for studying the impact of drunk driving laws. *Accident Analysis and Prevention*, 15, 415–428.

Ross, H.L. and R. McCleary (1984) Liberalization and rationalization of drunk-driving laws in Scandinavia. *Accident Analysis and Prevention*, 16, 471–487.

Ross, H.L., R. McCleary and T. F. Epperlein (1982) Deterrence of drinking and driving in France: An evaluation of the law of July 12, 1978. *Law and Society Review*, 16, 345–374.

Ross, H.L., R. McCleary and G.D. LaFree (1990) Can mandatory jail laws deter drunk driving? The Arizona case. *Journal of Criminal Law and Criminology*, 81, 156–170.

Rubin, D.B. (1974) Estimating causal effects of treatments in randomized and nonrandomized studies. *Journal of Educational Psychology*, 66, 688–701.

Rubin, D.B. (1977) Assignment of treatment group on the basis of a covariate. *Journal of Educational Statistics*, 2, 1–26.

Rubin, D.B. (1978) Bayesian inference for causal effects: The role of randomization. *Annals of Statistics*, 6, 34–58.

Rubin, D.B. (1980) Randomization analysis of experimental data: The Fisher randomization test comment. *Journal of the American Statistical Association*, 75, 591–593.

Rubin, D.B. (1990) Comment on "Neyman (1923) and causal inference in experiments and observational studies." *Statistical Science*, 5, 472–480.

Rubin, D.B. (2006) *Matched Sampling for Causal Effects*. Cambridge: Cambridge University Press.

Rubin, D.B. (2008) For objective causal inference, design trumps analysis. *Annals of Applied Statistics*, 2, 808–840.

Rubin, D.B. (2010) Reflections stimulated by the comments of Shadish (2010) and West and Thoemmes (2010). *Psychological Methods*, 15, 38–46.

Russell, B. (1918) *Mysticism and Logic and Other Essays*. London: George Allen and Unwin.

Said, S.E. and D.A. Dickey (1984) Testing for unit roots in autoregressive moving average models of unknown order. *Biometrika*, 71, 599–607.

Schlaifer, R. (1980) The relay assembly test room: An alternative statistical interpretation. *American Sociological Review*, 45, 995–1005.

Schmidt, F.L. and J.E. Hunter (1997) Eight common but false objections to the discontinuation of significance testing in the analysis of research data. Pp. 37–64 in L.L. Harlow, S.A. Mulaik and J.H. Steiger (eds.) *What If There Were No Significance Tests?* New York: Psychology Press.

Schnell, D., A. Zaidi and G. Reynolds (1989) A time series analysis of gonorrhea surveillance data. *Statistics in Medicine*, 8, 343–352.

Seidman, D. and M. Couzens (1974) Getting the crime rate down: Political pressure and crime reporting. *Law and Society Review*, 8, 457–494.

Schwarz, G. (1978) Estimating the dimension of a model. *Annals of Statistics*, 6, 461–464.

Shadish, W.R., Cook, T.D. and Campbell, D.T. (2002) *Experimental and Quasi-experimental Designs for Generalized Causal Inference*. New York: Houghton Mifflin.

Shahmanesh, M., V. Patel, D. Mabey and F. Cowan (2008) Effectiveness of interventions for the prevention of HIV and other sexually transmitted infections in female sex workers in resource-poor settings: a systematic review. *Tropical Medicine and International Health*, 13, 659–679.

Shils, E.A. and M. Janowitz (1948) Cohesion and disintegration in the Wehrmacht in World War II. *Public Opinion Quarterly*, 12, 280–315.

Shumway, R.H. and D.S. Stoffer (1980) An approach to time series smoothing and forecasting using the EM algorithm. *Journal of Time Series Analysis*, 3, 253–264.

Shumway, R.H. and D.S. Stoffer (2011) *Time Series Analysis and Its Applications: With R Examples*. New York: Springer.

Silverman, R.A. and L.W. Kennedy (1987) Relational distance and homicide: The role of the stranger. *Journal of Criminal Law and Criminology*, 78, 272–308.

Skyrms, B. (2000) *Choice and Chance: An Introduction to Inductive Logic*, 4th Edition. Belmont, CA: Wadsworth.

Snow, J. (1855) *On the Mode of Communication of Cholera*, 2nd Edition. London: John Churchill.

Spanos, A. (2013) Who should be afraid of the Jeffreys Lindley paradox? *Philosophy of Science*, 80, 73–93.

Spitzer, J.J. (1982) A fast and efficient algorithm for the estimation of parameters in models with the Box-and-Cox transformation. *Journal of the American Statistical Association*, 77, 760–766.

Suppes, P. (1970) *A Probabilistic Theory of Causality*. Amsterdam: North-Holland Publishing.

Tarran, B. (2015) In brief: A psychology journal bans p-values. *Significance*, 12, 6.

Thompson, S.P. (1914) *Calculus Made Easy*, 2nd Enlarged Editon. London: MacMillan.

Thompson, W.W., E. Weintraub, P. Dhankhar, P-Y. Cheng, L. Brammer, M.I. Meltzer, J.S. Bresee and D.K. Shay (2009) Estimates of US influenza-associated deaths made using four different methods. *Influenza and Other Respiratory Viruses*, 3, 37–49.

Tobías, A., J. Díaz, M. Saez and J.C. Alberdi (2001) Use of Poisson regression and Box-Jenkins models to evaluate the short-term effects of environmental noise levels on daily emergency admissions in Madrid, Spain. *European Journal of Epidemiology*, 17, 765–771.

Topsoe, F. and J. Stillwell (1990) *Spontaneous Phenomena: A Mathematical Analysis*. Boston: Academic Press.

Trafimow, D. and M. Marks (2015) Editorial. *Basic and Applied Social Psychology*, 37, 1–2.

Tsay, R.S. (1986) Time series model specification in the presence of outliers. *Journal of the American Statistical Association*, 81, 132–141.

Tsay, R.S. (2002) *Analysis of Financial Time Series*. New York: Wiley.

Van Bavel, J.J., Mende-Siedlecki, P., Brady, W.J. and D.A. Reinero (2016) Contextual sensitivity in scientific reproducibility. *Proceedings of the National Academy of Science*, 113, 6454–6459.

Veney, J.E. (1993) Evaluation applications of regression analysis with time-series data. *Evaluation Practice*, 14, 259–274.

Vitiello, M. (1998) Proposition 215: *De facto* legalization of pot and the shortcomings of direct democracy. *University of Michigan Journal of Law Reform*, 31, 707–776.

Wagner, A.K., S.B. Sournerai, F. Zhang and D. Ross-Degnan (2002) Segmented regression analysis of interrupted time series studies in medication research. *Journal of Clinical Research and Therapeutics*, 27, 299–309.

Walker, G. (1931) On periodicity in series of related terms. *Proceedings of the Royal Society of London, A*, 131, 518–532.

Webb, E.J., D.T. Campbell, R.D. Schwartz and L.B. Sechrest (1966) *Unobtrusive Measures: Nonreactive Research in the Social Sciences*. Chicago: Rand McNally.

Wei, W.S. (2006) *Time Series Analysis: Univariate and Multivariate Methods*, 2nd Edition. Reading, MA: Addison-Wesley.

Wilkinson, L. and Task Force on Statistical Inference, APA Board of Scientific Affairs (1999) Statistical methods in psychology journals: Guidelines and explanations. *American Psychologist*, 54, 594–604.

Windelband, W. (1894) *Geschichte der alten Philosophie: Nebst einem anhang: abriss der Geschichte der Mathematik und Naturwissenschaften*. In *Altertum von Siegmund Gunter*. Munich: Beck.

Wolf, J.R. (1848) *Nachrichten von der sternwarte in Berne*. Sonnenflecken Beobachtungen. Mittheilungen der naturforschenden gesellschaft in Bern, 169–173.

Wolfgang, M.E. (1958) *Patterns in Criminal Homicide*. Philadelphia: University of Pennsylvania Press.

Wong, M.L., K.W. Roy Chan, and D. Koh (1998) A sustainable behavioral intervention to increase condom use and reduce gonorrhea among sex workers in Singapore: Two-year follow-up. *Preventive Medicine*, 27, 891–900.

Wu, L. and H. Hayashi (2013) The impact of the great east Japan earthquake on inbound tourism demand in Japan. *Journal of the Institute of Social Safety*, 21, 109–117.

Yule, G.U. (1927) On a method of investigating periodicities in disturbed series with special reference to Wolfer's sunspot numbers. *Philosophical Transactions*, A226–267.

Zellner, A. (1971). *An Introduction to Bayesian Inference in Econometrics*. New York: Wiley.

Znaniecki, F. (1934) *The Method of Sociology*. New York: Farrar & Rinehart.

Zumbo, B.D. and A.M. Hubley (1998) A note on misconceptions concerning prospective and retrospective power. *The Statistician*, 47, 385–388.

Aaronson, D.E., 224
ABAB design, 200
Abadie, A., 23, 299, 305, 307
Abel, T.F., 335
abortion laws, 286
Abraham, B., 264
Agresti, A., 240
Aguinis, H., 22, 234
airline model, 130, 154
Akaike Information Criterion (*AIC*), 138
Akaike, H., 134, 138
Alberdi, J.C., 258
Alt, F.B., 252, 261
amoxicillin, 340
Anchorage precipitation, 123, 153
Anderson, D.M., 301
Anderson, D.R., 140
Anderson, R.M., 327
Andrews, D.W.K, 261
anti-smoking (Proposition 99), 298
antibiotics, 340
armed robberies, 252
Australian Family Law Act of 1975, 221, 230
Australian traffic fatalities, 130, 140, 153, 229, 250
autocorrelation function (*ACF* or ρ_k), 34
autocovariance function (γ_k), 26, 34
autoregressive (*AR*)
    mean, 98
    operator, 51

polynomial, 41
process, 31

Bacastow, R.B., 127
backshift operator (*B*), 50
backward substitution, 39
Bacon, F., 291
Baddour, L.M., 341
Baer, D.M., 212
Baghelai, C., 262
Baker, A.B., 335
Bal, D., 299
Balbach, E.D., 299
Barron, D.N., 256
Barron, J.L., 9, 17
Bayes factor, 139
Bayesian Information
    Criterion (*BIC*), 139
Bayesian vocabulary, 246
Beatty, J., 22, 233, 267
Bechtold, H.T., 316
Beck, L.W., 315
Becker, H.S., 291
bedtime disruptions, 259
Bell, W.R., 183
Benedetti, F., 218
Bergen, S., 17, 286
Berger, J.O., 249
Berlin, J.N., 244
Berry, C., 299
beta (β) particles, 88, 176
Beveridge, W.H., 5, 103

Bhattacharyya, M.N., 130
Binford, L.R., 337
Blum, N., 259
Bobula, J., 262
bounds
    invertibility, 41, 45
    stationarity, 41, 45
    system stability, 203
Bower, C.R., 328, 332
Box, G.E.P., 19, 45, 87, 104, 162, 186, 261
Box-Cox transformation function, 104,
    151, 162
Box-Steffensmeier, J.M., 149
Brady, W.J., 344
Brammer, L., 258
Brandt, P.T., 254
Breault, K.D., 322
Bresee, J.S., 258
British breathalyzer experiment,
    285, 339
British traffic fatalities, 208
Brock, A., 17, 286
Bunge, M., 289
Burnham, K.P., 140
Burns, D.M., 299

Calder, B., 287
Cameron, A.C., 256
Campbell's Law, 324, 336, 337
Campbell, D.T., 2, 10–15, 19, 22–25, 232,
    251, 274, 275, 280, 281, 289, 291, 294,
    296, 299, 312, 316–318, 333, 334,
    336, 340
Canadian homicide, 4
Canadian inflation, 95, 103, 145, 153
Caporaso, J.A., 215
Carpendo, C.M., 199
Carter, A.F., 127
causality, 288
    Aristotelian, 289
    counterfactual, 292
    Humean, 290
    Mill's method of agreement, 291
    Mill's method of difference, 291
    Mill's methods, 290
    Rubin, 23

Rubin's model, 292
Chan, K.W., 16
Chen., C, 258
Cheng, P.-Y., 258
cholera, 214
Chree, C., 5
Cincinnati Directory Assistance
    calls, 8, 189, 228
clindamycin, 340
CO_2, 127, 139, 153, 182
co-integration, 148, 301
co-proxamol, 17, 286
Cobb, L., 19
coin-flip random walk, 54, 179
Coleman, B.J., 241
Coleman, J.S., 255
Connecticut Crackdown on Speeding,
    281, 283
construct validity
    detection modeling, 328
    fuzzy onset as a threat, 325
    fuzzy response as a threat, 326
    periodicity as a threat, 321
    timeframe as a threat, 319
    worldview as a threat, 324
Cook, T.D., 2, 12–15, 19, 21, 23–25, 232,
    251, 274, 275, 287, 312, 316–318,
    333, 334
Cosler, J., 262
Couzens, M., 337
Cowan, D.W., 335
Cowan, F., 16
Cox, D.R., 104, 162
Cronbach, L.J., 11, 12, 315, 316
Crosbie, J., 260
Curtis, K., 122

Díaz, J., 258
Dao-Tran, T.K., 194
Daston, L., 22, 233, 267
Davidson, L.L., 258
Davis, B.R., 194
Davis, F., 211
Dayer, M.J., 341
Del Rosario, M.L., 287
Delampady, M., 249

Deutsch, S.J., 252, 261
deviance statistic, 137, 141, 199
Dhankhar, P., 258
diagnosis, 86
Diamond, A., 23, 299, 305, 307
Dickey, D.A., 135, 143, 144, 183
Dickson, W.J., 7
Diehl, H.S., 335
Dienes, C.T., 224
Dienes, Z., 233, 240
Dobrin, A., 322
Dollard, J., 6
donor pool, 302
Doob, L.W., 6
Durkin, M.S., 258

Edgington, E.S., 260
Edwards, A.W.F., 162
Edwards, W., 233
Efron, B.E., 237
Elton, C.S., 3
Emerson, M., 211
Enders, W., 149
endocarditis, 340
Engerman, S.L., 336
Engle, R.F., 301
Erlebacher, A.E., 280, 297
Erven, J.M., 279
estimation, 86
European wheat prices, 103, 141
Evans, R., 166
Evanston, Illinois, 281
Ewald, P., 215
expected value, 30, 67
Experimenting Society, 297

Falcon, A., 289
Fein, J., 101
Fernandes, C., 254
Finlay, B., 240
Finniss, D.G., 218
Fisher information ($I(\hat{\mu})$), 161
Fisher, R.A., 7, 23, 233–235, 237, 241, 245,
     266, 267, 307
Florence, P.S., 7

Fogel, R.W., 336
forecasting intervention analysis, 261
Fox, K.K., 16
Fox, R., 211
Franke, R.H., 192, 193, 277
Freeman, J.R., 149
Freeman, K.A., 259
Friedman, M., 166
Friesema, H.P., 215
Friman, P.C., 259
Fruhwirth-Schnatter, S., 254
Fukushima Daiichi disaster, 148
Fuller, W.A., 135, 143

Gallup Poll, 215
gambler's ruin, 55
Gardeazabal, J., 307
Gardener. R.S., 199
Garey, K.W., 194
Gentry, L.O., 194
geometric mean, 105
Geweke, J., 178
Ghosh, J.K., 249
Gigerenzer, G., 22, 233, 267
Gill, J., 244
Gilpin, E., 299
Girardi, L.M., 329
Glantz, S.G., 299
Glass, G.V., 1, 22, 25, 185, 281, 328, 332
Glymour, C., 292
Goldsmith, L., 211
Goldstein, G., 215
gonorrhea, 16
Goodman, C., 262
Goodman, J., 299
Goodman, S.N., 235, 244
Gottman, J.M., 1, 25, 185
Gotzsche, P.C., 218
Granger, C.W.J., 7, 19, 168, 185, 301
Gregory, A.W., 149
Griffiths, C., 17, 286
Gulledge, T.R., 184
gun control laws, 252
Gunnell, D., 17, 286
gunshot wounds, 321

Hájek, A., 240
Hacking, I., 245, 267, 315
Hainmueller, J., 23, 299, 305, 307
Hall, R.V., 211
Hallfors, D., 301
Hamilton, J.D., 142
Hansen, B., 301
Hansen, B.E., 149, 262
Harvey, A.C., 208, 254
Hattie, J., 221
Hawthorn experiments, 7, 192, 276
Hawton, K., 17, 286
Hay, R.A., 252, 261
Hayashi, H., 148
Heath, L., 287
Heimann, M., 127
Hennigan, K.M., 287, 288
Hepworth, J.T., 6
history, 275
Hitt, M.P., 149
Hoff, K.E., 259
Holland, P.W., 23, 292, 293, 295, 296
Homel, R., 220
Hovland, C.I., 6
Hróbjartsson, A., 218
Hu, T., 299
Hubley, A.M., 244
Hudak, G., 88
Huitema, , 260
Hwang, L.Y., 194

identification, 85
information criteria, 135
input-output diagrams, 36
instrumentation, 278
International Statistical Classification of
    Diseases, Injuries and Causes of Death
    (ICD), 280
intervention component $(X(I_t))$, 21
intervention model
    abrupt, permanent, 188
    complex, 221
    decaying impact, 214
    gradually accruing impact, 202
invertibility bounds, 45

Ioannidis, J.P.A., 344
Izenman, A., 3

Janowitz, M., 335
Japanese foreign visitors, 148
Jardine, L., 291
Jeffreys, H., 248
Jeffreys-Lindley paradox, 244
Jenkins, G.M., 19, 45
Johansen, S., 149
Jones, S., 341
Joo, H., 22, 234
journal
    Basic and Applied Social Psychology, 265

Kadane, J.B., 244
Kapur, N., 17, 286
Kaul, J.D, 192, 193, 277
Keeler, T.E., 299
Keeling, C.D., 127
Kellerman, A.L., 253
Kendall, M.G., 237
Kennedy, L.W., 4, 5
Kenny, D.A., 280
Kepka, E.J., 328, 332
Kerwin, M.E., 199
Khatapoush, S., 301
Kim, I.-M., 142
King, D.R., 88
Kirby, K.C., 199
Kmenta, J., 162
knife wounds, 321
Koh, D., 16
Korean War, 287
Koretz, D.M., 337
Kposowa, A.J., 322
Kramer, S., 120, 279
Kroeber, A.E., 3, 4, 115, 338
Krueger, J., 233, 249
Kruger, L., 22, 233, 267
Kruschke, J.H., 22, 234, 245, 267
Kuhn, L., 258
Kuhn, T.S., 10, 289, 290
Kullback-Leibler index, 138
Kuznets, S., 338

LaFree, G.D., 230
lag-k, 26
Lai, A., 215
Lai, D., 194
Langwell, K., 262
Layton, A.P., 130
Leek, J.T., 266
Legge, J.S., 286, 287
Lester, D., 322
Levine, W.C., 16
Lieberson, S., 291
Lin, B., 184
Lindman, H., 233
Lineberry, R.L., 215
Liu, L-M., 258
Liu, L.-M., 88
Ljung, G.M., 87
Lockhart, P.B., 341
Loftin, C., 322
logical positivism, 273, 315

Mabey, D., 16
MacCorquodale, K., 316
MacKenzie, D.L., 184
MacKinnon, J.G., 143
Maddala, G.S., 142
Manski, C.F., 313
Marks, M., 265
Marshall, C., 6
Masson, M.E.J., 249
matching, 281, 298
maturation, 276
Mauna Kea, 127
Mausner, J.S., 120, 279
maximum likelihood estimation, 154
May, R.M., 327
Mayr, E., 11
McCain, L.J., 185
McCleary, R., 2, 6, 9, 17, 19, 185, 205, 215, 222, 230, 252, 261, 276, 278, 279
McDowall, D., 2, 19, 122, 185, 252, 322
McSweeney, A.J., 8, 189
mean (μ_Y), 26
mean square forecast error ($MSFE$), 169
medical marijuana (Proposition 215), 301
Meehan, A.J., 337

Meehl, P.E., 315, 316
Meehl, P.W., 316
Meltzer, A., 262
Meltzer, M.I., 258
Mende-Siedlecki, P., 344
methadone maintenance treatment, 199, 228
Mill, J.S., 290
Miller, N.E., 6
Miller, R.B., 183
Mills, T.C., 5
missing data, 262
MMPI test, 6
Mook, W.G., 127
Moran, J.S., 16
Morgan, S.L., 292
Morgenstern, O., 324
Mosconi, R., 149
motorcycle helmet laws, 275
moving average (MA)
    mean, 100
    operator, 52
    polynomial, 41
    process, 31
Mowrer, O.H., 6
Murray, M.P., 149
Musheno, M.C., 224
Mushkatel, A.E., 325
My Lai, 337

Nakashima, A.K., 16
Naltrexone, 9
Nason, J., 149
National Center for Health Statistics (NCHS), 302, 324, 331
National Highway Traffic Safety Administration (NHTSA), 275, 302, 324, 331
National Institute for Health and Clinical Excellence (NICE), 340
natural experiment, 296
Nerlove, M., 62, 122
nested model, 136
Neter, J., 240
New Hampshire Medicaid prescriptions, 196, 202, 228

Newbold, P., 168
Neyman, J., 233, 234
Ng, S., 144
Nicholson, M., 3
Nickerson, R.S., 233
Nielsen, B., 149
Nienstedt, B.C, 279
noise component $(N(a_t))$, 20
Norpoth, H., 215
Northwestern University, 281

O'Grady, K.E., 7
one-shot case study, 5
Open Science Collaboration, 344
opiate blocker, 9, 17
outliers, 253
Owen, M., 211
Ozdowski, S.A., 221

Padia, W.L., 328, 332
Pandiani, J.A., 329
Parsonson, B.S., 212
Patel, V., 16
Patterson, K., 142
Pawitan, Y., 155, 157, 162, 165, 267, 272
Pearson, E.S., 233, 234
Pearson, K., 92
pediatric trauma admissions, 101, 138,
     156, 178
Peng, R.D., 266
Perron, P., 144
Peterson, R., 6
Pevehouse, J.C.W., 149
Phillips, P.C.B., 144
physician expenditures, 262
pi-weights (π), 171
Pierce, D.A., 87
Piper, S.C., 127
Pitcher, B.L., 278
placebo
     control group, 339, 340
     effect, 17, 217, 218, 229, 335
     impact, 219
     patient, 218, 229
     test, 306, 307

Poisson process, 254
Polyson, P., 6
Porcia, E., 211
Porter, T., 22, 233, 267
portmanteau statistic, 87
Prendergast, B., 341
presidential popularity, 215
Price, D.D., 218
productivity, Hawthorn experiments,
     192, 228
psi-weights (ψ), 169
psychiatric readmission rates, 329
public drunkenness arrests, 224
pulse function (∇I_t), 216
purse snatchings, 253

Q-statistic, 87
Quandt, R., 262

Raftery, A.E., 248, 249
reactivity, 334
Reed, D.R., 253
Rees, D.I., 301
regression, 280
Reichardt, C.S., 316
Reinero, D.A., 344
Reynolds, G., 16
Richardson, J., 3, 115
Riggs, J.E., 222
Rindskopf, D., 22, 239
Rivara, F.P., 253
Roeloffzen, H., 127
Roethlisberger, F., 7
Romeri, E., 17, 286
Rorschach test, 6
Rosbrook, B., 299
Rosenwasser. B.J., 199
Ross, H.L., 205, 220, 230, 276, 281, 285
Ross-Degnan. D., 196
Rubin, D.B., 23, 280, 292–294
Russell, B., 273, 315

Saez, M., 258
Said, S.E., 144
Samanta, T., 249

Savage, L.J., 233
Schlaifer, R., 277
Schnell, D., 16
Schnoes, C., 259
Schwartz, R.D., 336
Schwarz, G., 139
score function ($S(\mu)$), 160
Sears, R.R., 6
seatbelt laws, 204, 205, 208, 248
Sechrest, L.B., 336
Seidman, D., 336
selection, 283
self-injurious behavior, 9, 217, 229
sequence
    arithmetic, 75
    definition, 72
    geometric, 77
series
    comparison test, 82
    necessary condition test, 80
Shadish, W.R., 2, 13–15, 19, 23, 24, 232,
    251, 274, 294, 312, 317, 318, 333, 334
Shahmanesh, M., 16
Shay, D.K., 258
Shils, E.A., 335
Shumway, R.H., 262, 263
Silverman, R.A., 4, 5
Silverthorne, M., 291
Simkin, S., 17, 286
skirt widths, 3, 115, 139
Skyrms, B., 267, 290
Slutzky, E., 44
Smith, K.L., 17, 286
Snow, J., 214
Sournerai, S.B., 196
South Carolina homicides, 88
Spanos, A., 244
Spitzer, J.J., 164
Stanley, J.C., 1, 2, 5, 7, 11, 15, 22, 23, 274,
    275, 283, 292, 294, 299, 316, 333, 334,
    340
Stata *synth*, 305
stationarity bounds, 45
statistical power
    Dickey-Fuller test, 146
    functions, 243

Neyman-Pearson hypothesis test, 237
Quandt-Andrews method, 262
sample *ACF*, 212
threat to statistical conclusion validity,
    232
threshold at $N = 120$, 320
step function (I_t), 187
Stillwell, J., 88
Stouffer, D.S., 262, 263
sudden infant death syndrome (SIDS),
    280
suicide, 286
Sung, H., 299
sunspot numbers, 111, 136
Suppes, P., 290
surgical site infection rates, 194, 228
SUTVA, 313, 317
Swijtink, Z., 22, 233, 267
synthetic control time series, 298

talking out incidents, 211, 229
Tarran, B., 266
Taylor, D.V., 9, 17
test
    τt-statistic, 145
    $\tau \mu$ statistic, 144
    Kolmogorov-Smirnov (KS)
        goodness-of-fit, 87
    Augmented Dickey-Fuller, 143
    Bayesian hypothesis, 244, 267
    Dickey-Fuller, 143
    Fisher's significance, 234, 267
    likelihood ratio, 142
    modern hybrid hypothesis, 238, 267
    Neyman-Pearson hypothesis, 236,
        265, 266
    Pearson goodness-of-fit, 92
    Phillips-Perron, 144
    robustness of synthetic control
        contrast, 309
    unit root, 142
    unknown intervention time-points, 261
tetanus immunization, 326
Thompson, S.P., 25
Thompson, W.W., 258
Thornhill, M.H., 341

Tiao, G.C., 19, 186, 261
Tobías, A., 258
Topsoe, F., 88
Touchette, P., 9, 17
Trafimow, D., 265
Trivedi, P.K., 256
Tsay, R.H., 87, 258
Tucson burglaries, 279

U.K. GDP growth, 99, 157, 181
U.K. traffic fatalities, 248
U.S. birth rates, 183
U.S. diabetes mortality rates, 279
U.S. gonorrhea cases, 16
U.S. tuberculosis cases, 118, 146

validity, 10
    construct, 14, 315
    external, 15, 333
    internal, 14, 273
    statistical conclusion, 14, 231
Van Bavel, J.J., 344
variance (σ_Y or γ_0), 26
Veney, J.E., 326
Vietnam War, 276, 337
Vitiello, M., 301

Wagner, A.K., 196
Walker, G., 108
Wasserman, W., 240
Watt, D.G., 149
Webb, E.J., 336
Wei, W.M., 87
Weintraub, E., 258
West, S.G., 6

Wharton, J.D., 287
white noise, 2
    hypothesis tests, 91
    process, 28
    serial independence, 29
Whiteman, C., 178
Whitmore, G.A., 240
Whittington, W.L., 16
Whorf, T.P., 127
Wiersema, B., 322
Wiggins, C.D., 241
Wilkinson, L., 22
Willard, D., 211
Williams, J.T., 254
Willson, V.L., 1, 25, 185
Wilson, L.A., 325
Windelband, W., 11
Winn, D., 299
Winship, C., 292
Wolf, J.R., 3
Wolfgang, M.E., 322
Wong, M.L., 16
Woods, D.W., 259
Wu, L., 148

Yantek, T., 215
Yule, G.U., 3, 44, 108, 111
Yule-Walker equations, 108

Zacks, S., 19
Zaidi, A., 16
Zellner, A., 178
Zhang. F., 196
Znaniecki, F., 291
Zumbo, B.D., 244